111127 $9.75

measurement in physical education

FOURTH EDITION

Donald K. Mathews, D.P.Ed.

Professor in Physical Education and Physiology;
Director of Exercise and Physiology Research Laboratory
The Ohio State University, Columbus, Ohio

illustrations and original cover artwork by Nancy Allison Close

W. B. Saunders Company
Philadelphia   London   Toronto

W. B. Saunders Company: West Washington Square
Philadelphia, Pa.   19105

1 St. Anne's Road
Eastbourne, East Sussex BN21 3UN, England

833 Oxford Street
Toronto, M8Z 5T9, Canada

Measurement in Physical Education   ISBN   0-7216-6177-7

Print No.: 9   8   7   6   5   4

preface

Helping you, the student, become a better physical education teacher is the prime mission of this text. Consequently you, rather than your professor, had to be foremost in my mind as I wrote. Today physical education enjoys a prestigious posture among educational programs. Research findings in medicine and the behavorial sciences attest to the value of our great profession: These findings show that children may be physically and socially handicapped without adequate physical education programs.

Your mission is the most important of all: to conduct a physical education program which will benefit every child. Success is necessarily dependent upon understanding the philosophy and measurement unique to physical education. Measurement is fundamental to critical analysis in physical education. Mastery of the subject matter in this course will enable you to: (1) determine pupil status; (2) design an effective program; and (3) measure progress. The ability to analyze critically is a necessary attribute of the professional person. It is almost a guarantee that each child will receive a rewarding physical education experience.

In order for me to assist you in arriving at our goal, I kept the following three aims in mind while writing this text:

1. To present the measurement materials with emphasis on techniques of test administration and application of results to the program.

2. To discuss only essential statistical methods so that the student may scientifically evaluate the tests and analyze his data for application to the program.

3. To illustrate and describe accurately most of the tests in such a manner that they may be administered directly from the textbook.

If these purposes have been accomplished, the professional student will discover that the scientific approach to physical education can be a valuable way in which to stimulate pupil and teacher and to show why administrators and parents should hold the physical education profession in high regard.

It is with sincere gratitude that I acknowledge the assistance and encouragement that came from so many quarters in the preparation of this book. Particular thanks are extended to Dr. Karl Bookwalter of Indiana University, who read the complete manuscript and offered many excellent suggestions; to Dr. Mary Kientzle of Washington State University for her fine work in editing the statistical materials; to Dr. Marion Broer of the University of Washington for her valuable suggestions pertaining to the area of knowledge testing; to Professor Virginia Shaw for editing, as well as for contributing much of the material on evaluation of body mechanics; and, finally, to Professor Ruth Slonim of the English Department at Washington State University, who deserves a meritorious citation for her guidance in literary expression. To these people and to the authors of the numerous tests appearing in this text I am deeply grateful, for without their kind assistance the completion of this book would have been impossible.

DONALD K. MATHEWS

contents

chapter 6

general motor ability 157

chapter 7

sports skill testing 204

chapter 8

cardiovascular tests 229

chapter 13

marking in physical education   374

chapter 14

organization and administration of the measurement program   391

appendix A

table of square roots of numbers from 1 to 1000   405

appendix B

suggested laboratory exercises   416

appendix C

the New Britain system   420
    BY CHARLES T. AVEDISIAN AND JOSEPH A. BEDARD

appendix D

norms for AAHPER youth fitness test   428

appendix E

norms for Kirchner motor fitness test   452

appendix F

norms for Oregon motor fitness test   456

index   463

chapter 1

approach to measurement and evaluation

Indeed, the application of scientific knowledge to determine the kind and amount of physical activity needed to meet the individual child's needs is imperative to the further improvement of physical education programs.

Ellis Champlin

Why a course in tests and measurements? This is a logical question and deserves a complete answer. As a physical educator you are going to be entrusted with the most priceless product on earth, children. The pupils under your guidance are individuals and as such require specific attention. A child is extremely complex in make-up and decidedly unique in many respects. He has varying abilities in the numerous physical and mental skills required of him by the culture he has inherited, and he has certain physiological limitations. In some skills he will excel; in others he will lack ability. Since it is acknowledged that some pupils can handle a more difficult course of instruction than others, how does the teacher select the proper program for each pupil? He does this through the use of evaluation and measurement techniques.

Evaluation implies the judgment, appraisal, rating, and interpretation so fundamental to the *total* educational process. Such qualitative methods and instruments as teacher observation, judgments, surveys, anecdotal records, check lists, score cards, and questionnaires are employed to consider evidence in the light of value standards and in terms of the particular situation and the goals of the group or individual. Evaluation is a continuous process dealing with the overall goals of education.

Measurement is a part of evaluation; it is a quantitative procedure using tools or instruments, such as a dynamometer to measure strength, a scale to determine weight, or a knowledge test to evaluate comprehension of subject matter. Measurement deals with an immediate objective, such as one's skill in or knowledge of badminton, whereas evaluation includes the results of measurement in appraising the progress of the individual or group toward the goals of education. Oberteuffer and Beyrer[14] state: "Measurement focuses on specific knowledge or skills of the moment; evaluation is an ongoing process aimed at judging the amount of change (preferably improvement) over a period of time." These authors make the point that measurement is most concerned with knowledge of subject matter whereas evaluation is concerned with how the knowledge affects the total behavior of the individual or group. It is the application of measurement and evaluation to the program and to the pupil which forms the scientific basis for the practice of physical education.

Measurement truly diminishes error in programming, thus assuring the most direct route between pupil status and the proposed educational objectives. Let us stop for a moment to consider the general whose objective is the immediate eradication of a particular enemy outpost. In order to arrive at this objective in the shortest possible time and over the least hazardous way, the general and his staff must carefully study a map of the area to plan the most advantageous route. By comparison, the teacher uses measurement in place of the map to aid him in understanding the needs of the child. In this manner the most efficient program may be initiated to aid the child in arriving at the teacher's stated objective. One should take note here that failure on the part of the teacher to employ measurement may be just as disastrous as the failure of the general to use a map. It is more than likely that neither would arrive at his planned objective.

It should be noted that measurement is actually founded upon philosophy, for from our educational philosophy are derived the objectives that we set in physical education. In order to determine the extent to which these objectives are met, it is necessary to measure. Information on the status of the individual relative to the proposed objective may be determined through measurement and evaluation. This information may then be interpreted in light of the stated objectives so that the most effective program to meet the individual's needs may be presented. It is important here to point out that measurement and evaluation are *a means to an end, not an end in themselves*. It also should be made clear at this time that professional progress rests primarily with the philosophers. These people help us to understand and interpret the broad purposes of education. These purposes are referred to as goals or aims of education, whereas the more specific steps that must be taken to reach the goals are called objectives. Borrowing again from the military, the broad aim or goal of the general is to win the war, whereas the capture of an outpost is one of the numerous objectives that must be reached before the final goal is within grasp.

Since the primary function of measurement is to evaluate the effects of instruction in the light of educational outcomes, it is necessary to review the purposes and objectives of the physical education program.

Purpose and objectives of physical education. Physical education may simply be defined as *education* through or by means of the physical. This implies that the aims or goals of physical education are the same as those of general education. Thus the physical educator strives to achieve the aims of education through or by means of large muscle activity.

As the goals or aims of education are stated in somewhat general terms and apply to the total contribution of education in its broadest concept, it is necessary to be more specific in indicating the contribution of physical education in terms of helping the pupil to reach the aims of education. These specific contributions of physical education are referred to as *objectives,* and may be thought of as guideposts in helping to direct the physical education program toward achieving the aims of education. The objectives of physical education are the foundation of program construction and for several important reasons they should color every professional move the physical educator makes.

First of all, objectives in physical education are tangible. They can be adequately observed and, for the most part, objectively measured. Second, the objectives of physical education can be substantiated on the basis of present-day findings in the research literature. Third, the primary objectives of physical education, when accomplished, result in attributes vitally necessary for complete growth and development of youngsters. Next, these objectives, by their very nature, help the lay person, as well as the professional, to understand the place of physical education in the over-all educational program. Finally—and so important—professional objectives, when completely comprehended, give the physical educator his professional insight and direction. Complete understanding and use of objectives in physical education, when teaching, are the true mark of the professional.

When reading the professional literature, one finds authors using varying terminology in listing objectives. One should not be alarmed by the fact that each writer has apparently made up his own terms independently. Actually, physical educators basically agree on objectives even though as authors they may state them in somewhat different forms.

As an illustration, Nash[13] expresses physical education objectives under the following four headings:

1. Organic development.
2. Neuromuscular development.
3. Interpretive development.
4. Emotional development.

Brownell and Hagman[1] list the objectives in the following manner:
1. Physical fitness.
2. Social and motor skills.
3. Knowledges and understandings.
4. Habits, attitudes, and appreciations.

Williams[19] claims that physical education makes four possible contributions to the education of the individual:
1. Development of organic systems.
2. Development of neuromuscular skills.
3. Development of interest in play and recreation.
4. Development of standard ways of behavior.

Bucher[2] lists the following as physical education objectives:
1. Organic development.
2. Neuromuscular development.
3. Interpretive development (includes knowledges, judgments, and appreciations attending the performance of physical activities).
4. Personal-social development.

Regardless of the terminology, the essential contributions of physical education to the established purposes of education are agreed upon by the profession. These objectives must be thoroughly understood and kept constantly in mind, for, as we stated earlier, the major purpose of measurement and evaluation is to determine whether or not the program has been successful in meeting these desired outcomes. For the purposes of this text, the following terminology for objectives has been selected: physical fitness, recreational fitness, and social fitness.

Physical fitness. This term has been an elusive one to define objectively. The simplest definition is: the capacity of an individual to perform given physical tasks involving muscular effort. In order to ascertain how the leading authorities in medicine as well as physical education define physical fitness, a number of definitions made during a period of sixteen years were analyzed. This analysis revealed that the term "fitness" was most generally interpreted in its broadest concept, that of total fitness, and includes the following four components:
1. Psychological fitness:
   a. The emotional stability necessary to meet the everyday problems characteristic of one's environment, and
   b. Sufficient psychological reserve to handle a sudden emotional trauma.
2. Health, or normal physiological function.
3. Body mechanics, or efficient performance in skills, from the common everyday skills of standing, walking, and sitting to the most complex, such as that manifested by a football player executing a perfect block, or the performance of an intricate pattern of movement by a dancer.

4. Physical anthropometry, a type of fitness reflected in body contour as a result of good muscular tonus as well as proper body weight.

In a statement prepared by 100 delegates to the AAHPER Fitness Conference in September, 1956, at Washington, D.C., the group put forth the following components as those an individual must possess in order to function efficiently in satisfying his own needs as well as in contributing his share to the welfare of society:

1. Optimum organic health consistent with heredity and the application of present health knowledge.
2. Sufficient coordination, strength, and vitality to meet emergencies as well as the requirements of daily living.
3. Emotional stability to meet the stresses and strains of modern life.
4. Social consciousness and adaptability with respect to the requirements of group living.
5. Sufficient knowledge and insight to make suitable decisions and arrive at feasible solutions to problems.
6. Attitudes, values, and skills that stimulate satisfactory participation in a full range of daily activities.
7. Spiritual and moral qualities that contribute the fullest measure of living in a democratic society.

As a primary objective of physical education, the attainment of total fitness has overwhelming implications for growth and development of youth. As the definition implies, a child who is fit enjoys robust health, a fine-looking physique, a satisfactory level of social and emotional adjustment, and a proficiency in the basic skills of movement.

Such a comprehensive definition of total fitness permits us to identify in a general way the prime responsibility to children we as physical educators have inherited. However, as our objective is to *measure* and reflect to a reliable degree the status of children in terms of fitness, we must note in a more precise manner the tangible qualities that can be evaluated. The term *physical fitness* is somewhat exact in its meaning, indicating to us specific components we might measure to reflect a person's fitness status. The sensible organic ingredients of physical fitness include muscular strength, muscular endurance, muscular power, muscular flexibility, cardiovascular or cardiorespiratory fitness, and neuromuscular coordination.

Muscular strength. Muscular strength is defined as the force that a muscle or group of muscles can exert against a resistance in one maximum effort. It is measured in units of pounds. A person possessing satisfactory muscular strength usually exhibits a nice-looking physique and may possess a better than average proficiency in sports. Onset of fever or disease causes a decline in strength, whereas chronic substrength may be a predisposing factor in slow motor learning and poor posture.

Muscular endurance. The ability of a muscle to work against a moderate resistance for long periods of time is termed muscular endurance. It differs from muscular strength in that it reflects the ability of a muscle to contract and relax continuously over a period of time. The officer directing traffic, the act of walking, and the performance of light calisthenics that use many repetitions are good examples of muscular endurance events.

Muscular power. Power movements include such events as the high jump, broad jump, 100-yard dash, and those activities requiring quick starts, as in football, ice hockey and basketball. One's ability to get his body mass moving in the shortest period of time is a measure of power. The physiologist refers to such events as being anaerobic (without oxygen), i.e., they are performed in such a short period of time that oxygen is not required in producing the necessary energy.

Muscular flexibility. Flexibility is usually interpreted as the range of motion at a particular joint, measured in degrees. Extensibility of the soft tissue, ligaments and especially of the muscle and the anatomical structure of the joint help to determine the degree of flexibility. Flexibility is specific to the movement and there is little relationship of flexibility measures to sex and age. Specialized forms of physical activity appear to develop specific patterns of flexibility. There is probably an optimum range of flexibility which would aid performance and act as a preventive of muscular injury. Extreme flexibility may be a predisposing factor in joint injuries; less than normal flexibility may result in tearing of connective tissue. George Holland[7] has prepared an excellent review of the literature dealing with the physiology of flexibility.

Cardiovascular fitness. Sometimes called cardiorespiratory fitness, this type of high-level fitness is possessed by the participants in long-distance track and swimming events. Excellent cardiorespiratory condition reflects a strong heart, good blood vessels, and properly functioning lungs. Such gross body activities performed over long periods as walking, long-distance hiking, bicycle riding, running, and swimming improve cardiovascular condition. Perhaps the marathoner, who runs twenty-six miles in approximately two and one-half hours, is the athlete who best exemplifies excellent cardiovascular fitness. An event in which the person works submaximally over a period of time is termed aerobic (with oxygen). Events that take longer than four minutes to perform require oxygen to produce the needed energy. The individual running two miles or further would derive his energy predominantly through aerobic metabolism; in runs of less than a mile, anaerobic metabolic pathways would be the primary means for deriving the necessary energy. Thus, we might consider *aerobic capacity* or aerobic fitness (the ability of a person to maximally employ the oxygen metabolic pathway) to be a better term than cardiovascular-cardiorespiratory fitness.

Neuromuscular coordination. The mere ability of a person to manipulate his body physically connotes some degree of this type fitness. The ballet dancer, the person performing on a trampoline, the diver, and the gymnast all possess a high degree of neuromuscular coordination. Two terms have been widely used in physical education to earmark neuromuscular coordination: general motor ability, and motor fitness. The former might be used interchangeably with general athletic ability, or one's proficiency in a wide variety of sports, whereas the latter most directly infers one's ability to perform work details, or to perfect skills. Running, jumping, carrying, lifting, pushing, pulling, climbing, dodging, and balancing would be the more fundamental factors used to reflect motor fitness ability. The fundamental mechanism contributing to our understanding as to how a person learns new skills (develops motor ability) has been elusive. Recent research has shed new light on this very important area, and is discussed in Chapter 4.

It is easy to see that all five of the components of physical fitness are intricately related but at the same time reflect, each in a special way, some aspect of general organic fitness. Hence reference to the low-fit child does not necessarily imply that he needs to run an obstacle course to raise his fitness level. It does mean, however, that there could be numerous factors causing low fitness, such as poor nutrition, emotional problems, organic drains, orthopedic deficiencies, low strength, insufficient muscular endurance, lack of flexibility, and others. One of our problems, then, will be to recognize, through measurement, the sub-fit child and then to find the cause or causes *before* a program for amelioration of the condition is decided upon.

Frequently the question, "Fitness for what?" is asked. The answer may simply be stated as: sufficient fitness for performing daily tasks without undue fatigue at the day's end. Fitness above and beyond that required in daily living, as needed in various sports, is another matter. And also, an athlete may be fit for throwing the javelin, but not fit for distance running. Recognition of these specialized types of condition should not be the major concern of the physical educator. The type of *total fitness* required for daily living should be of first importance. Just making an individual fit for the sake of being fit is not sufficient. In order to realize completely the attainment of this primary objective, the physical educator must include in his program the reasons for maintaining a fit body as well as the most effective methods for its development.

Once a pupil has reached a satisfactory level of fitness and has an appreciation of how fitness is vital to his full growth and development, the effect of the fitness objective is more completely realized.

Recreational fitness. A pupil is recreationally fit if he possesses sufficient skill in a variety of activities to enjoy participating in them. Here the emphasis may be placed upon such neuromuscular skills as badminton, tennis, bait and fly casting, canoeing, sailing, or camping; for it is in these activities that the carry-over into adult life most frequently takes place.

The skills must be carefully taught and used to motivate continued participation in physical education activities. The physical educator who raises the performance standard from low mediocrity to a level of enjoyment of activity has rendered an invaluable service both to children and to society.

Social fitness.   This objective encompasses the ability of an individual to get along with people. Although the definition is brief, the complexity of factors related to social fitness complicates the problem of measurement. Such elements as attitudes, sportsmanship, appreciations, leadership ability, command of social graces, and many other desired outcomes of physical education are included in this broad category of social fitness. It is here that ideals and behavior, the basis of democracy, may be taught and developed.

The coeducational program allows for teaching and practice of social skills. In the games and sports area we find one of education's best laboratories for democratic experiences. The pupil must learn to respect rules, to cooperate with teammates, and to treat opponents fairly and with the courtesy due good sportsmen. Leadership is developed through leaders' corps and team captains.

The objectives of physical education are logically served in varying degrees through the activity program. For example, if we concentrate on one objective, say physical fitness, our greatest results should be expected in terms of fitness. But at the same time we should attain progress toward the other objectives, for the youngster is a total being and what affects any part affects the whole. This factor must be recognized if we are to understand fully the place of measurement and evaluation in the total program. If the group as a whole stands high in fitness, emphasis may then be directed more toward the social or recreational objectives, at the same time keeping in mind the need for maintaining this achieved state of fitness.

Classification of testing instruments.   Now that we understand what physical education instruction can hope to accomplish in terms of objectives, we must look to measurement to help identify the child's needs and to determine whether or not we have been successful in meeting them. Quite obviously, it appears that we should select a test or tests under each of the three major objectives.

It then follows that the tests selected could logically be presented under the headings of the objectives; i.e., all the tests measuring physical fitness in one chapter, those measuring social fitness in another, and a third chapter containing tests of recreational ability. However, because of the numerous subdivisions under each objective—for example, in the area of physical fitness—such classification becomes much too broad for purposes of study. Furthermore, a test that measures some aspect of fitness may also measure a phase of athletic ability, adding further confusion to such general classification. In order to present a bird's-eye view of measurement and evaluation, the following classification of testing materials is offered in hopes that the reader will easily comprehend the more minute aspects of measurement, but will, at the same time, keep in mind their application in terms of the overall objectives of physical education. One might say, "Here are the trees; beware, however, of losing sight of the fact that they make up a forest."

Strength tests. This type of measurement is used to reflect certain aspects of total fitness as well as to measure athletic ability. These tests consist, for the most part, of the subject applying a force that is measured by some type of scale or dynamometer. In this way the strength of the muscle group is recorded in pounds of pull. Muscular endurance tests, which are usually classified as strength tests, make use of the weight of the body parts as the resistance for the muscle group to work against. For example, in pull-ups or push-ups, the body weight is the resistance for the muscles of the shoulder girdle to overcome. So, too, in executing a sit-up, the upper trunk might be regarded as the resistance that the abdominal muscles must overcome in order for the individual to sit up.

Cardiovascular tests. Cardiovascular or cardiorespiratory tests are used to determine the efficiency of the heart and blood vessels. Generally speaking, these tests usually require the subject to perform some specified exercise, such as stepping up and down on a bench, or running in place. Before exercise, immediately following exercise, and for a certain period thereafter, the pulse rate is counted. The object is to determine the ability of the cardiovascular system to adjust to the exercise, and it is recorded in terms of the pulse rate. In the more complex tests, the blood pressure as well as pulse rate is recorded, before and after the exercise period. The scores are placed in a formula and an index of efficiency is then computed. More recently, measurement of a person's aerobic capacity has been accepted as the most valid manner in which to reflect this type of fitness. The ability of a person to maximally consume oxygen during exhaustive work is termed his maximal oxygen consumption. Values for an adult may range from 2.5 to 6.5 liters per minute, depending upon the size and aerobic capacity (cardiovascular fitness) of the individual. Treadmills, gas analysis equipment and trained technicians make such measurements impractical for a school situation. Nevertheless, your knowledge of this manner of measurement is essential to understanding the more practical tests which could be used in your school for appraising aerobic capacity.

Muscular power tests. Accurate measurement can be made of the athlete's ability to perform explosive events. The broad jump as well as the vertical jump are aids in such appraisal. Using a timer, the speed with which a person can propel himself up a given number of stairs has provided an excellent quantitation of power output. The time in the 50-yard dash with a running start has also proved a valid measure of power.

Motor ability tests.   Motor ability may be taken as synonymous with general athletic ability, and the motor ability tests measure the immediate capacity of a person to participate in a variety of sports. If, for example, a person scored exceptionally high on a motor ability test, it would indicate that he had a high degree of present ability for most sport activities. Track and field skills are often measured to determine athletic ability, for they are fundamental to proficiency in sports. Included are such activities as shot put, high jump, dashes, rope climb, broad jump, and basketball and baseball throw for distance.

Perceptual motor tests.   This method of measurement and evaluation is finally receiving widespread use and study in our field. Assaying the child's facility with his body is essential if proper growth and development of that youngster is to be assured. There is increasing scientific evidence that the higher thought processes are intricately related to the amount of movement explorations a child experiences during his growth. Vision, sensory perception, strength and motor development are among the attributes positively modified through movement experiences. Performing on a balance beam, skipping, jumping, maneuvering through physical mazes and numerous other activities requiring kinesthesia allow measurement and evaluation of a child's perceptual motor status.

Motor fitness tests.   Tests falling within this classification were used during World War II for evaluating the type of fitness thought necessary for military personnel. Motor fitness is a phase of motor ability. The tests used in its evaluation contain such basic components as strength, speed, agility, endurance, balance, power, and flexibility. The primary purpose of the tests is to determine the fitness of the body for strenuous work, particularly for the vigorous type of activity required of military personnel. The items most used in these tests are pull-ups, push-ups, sit-ups, dashes, squat thrusts, squat jumps, and broad jump.

Skill tests.   These tests are used for measuring the ability of a pupil in specific sports, such as basketball, baseball, archery, or golf. Skill tests usually involve a combination of the most essential skills required to play the particular sport. For instance, a tennis test might utilize volleying a ball against a wall for a specified period of time; a soccer test would most likely include dribbling through a maze against time, as well as kicking for distance and accuracy.

Body mechanics.   These tests attempt to evaluate the functional efficiency of the body in terms of standing, walking, and sitting skills. Tests for standing posture, as well as evaluation sheets for performance in certain selected skills, such as lifting and lowering weights, climbing and descending stairs, are employed to ascertain deviations from normal.

Nutritional testing.   As the name implies, through nutritional testing the nutritional status of the child is evaluated, taking into consideration the body build. Such items as hip width and chest width and depth are measured by calipers in order to predict the body weight for that particular structure. Such tests attempt to take into consideration individual structural differences that the common age, height and weight tables do not.

Social fitness tests.   Employed in this area are written tests, rating scales, and sociographs to evaluate sportsmanship, attitudes, conduct, and other factors. Although the physical education program seemingly has much to offer in developing the social fitness of the child, a great deal needs to be done to expand this area of evaluation.

Knowledge tests.   Sports and health knowledge tests are essential to the measurement program. The understanding of skills, techniques, rules, and strategy may be evaluated by use of paper-and-pencil tests. Health knowledge, practices, and attitudes must be determined through knowledge tests. The information gleaned from the written test may be used for determining pupil status, for measuring progress, for marking, and for indicating possible instructional weaknesses.

Why Measure?

As the Physical Education Director, you are seated in the auditorium of a high school, observing your graduating seniors as they receive their diplomas—pupils who, for a number of years, have been subjected to the disciplines and pedagogy of modern education. They have been under an educational regimen subdivided into various categories, such as English, dramatics, music, history, and physical education, all contributing to the development, growth, and happiness of the individual pupil.

You might well ask yourself, "Has my program contributed its share to the development of this graduating senior? Does he have the characteristics that show that he is *physically educated?*"

Some characteristics of the physically educated pupil.   Just what are the basic criteria for determining whether or not the pupil is physically educated? Obviously the evaluating criteria must consist of the objectives of physical education. Specific questions relative to the objectives of physical education, which you, as the director, might ask yourself, may include:

1. Is the pupil physically fit?

2. Does he realize the importance of general fitness and its relationship to his health and happiness?

3. Does he understand the basic physiological principles involved in the development and maintenance of fitness?

4. Is he equipped with sufficient recreational skills to enable him to participate in a variety of activities well enough to enjoy himself?

5. Does he have knowledge and understanding of recreational facilities available in his home state, as well as the skills to take advantage of these facilities?

6. Can he participate effectively in mixed groups?

7. Does he have skill in social graces?

8. Does he have poise and grace in the fundamental movements of standing, walking, and sitting?

If, as the Director of Physical Education, you can answer "yes" to these questions, in all probability you have been successful.

Physical fitness, recreational fitness, and social fitness, as mentioned previously, are the basic objectives of physical education. Although these may be further subdivided into more specific objectives, for our purposes the more general listing will serve satisfactorily.

Provided the above objectives can be effectively met, it is easy to comprehend the great potential that physical education possesses in contributing to the growth and development of our children. As one studies the research materials in physical education and in professions such as medicine and psychology, closely allied to our profession, one becomes quite enthusiastic about the possibilities inherent in a well-conducted program of physical education.

As an illustration of what a good physical educator with a good program can do for a youngster, the following incident comes to mind.

While a physical fitness testing team was helping a school to establish a measurement program, a freshman high school boy, whom we shall call Bill, was found to have an extremely low score on his fitness test. The background of this pupil was immediately investigated. It was found that his academic grades were low; the guidance department stated that the boy presented a serious behavior problem; the physical education director said that he was constantly forgetting his gym equipment, among other things. It looked as if this boy was rapidly becoming a "juvenile casualty." After collecting all pertinent information about Bill, the physical education director of the school called him in for an interview and gained some interesting information. Because of his low fitness, it was difficult for Bill to learn the skills that were being taught in gym class. For example, one day the group was performing skin-the-cat on the horizontal bar. The boys were standing in line, and when it came Bill's turn, he did not have the arm strength to pull himself up. Immediately his classmates began to chide him. This, of course, was quite an emotional jolt for Bill. The experience was repeated on a number of occasions when the class was working on apparatus, stunts, or tumbling; Bill just didn't have the basic strength that would allow him to learn the skills. What would you have done if you were this pupil? Probably just exactly what Bill did. In order to receive recognition among his own group and to prove he was not a "weakling," he reacted in such a manner that he presented a serious behavior problem.

At the conclusion of the interview, Bill and the physical education director decided on a special strengthening program. Bill would attend the regular physical education class on the days that he could perform with some degree of proficiency. In the meantime, a special twice-a-week period was established during which Bill began working to improve his low fitness score.

One year later, when the physical fitness testing team was again helping this same school with its testing program, and while its members and the physical education director were reviewing the score cards, there was a knock at the door. The intruder proved to be Bill, who had been anxiously "waiting it out" to find how he had done on this year's fitness test. His score had risen from 65 (100 being average) to 135, an increase of 108 per cent. After Bill had been told the results and congratulated on his great improvement, the director told the testing team how, within the last year, Bill's entire personality had changed. The boy was doing so well scholastically that his teachers had commented to the physical education director on what a radical change had occurred in the youngster's behavior. Bill became so outstanding within one year that the hometown newspaper published a story about him.

Over a period of ten years the author has encountered numerous similar examples of youngsters with low fitness scores who were greatly helped by the physical educator. It is apparent that, in order for most youngsters to feel a part of their group or have acceptance by the group, fitness and skill should be developed. If the pupils do not possess sufficient strength to learn these skills, or do not have good instructional opportunity for their mastery, they will, in many instances, deviate from normal behavior patterns in order to achieve some recognition.

What measurement does for the program.   Going back to the illustration of the physical director observing his graduating seniors, it is obvious that in order for a student to be physically educated he must possess the characteristics that the objectives of physical education purport to accomplish. The only way a director can know that objectives have been accomplished is to *measure*. Four specific ways in which a good measurement and evaluation program will help the physical educator are, by classifying students, by determining student status, by measuring progress, and by providing objective means for marking.

Classifying students.   Measurement enables the teacher to place pupils of like ability in the same group. Because much of the physical education program is made up of team activities, it is necessary that pupils on the same level of skills participate together.

Homogeneous grouping facilitates teaching and also creates a much more desirable social atmosphere for the instructional classes than does heterogeneous grouping. As an example, if you were proficient in basketball, you certainly wouldn't enjoy a class composed of dubs. Much more important, if you were a dub, you certainly would feel inadequate in a class of highly skilled players.

The physical educator, because of his well-trained body, frequently fails to recognize the feelings of a poorly coordinated youngster in the physical education class. It is logical that a pupil will be more at home in a class where the majority of the students are of the same general athletic ability.

Determination of student status.   This implies the present standing of the youngster in terms of the physical education objectives. What is the status of his fitness, his proficiency in skills, his ability to get along with others? The only way to determine objectively where the pupil stands in each of these areas is to measure and evaluate.

Once the student's abilities are understood, it becomes possible to construct a program based upon his needs. Too frequently a program made up of seasonal activities is conducted without consideration of each individual student's present ability to participate. For example, in a tennis class, varsity-caliber pupils would not be given the same lesson prepared for beginners. Also, one shouldn't concentrate on strengthening and conditioning activities for a group of youngsters possessing a high degree of fitness. In each case, one must, in order to do an efficient job, evaluate the status of the pupil *before* constructing the program. Measurement and evaluation serve as the basis for scientific program construction.

Measurement of progress.   A large Eastern industry has as its slogan "Progress Is Our Most Important Product." The significance of this quotation has strong implications for the physical educator, since improvement motivates both the pupil and the instructor.

By measuring at the beginning and the end of the school year it is possible to compare individual scores, to show progression or retrogression. This difference in scores serves as a stimulation for the pupil to improve his record. He has something tangible to shoot for.

The measurement of progress serves as a stimulus to the instructor and also gives him insight as to the effectiveness of the teaching methods employed. For instance, if the major portion of the class is remaining static, there is a possibility that the teacher's method is at fault. It is impossible to follow objectively the progress of the student and the program without measurement.

Providing objective means of marking.   For a long time, grading has been a thorn in the side of physical education. Most likely two of the best reasons for this are the large number of pupils that must be taught by the physical educator, and the complex nature of the program. That is to say, physical education is a program in itself, made up of many courses.

It is somewhat difficult to mark on each skill and, at the same time, to weigh each in terms of its contribution to the total grade. Objective tests and wise use of evaluative techniques enable the instructor to grade accomplishments so that the mark is meaningful to pupil, parent, and administrator. In addition to the pedagogic values inherent in grading, a child's mark may be valuable as an instrument in public relations for the physical educator. Chapter 13 is devoted entirely to suggestions that may be taken into consideration when a marking system is being established.

How Measurement Applies to the Program

In administering any test, whether it be in spelling, in arithmetic, or in physical education, the scores generally will be distributed along a continuum from low to high. A small percentage will fall on the low end of the distribution, a small number will be exceptionally high, and the greater portion will be average or near the mean for the group.

If the test should be one in spelling, those pupils on the low end of the distribution would naturally be the poorer spellers, while the more expert spellers would score at the top. Obviously, the abilities of these two groups in terms of spelling is quite different. Hence the teacher would be guided by the test results in planning lessons for these pupils.

This same general reasoning applies when, for example, a test of physical fitness is administered. On the basis of the test results, the pupils will fall into groups with similar needs, depending, of course, upon the test administered. Figure 1 portrays in a basic manner how measurement generally is tied into the physical education program. This skeleton outline might be compared to the sailor's compass, as he sets sail to a strange land. Because of his unfamiliarity with the new places that he will encounter, it is necessary for him to use a compass as a point of reference to prevent him from becoming confused.

Like the sailor, you, too, are embarking upon a journey that will offer many new experiences as you study the materials in measurement. Thus you will need a point of reference to prevent you from becoming lost in a maze of tests that will be presented. A basic outline (Fig. 1) should be kept in mind to help you to understand where and how the particular instrument you are studying applies to the program. Let us emphasize the importance of constantly keeping in mind the relationship between the measuring instrument and the program, for measurement is meaningless unless we make application of the results in the construction of our physical education program.

To visualize more completely how measurement serves in relationship to the physical education program, let us briefly discuss each phase of the basic outline appearing in Figure 1.

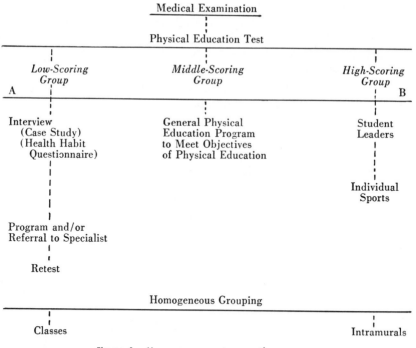

Medical Examination

Physical Education Test

Low-Scoring Group	Middle-Scoring Group	High-Scoring Group
A		B
Interview (Case Study) (Health Habit Questionnaire)	General Physical Education Program to Meet Objectives of Physical Education	Student Leaders
		Individual Sports
Program and/or Referral to Specialist		
Retest		

Homogeneous Grouping

Classes   Intramurals

Figure 1. How measurement serves the program.

Medical examination.   Before any strenuous tests are used to measure the general fitness of the pupils, a medical examination is desirable. This medical examination, among many other things, is valuable in that it is the physician's stamp of approval for the pupil to participate in the regular physical education program. By this means, children with orthopedic deficiencies, cardiac impairment, tendencies toward hernia, and other medical problems, whose health would be jeopardized in taking the test, are screened out. Some school systems do not afford the opportunity for each child to be examined by a medical doctor. In such situations the public health nurse and classroom teacher may be of considerable assistance in locating any children whose health might be endangered by taking the general fitness test.

The medical examination is also of value to the physical educator insofar as it may detect those children who would benefit by an individual program. As an illustration, the physician may find a child with a severe scoliosis and prescribe a corrective program of exercises. The exercises could be administered by the physical educator under the physician's supervision. This is a clear-cut and practical example of how the coordinated efforts of the physician and physical educator can achieve great benefits for the child. As the cooperation of the medical doctor and the physical educator is of utmost importance in working with the sub-fit child, a more complete discussion of this desirable relationship appears in Chapter 14.

Physical education test. Following the medical examination, the physical education test is administered. This test should separate the pupil population into at least three classifications based upon general fitness: the low group, the middle group, and the high group.

The low group. The low group, for the most part, constitutes those pupils requiring special attention in terms of general fitness. Usually 20 per cent of the children tested fall into this classification. The major problems of these sub-fit children include obesity, malnutrition, orthopedic defects, sub-strength levels, emotional disorders, and poor neuromuscular coordination. You certainly can recall these types of youngsters from your own physical education class in junior and senior high school— little Mary, so fat she could hardly jump rope; and Tommy who always had an excuse why he should not be dressed for class. Perhaps Tommy never had a feeling of accomplishment in the various skills taught, and, as a result, avoided gym like the "seven-year-itch." Then too, there are always a few children actually fearful of body contact sports. For the most part, the behavior we observe among these youngsters may be the result of more complex problems. To determine the specific causes of such problems requires that the physical educator investigate all materials available in the school that might have an important bearing upon the child's low fitness. Such records would include the report of the medical examination, the academic record, and evaluative materials that the guidance director might possess, as well as the information that could be obtained from a visit with the classroom teacher. Because of the complex nature of fitness, every resource available in the school should be tapped in order to discover the possible cause or causes of low fitness.

Following collection of this information, the child is summoned for an interview. As can be seen from Figure 1, the case study form and the health habit questionnaire (which appear on pp. 397–399) may be used to make available other information that may give more insight into the child's condition.

The physical educator should now be in a position to determine the type of program that the child needs. If the cause of low fitness is not immediately apparent, the child should be referred to a medical specialist for more complete evaluation.

We might pause for a moment here to consider the knowledge you have gained from such courses as anatomy, kinesiology, physiology, body mechanics, the atypical child, and fundamentals of movement. In working, particularly with the low-fit group, you will be required to draw heavily on the knowledge obtained in these courses. And furthermore, the continued practical application of this scientific knowledge will develop not only self-confidence but also a great respect for what you and your profession have to offer in terms of contributing to the growth and development of children.

Once the cause or causes for the low fitness are determined and the individual program is initiated, the child's progress should be followed by retests four to six weeks apart.

The middle group. The middle group is by far the largest of the three groups and should constitute 60 to 70 per cent of the pupils. These children's needs are served for the most part by the regular program, and the average test score, for example, in terms of general fitness, gives the status of the group as a whole. Thus the instructor knows how his student body stands relative to this objective. Obviously, if the group is low in fitness, the instructor should plan to elevate the group's status by including more activities of a strenuous nature. If the score of the majority of the children is high, then stress may be directed toward the recreational and social fitness objectives.

The high group. The characteristics of the high-scoring pupils, in general, will be quite a contrast to those youngsters on the low end of the scale. The high-scoring pupils are generally adept in skills, have a nice-looking physique, and thrive on sports activity. These individuals have certain needs that must be met by the physical education program. Actually, the primary purpose of the athletic program is to create a situation to challenge these highly skilled youngsters in a variety of sports. It is probably best to stress such activities as tennis, golf, and bait and fly casting, which have great carry-over value into adult life. These pupils also may serve effectively as student leaders, as a result of their high degree of competency in skills. When these youngsters are used as leaders, they are an asset to the physical education program, and have as well an opportunity to develop desirable leadership qualities.

It should be apparent by now that we can expect the three groups to be quite different in terms of general fitness, and, because this is true, each group should have a program planned for its particular needs.

Homogeneous groups. Classifying youngsters into groups of like ability according to certain traits is referred to as homogeneous grouping. A good testing program should enable the instructor to classify his pupils into like groups for participating in the classroom, as well as for equating teams in the intramural program.

History of Measurement

A brief survey of the history of tests and measurements will not only aid us in appreciating the efforts of our professional predecessors, but also afford us a better understanding of this feature of our profession.

It wasn't until the latter part of the 1880's that measurement was given much attention. However, once objective measures of pupil status and progress were introduced, the field grew rapidly. As Van Dalen, Mitchell, and Bennett[18] state: ". . . particularly after 1920, methods in physical education were enriched by the widespread use of tests and measurements and tools of evaluation."

We may conveniently classify the development of this field into the following general areas: (1) Anthropometry; (2) strength; (3) athletic achievement (i.e., running, throwing, and jumping events); (4) sport skills; (5) classification (tests for the purpose of placing pupils into groups of similar ability); (6) personal and social adjustment; (7) cardiovascular fitness (i.e., condition of heart, lungs, and blood vessels); (8) knowledge; and (9) motor fitness.

Anthropometry.   Anthropology deals with the study of man; that is, the study of body and mind and their interrelationships. *Anthropometry* is the science of measuring the human body and its parts. It is used as an aid to the study of human evolution and variation. Between 1885 and 1900 anthropometric measurement in physical education flourished. Dr. Hitchcock at Amherst and Dr. Sargent at Harvard performed some forty such measures, including age, height, weight, chest girth, and lung capacity, as well as girths and lengths of body appendages. During this period Dr. Sargent published a number of articles, including a manual on the physical measurements of outstanding athletes and norms typifying the physical measurements of the American college man and woman.

Strength tests.   In 1699, De La Hire compared the strength of men in lifting weights and carrying burdens with that of horses (Hunsicker and Donnelly)[8]. For some 270 years man has been concerned with the measurement of strength and its relationship to health and athletic prowess.

Sargent,[16] in 1873, while still a medical student at Yale, formulated the intercollegiate strength test. This test measured back and leg strength on a dynamometer; right and left grip with a manuometer; lung capacity with a wet spirometer; and arm strength by the number of pull-ups and dips that could be performed by the subject. Dipping was followed almost immediately by chinning, in order to test muscular endurance. Sargent felt that the primary object of physical training was to develop all-round muscular power for strengthening and improving the structure and functions of all parts of the body. In 1880, he introduced his test at Harvard to evaluate the physical condition of the students. Fifteen colleges and universities adopted the test in 1897.

Kellogg[9, 10] and Martin[12] made extensive contributions in the area of strength testing. After ten years of study, Kellogg developed the Universal Dynamometer with which he could test twenty-five muscle groups. Kellogg viewed exercise from the standpoint of its importance as a therapeutic measure. It had been hypothesized that types of exercise could be prescribed on the basis of muscle size. Seaver and Sargent, however, soon recognized that body size and measures of muscular strength alone did not contribute enough data upon which to base judgment of a man's power and working capacity. Seaver[17] stated that a "large man is not always the strong man, and with equal truth it may be said that the strong man is not always the man of high endurance."

Around 1905, strength tests were discarded because it was felt that they did not take into account measures of endurance and heart and lung development. The fallacious idea that men became muscle-bound by strength exercises and that the tests ruined them for interscholastic competition became prevalent among the athletes. Then too, violation of the rules employed in intercollegiate competition resulted in a wane of interest. For these reasons, strength testing declined during the first part of the twentieth century.

In 1915, while studying the aftereffects of the Vermont polio epidemic, Martin recognized the need for a type of strength test which could be used for comparing normal and involved muscle groups. The principle of resistance to a pull rather than actual strength exertion was introduced by Martin. The resistance to a pull or the "break technique," which it was later called, was recorded by means of a spring scale.

Rogers[15] revived strength testing in 1925 with the publication of his dissertation. He improved upon Sargent's intercollegiate test through construction of norms and statistical validation studies. As a result of these studies the Physical Fitness Index (PFI) and the Strength Index (SI) were developed.

More recently, Clarke[4] developed strength tests to measure muscle groups responsible for thirty-eight joint movements. The tests are highly objective, with coefficients of correlation ranging from .74 to .99. The proper position of the joint for the application of the pulling force is specified in each of the thirty-eight tests. A goniometer is utilized to determine the proper joint angle—the angle at which the muscle group can exert its greatest pulling force. The tension which results from the muscular exertion on the cable is measured in tension pounds with a tensiometer (see Figure 11). The tension pounds can be converted into actual pounds' pull by means of a calibration chart. A more detailed description of these tests appears later in this chapter.

In 1954, Kraus[11] published a number of minimal muscular fitness tests along with data that showed that American children were physically inferior to their European contemporaries. As can be imagined, renewed interest in the field of measurement became manifest, particularly in the elementary, junior, and senior high schools.

Athletic achievement tests.[6, 18]   Gulick formed the Public Schools Athletic League in New York City and introduced achievement tests for elementary schools in 1904. Similar means of measurement were begun in the Baltimore schools during 1908. The popular Athletic Badge Test, published in 1913, had accompanying norms which established minimum standards for every boy. Test items included running, high jump, pull-ups, short dashes, standing high jump, rope climb, push-ups and shot-put. Basketball throw, short dashes and vaulting comprised events for girls. From 1918 through 1920, the Universities of California, Oregon, and Ohio State used such tests for appraising the health and physical efficiency of university students. In 1907, Dr. George Meylan of Columbia University employed the first college achievement tests that measured knowledge of physical fitness, body mechanics, and swimming.

In 1920, Dr. C. H. McCloy published his athletic scoring tables—one of the first applications of statistical procedures to physical education. Meanwhile, at Harvard, Dr. Sargent introduced The Physical Test of a Man. The test measures the explosive power of the legs, and is significantly related to track and field ability. This test, commonly referred to as the Sargent Jump, remains worthwhile today.

The National Recreation Association (1929) developed National Physical Achievement Standards for boys in track and field, games, gymnastics, and aquatics.

Brace in 1927 and Cozens in 1929 published standards for athletic achievement.

A survey conducted in 1920 indicated that the most frequently used tests for boys were: running, high jump, pull-ups, short dashes, standing and running broad jump, rope climb, push-ups, three standing broad jumps, and shot-put. For girls, these tests were: basketball distance throw, short dashes, rope climb, and vaulting.

Sport skill tests.   Brace, in 1924, was the first to use the T-scale method for constructing norms. He used the method to establish norms or standards in a basketball test for girls. The construction of such tests to measure playing ability in particular sports increased rapidly. In 1938 Glassow and Broer published a compilation of skill tests. Today the AAHPER is sponsoring the development and publication of skill tests for fifteen sports. The primary purposes of the AAHPER Sports Skill Tests Project (under the chairmanship of Frank Sills) are as follows: improved grading, better teaching, and greater motivation for pupil improvement.

Classification tests.   Rielly in 1917, followed by McCloy, Rogers, and Brace around 1927, devised tests based primarily upon age, height, weight, strength, and sex for the purpose of placing pupils in homogeneous groups for physical education classes.

Personal and social adjustment.   Luther Van Buskirk in 1928 introduced a character rating scale in physical education. His work was followed with the publication of such a scale by McCloy at Iowa and more recently by Cowell at Purdue.

Cardiovascular tests.   In 1890, Mosso, an Italian physiologist, aroused interest in cardiovascular testing through the invention of an ergograph (an instrument to measure work). In 1905, Crampton devised one of the first cardiovascular tests. This test was followed by McCurdy's test in 1910 and Schneider's test for evaluating the cardiovascular condition of British pilots during World War I. In 1930, Tuttle published his pulse ratio test. Work at the now extinct Harvard Fatigue Laboratory in the 1940's by Brouha and others resulted in the construction of the Harvard Step Test, an instrument widely used today.

Knowledge tests.   By 1925, Brace had published a knowledge test for basketball and Beall had published such a test for tennis. Later work in the 1940's by Scott, French, and Broer contributed much toward establishing this phase of evaluation in physical education.

Motor fitness.   In 1941, at the outbreak of World War II, a large number of these tests, which included pull-ups, push-ups, running, and sit-ups, were developed for every branch of the armed forces. In accordance with valid statistical procedures, norms were established to permit reliable means of appraising fitness of personnel. Today this type of test is quite popular in both public schools and colleges. The AAPHER test is one of the most recent developments in this area of measurement.

In concluding this brief historical outline, we might mention that today the field of measurement and evaluation is well established. All good programs employ instruments of testing and measurement. The scientists in the rapidly increasing number of physical education research laboratories in colleges and universities continue to develop better methods by which we can evaluate the progress of teacher and pupil alike.

Summary and Conclusions

Whatever tests you employ in working with children, it is necessary to make application of the results to your program. If you do this, your pupils, when they graduate, will be indeed physically educated. They will be proficient in recreational activities, possess nice-looking physiques, appreciate the meaning of fitness, and have the necessary skills to function effectively and harmoniously within a group.

This chapter has given a somewhat general orientation to the field of tests and measurements. The purpose and objectives of physical education have been reviewed with the idea of showing the relationship of measurement to objectives, and the general classification of testing materials has been presented.

Measurement has been defined as that part of evaluation which deals with an immediate objective, whereas evaluation is a continuous process over a longer period of time, and involves the goals of the total program as affecting the individual group.

The brief historical outline has oriented us in regard to the beginning of measurement as well as to the present and future directions of this area of physical education.

In conclusion, it seems reasonable to suggest several objectives that the student might hope to achieve during the course in tests and measurements:

1. An understanding of the vital relationship that exists between measurement and evaluation and the objectives of the program. When you have succeeded in achieving this objective, the program, the pupil, and the teacher will benefit.

2. An appreciation for and knowledge of the principles in organizing and administering efficiently the measurement schedule in the physical education program. Efficient administration of the selected tests results in more reliable test scores and greater respect for the measurement schedule by pupils and colleagues.

3. A comprehension of basic procedures in analyzing the data collected from the testing program. In order to use effectively the results of the tests, you must understand elementary statistical procedures.

4. An understanding of the basic principles underlying the application of measurement results to the program. Regardless of the tests you select to administer, there are basic principles in applying the test results to your program. If these test results are not used, it is better not to test at all.

5. An acquaintance with the more pertinent tests in the field of measurement and evaluation. You should become sufficiently familiar with this field to know the best tests available for your particular needs. Furthermore, as a professional person, you should not only be conversant with them, but be able to evaluate these tests scientifically in terms of their utility in the program.

BIBLIOGRAPHY

1. Brownell, Clifford L., and Hagman, Patricia (Eds.): Physical Education—Foundations and Principles. New York, McGraw-Hill Book Company, 1951, Chapter 8.
2. Bucher, Charles A., Koenig, C., and Barnhard, M.: Methods and Materials for Secondary Physical Education. 2nd ed. St. Louis, C. V. Mosby Company, 1965, pp. 39–42.
3. Chamberlain, C. G., and Smiley, D. F.: Functional Health and the Physical Fitness Index. Research Quart., Vol. 2, March, 1931.
4. Clarke, H. Harrison: Application of Measurement to Health and Physical Education. 4th ed. New York, Prentice-Hall, Inc., 1969, p. 141.
5. Good, Carter V.: Dictionary of Education. 2nd ed. New York, McGraw-Hill Book Company, 1959, p. 209.
6. Hackensmith, Charles W.: History of Physical Education. New York, Harper and Row, Publishers, 1966.
7. Holland, George: The Physiology of Flexibility: A Review of The Literature. Kinesiology Review, 1968, pp. 49-62.

8. Hunsicker, Paul A., and Donnelly, R. J.: Instruments to Measure Strength. Research Quart., Vol. 26, December, 1955, pp. 408–420.
9. Kellogg, J. H.: The Measure of Man. Battle Creek, Michigan, Battle Creek Sanitarium, 1910.
10. Kellogg, J. H.: The Value of Strength Tests in the Prescription of Exercise. Modern Medicine Library, 1896, Vol. 2.
11. Kraus, Hans, and Hirschland, Ruth P.: Minimum Muscular Fitness Tests in School Children. Research Quart., 25:177–188, 1954.
12. Martin, E. G.: Tests of Muscular Efficiency. Physiol. Rev., 1:454, 1921.
13. Nash, Jay B.: Physical Education: Interpretations and Objectives. New York, A. S. Barnes & Company, 1948.
14. Oberteuffer, Delbert, and Beyrer, M.: School Health Education. 4th ed. New York, Harper and Brothers, 1960, p. 247.
15. Rogers, Frederick R.: Physical Capacity Tests in the Administration of Physical Education. (Contributions to Education No. 173.) New York, Teachers College, Columbia University, 1925.
16. Sargent, D. A.: Intercollegiate Strength Tests. Amer. Phys. Ed. Rev., 2:108, 1897.
17. Seaver, J. W.: Anthropometry and Physical Education. New Haven, A. O. Dorman Co., 1896.
18. Van Dalen, D., and Bennett, B.: A World History of Physical Education. New York, Prentice-Hall, Inc., 1971, p. 468.
19. Williams, J. F.: Principles of Physical Education. 8th ed. Philadelphia, W. B. Saunders Company, 1964, p. 38.

chapter 2

test selection

Once you have signed your first contract to teach, in addition to celebrating, you will in all probability do three things: obtain an inventory of available facilities and equipment from the school; procure your teaching schedule; and plan an outline of your physical education program for the coming school year in the light of your class schedule, facilities, and equipment.

Incorporated into the program outline should appear the measuring instruments you have selected to use. Certainly you will want to choose the best tests for the particular task in mind, whether they be skill tests, fitness tests, or orthopedic screening tests. Because there are in physical education numerous testing instruments from which to make a choice, it is necessary to weigh carefully the merits of each in making a selection. A primary purpose of this chapter is to help you to do a better job in selecting the testing instruments. This can be accomplished through the application of three general evaluative criteria: scientific authenticity, administrative feasibility, and educational application.

Test Evaluation

Scientific authenticity.   Before a test can even be considered for use in the program, we should make certain that it has been scientifically constructed and that it does an accurate job of measuring what it was designed to measure. The criteria used to evaluate a test, in terms of its scientific worth, are reliability, objectivity, validity, and norms.

Reliability and objectivity.   Reliability and objectivity simply refer to the consistency of the measurement for any given test. That is, if a test were administered to a group of pupils today, we should expect the same results from the test if it were administered to the identical group at another time. It is understood, of course, that in the meantime nothing is done by the group that would cause its members to be better or worse relative to the factor being measured.

Specifically, if one wished to determine the *reliability* of a badminton skill test, he would proceed in the following manner. First, the test would be administered to, say, thirty or forty pupils in the ninth grade, by one examiner. The test scores would then be recorded, and at another time, perhaps a week later, the same test would be administered to the identical pupils by the same examiner. There would then be two sets of data collected on the same group by one instructor. If the individual pupils obtained identical or very similar scores each time the badminton test was administered, we would conclude that the test scores were reliable. That is, they measured consistently the ability of the pupils in terms of the test. To be sure in this study of reliability, we must assume, as was mentioned before, that nothing has been done between tests to change the status of the group or its members in terms of what the test measures.

Reliability of the scores for a standardized paper-and-pencil test is determined in a similar fashion, with one exception. In order to have a test-retest as in the above badminton example, the researcher must construct alternate forms of the same test. Take, for example, a test that measures some phase of social fitness. In order to determine reliability, the author of the test would construct two forms that would measure the same phase of social fitness but with slightly different wording of the questions on each of the two tests. One form of the test would be administered to the group at one time, then at a later date the second form would be administered. If the pupils scored similarly on the two tests, the author would accept the test scores as being reliable.

Objectivity is almost identical in meaning to reliability, with the exception that two or more examiners are involved in collecting the data. It depends upon the ability of different examiners to agree when using the same test on the same group. As an illustration, in the above example in which reliability of the badminton test was being determined, only one examiner collected the two sets of data. To determine the test's objectivity would require at least two examiners, one gathering the first set of scores and the other collecting the second set of data from the same subjects. If the two sets of data agreed, it would be concluded that the test was objective.

Thus in these two sets of "measurement consistency," reliability refers to only one examiner repeating the same test on the same group of subjects and then comparing his own results, while objectivity refers to two or more examiners comparing their results. Naturally a test of objectivity is a better way to conduct this study of "agreement." This is true because, in reliability, where only one examiner is involved, he could consistently be repeating a measurement error that would not necessarily be revealed. It would be unlikely that two or more examiners would make identical mistakes.

Validity.   A test has validity if it measures what it purports to measure. For example, in a test of badminton playing ability, one would want to know how well the obtained test scores agreed with the ability of the group to actually play badminton. In order to determine this relationship one would first administer the test to a group of pupils. The pupils would then play a round-robin tournament, each person playing every other person. If those pupils who scored high on the test also won the most games in the round-robin tournament, one would accept the test as being valid.

Since validity is such an important criterion of a test it might be well to illustrate how a test for a team sport, say basketball, might be validated. First a group of players would be put through a given test of basketball playing ability. Next, a group of coaches thoroughly familiar with the game and the players would subjectively rank the subjects in terms of their playing ability. Then, if the coaches' judgments and the test scores agreed—that is, if those who scored high on the test were also ranked as better players by the coaches—it could be concluded that the test was valid. In other words, the test is measuring what it purports to measure, namely, basketball playing ability. It should be remembered that a test can be no better than its validity, regardless of its reliability and objectivity.

Correlation coefficient.   How are reliability, objectivity, and validity reported? Or what does one look for in the write-up of a test to determine how well the test stands up to its scientific authenticity? The degree of agreement between two variables (a variable being anything that a score may be assigned to, i.e., height, weight, speed, or any test score) is reported as a coefficient or correlation. A coefficient of correlation is used to report reliability, objectivity, and validity. For example, in the study of reliability or objectivity of the badminton skill test, a coefficient of correlation would be reported indicating the degree of agreement between the two sets of data that were gathered on the one group of ninth graders. So too, in the example of the study of validity, a coefficient of correlation would be reported indicative of the degree of relationship between the scores from the test of badminton playing ability and the number of games won by each participant in the round robin tournament.

A coefficient of correlation is computed mathematically, and is designated by the symbol r. If there is perfect agreement between two variables (and this rarely occurs), the r equals 1. If there is perfect agreement between two variables, but in the opposite direction (i.e., one variable becomes larger as the other becomes smaller), the correlation coefficient is assigned a negative value, and the r equals -1. An example of a negative correlation could be the relationship between time in running and leg strength, assuming that the stronger a person's legs are the faster he will be able to run. A greater amount of leg strength is reflected by a higher score, whereas the faster a person runs, the lower his time score, hence a negative correlation. Coefficients of correlation, degrees of agreement between two variables or tests, are usually reported in hundredths from $+1.0$ to -1.0, e.g., .96, .90, .89, .39, $-.46$, $-.97$.

A standard for evaluating tests. When a test is reported in the literature, there will be listed, through a correlation coefficient, the reliability, objectivity, and validity of the test. In order to help determine whether a coefficient or correlation is sufficiently high to state that the test is objective, reliable, or valid, a standard of evaluation has been worked out. Establishing such a standard has its faults, as there are certain exceptions that cannot be taken into consideration by a single scale. However, for practical purposes in evaluating tests for physical education classroom use, the scale should prove useful. In Chapter 3, where a little more attention is given to the correlation coefficient and to its interpretation, we will gain a better understanding of the reasons for selecting the following correlational ranges.

$r = .90$ TO .99. A correlation falling in this range indicates excellent agreement between the variables. Most tests in physical education should show *reliability* and *objectivity* within this range. Such variables as strength, speed in dashes, high jump, broad jump, and throws for distance are objective in nature and as such should give highly consistent results when being measured. Therefore, when evaluating tests in terms of reliability and objectivity, containing such objective measurements, one should expect the coefficients of correlation to fall within this range in order to be acceptable.

$r = .80$ TO .89. Objectivity or reliability coefficients reported within this range, in most cases, would be considered fair. However, validity coefficients may be interpreted as very good from .80 to .85 and excellent above .85. As validity indicates the ability of the test to measure what it purports to measure, one cannot expect as high a coefficient as might be found for reliability and objectivity. Seldom do we obtain a higher than .89 validity coefficient.

$r = .70$ TO .79. Many tests of psychology and education show reliability and objectivity coefficients within this range. In physical education activity tests, this range would be considered only poor to fair for reliability and objectivity. However, quite a number of acceptable validity coefficients may appear in this range. Their worth is dependent upon the complexity of the variables involved. As an illustration, if one were validating a test of general physical fitness, by correlating the obtained scores with a subjective medical examination, the resulting r could not be expected to be high because of the numerous factors involved. One factor that might cause a low correlation, in this particular situation, would be the questionable consistency of various physicians in appraising accurately the health status of the subjects in terms of the medical examination.

$r = .60$ TO $.69$. Generally speaking, this range of correlations, and those below, would be considered poor. However, as was stated above, in the more complex tests, such as those for general physical fitness, a validity coefficient falling within this range might be considered acceptable.

Norms. A norm is a standard to which an obtained score may be compared. Tests that have an accompanying set of norms are much more useful than those that do not. For instance, when a pupil receives a score on a given test, he wants to know how good this obtained score is, or how well it compares with other scores made by youngsters of the same size. Reference to the norm table, which is usually based upon age, height, and weight for a given sex, enables one to find the score that this particular pupil should have obtained for his body size. Thus, if the youngster scored a 60 and his norm were 55, it becomes apparent that he did better than would be expected for a child of comparable age and size.

Greater understanding of norms may be achieved by knowing something of their origin. As an example, let us assume that we wish to construct a set of norms for a test that measures athletic ability. Our first step would be to test a large group of youngsters for whom we want the norms to apply. Let us say that the norms are to be used for junior high school pupils; not only would we have to test a large number, but we should also have to obtain the scores from a random selection of such youngsters. Samples would have to be taken from urban as well as rural schools. If the norms were to apply nationally, the random selection should be extended throughout the country.

Once these data have been gathered, the norms may be computed. This is done by finding the average score for a particular body size. For example, if the norms were to be based upon age, height, and weight, the average score of all pupils of a given age in a particular body classification would constitute that norm. In this manner, a complete set of norms for the various ages and body sizes of junior high school pupils would be constructed for the test of athletic ability.

Norms may be evaluated on the basis of two criteria: (1) that a sufficient number of subjects have been tested to guarantee reliability of the normed scores, and (2) that the data have been obtained from a random population. It is easy to see that, if a sufficient number of subjects have not been tested, the norm might either be too high or too low. Also, if the data to be used in constructing the norms were predominantly gathered from exceptionally good athletes or from extremely poor ones, the norms would be an unfair representation of average ability.

Few tests in physical education have a good set of norms. The service tests, such as the Army, Navy, and Air Force tests, have norms collected on several hundred servicemen. Certain skill tests also have norm tables, the data for their construction being collected from subjects conveniently at hand. It is necessary to emphasize that one must be cautious in applying norms to a group of pupils for which the norms were not originally intended. If one is doubtful as to the value of using a given set of norms, it is better not to use them at all. Rather, one should construct his own norms from the pupils in the situation for which they are to be applied. Constructing norms by use of scales is a simple procedure and can prove of practical worth to the physical educator. Chapter 3 contains a detailed discussion of the methodology of computing norms.

Administrative feasibility.   In order for a test to be practical, it must be economical in terms of cost and time required for administration. One cannot specifically state the proportion of a budget that should be spent on equipment for testing, because of the obvious variation in accessible funds from school to school. You can be sure that it is a rare day when the administration volunteers funds, unless it can be proved that worth-while returns will be forthcoming. However, if the purchase of a piece of equipment can be substantiated on the basis of its contribution to the growth and development of children, it is worth while. Never feel ashamed of fighting for instruments that will benefit your pupils, for they are part of the very reason for which the school exists. By selecting tests that require little equipment—and there are a number of such tests—the measurement and evaluation program can be launched. The results of such a testing program can be the very basis for arguing your point if more expensive equipment is needed.

The amount of time one should devote to testing is moot. Some authorities state that it should be 10 per cent of the entire time allotted; the basis for this particular estimate is vague. For example, a test of general fitness may be given once in the fall and again in the spring, taking a total of six days for its administration. Obviously the time of administration depends upon the type of test, the amount of help, and the number of pupils tested. If the school meets 180 days, the six days of testing would represent approximately 3 per cent of the total attendance days. Some tests that may be administered are functional, that is, a basic objective is being strived for while, at the same time, scores are recorded. The author immediately thinks of a motor fitness test that perhaps contains pull-ups, a 300-yard run, and sit-ups for two minutes. Such a test is functional because the pupils are being conditioned in terms of fitness while they are being measured. The same consideration to a skill test, which usually involves executing a basic skill of a game consistently over a specified period of time. This too is functional, for the pupil is becoming more efficient in terms of that specific sport while he is being evaluated. It becomes apparent that it is almost impossible to state the specific amount of time that should be allotted for testing, as measurement and evaluation should be a continuous process. To separate evaluation and measurement from teaching is difficult and perhaps illogical. One should keep in mind, however, that tests are not made for the sake of testing. The testing schedule is designed to improve instruction and hence learning. This might be a more prudent criterion to apply in determining the amount of time that should be devoted to testing, rather than relying on a fixed percentage of program time.

Educational application. In selecting tests, it should be noted that the type of program to be offered during the school year, to a great extent, dictates the type of tests to be employed. Usually the program will be dependent upon the available facilities as well as climatic conditions and other such limiting factors. The area of testing most affected by such limitations will be in the program of sport skills. Generally speaking, it is desirable to administer a test of skills in each of the major recreational sports offered. Thus, tests should be selected that can be most useful in serving the program.

In addition to evaluating the status and progress of pupils in sport skills, the physical educator should include tests of physical fitness and also some means of evaluating social fitness.

Under the objective of physical fitness, a test reflecting general body condition, as in the area of strength, motor fitness, or cardiorespiratory endurance, could be selected. The variables involved in these tests reflect to a greater extent the general fitness of a pupil than do the tests of sport skills. In this way the sub-fit pupils can be discovered and the proper program to ameliorate the cause or causes of their lower achievement can be initiated. Also, a screening test in the field of body mechanics is a necessity to locate, at the earliest possible time, pupils having orthopedic deviations. Early diagnosis and the ensuing program will significantly diminish the number of pupils requiring corrective therapy in later years.

To round out the measurement schedule for the general program, tendencies toward emotional maladjustment should be evaluated continuously. Although there are not a great number of practical measuring instruments to select from in the area of social fitness, the very characteristic of the physical education program permits an excellent opportunity to observe and record tendencies toward maladjustment. The attitudes of the pupil in the various dynamic situations created by competition, in group games, and in the coeducational program become apparent, and can thus be noted and recorded by the alert educator. For example, the child who withdraws from group games or body contact sports, the youngster who bullies his smaller counterpart, the pupil who constantly forgets his uniform, and the "side-liner" all present symptoms that are usually products of deeper problems. Through determining its cause or causes, the basic problem may be discovered and ameliorated, resulting in tremendous benefit in terms of the child's growth and development.

Summary and Conclusions

The purpose of this chapter has been to help you to select tests for use in your program. The tests under consideration for use should be reliable, objective, and valid. Tests that have been scientifically constructed will include a statement, usually in the form of a coefficient of correlation, relative to the criteria mentioned.

A test for which a scale of norms is provided is very useful because it permits comparison of an achieved test score with an average score obtained from a number of pupils of comparable body size. These norms should be constructed from a large and random sample of subjects. They should be used only on subjects for whom they were intended.

Measurement and evaluation methods should be selected on the basis of the program and its objectives. Essentially, the broad objectives, of physical fitness, recreational fitness, and social fitness designate the areas in which tests should be chosen. Thus skill tests, a test of general fitness, an orthopedic test, and a means of evaluating social fitness are essential tests for the physical education program.

The application of the testing results to the general program includes: (1) determination of youngsters who are below par in terms of test findings; (2) diagnosis for failure or deviation from normal; (3) construction of a program based upon the child's needs; and, finally, (4) retesting to determine if improvement has taken place.

chapter 3

analysis of test scores

To prepare a delicious dinner, set the table, and fail to sit down to enjoy the meal is just as ridiculous as failing to analyze the measurement data after the test has been administered. In the following pages we will attempt to explain the analysis of test data.

The statistical know-how required for the necessary analysis of test scores for use in a physical education program is not difficult. Even if, as a youngster, you were frightened by an integer, the phobia should not prevent you from comprehending the statistical analyses presented in this chapter. In order to obtain from the data an adequate realization for the effort spent in its collection, the scores must be analyzed. There are answers to perhaps five questions that we might want to derive from these data:

1. How did the group as a whole do on the test?
2. How does each individual stand in relation to the group?
3. How can we homogeneously group the pupils?
4. How can we use these scores for grading purposes?
5. How do we go about constructing norms?

The following approach to analysis of test data places emphasis upon the interpretation of test scores rather than upon explanation of theory and derivation of techniques employed. The specific steps to the final answer are outlined in detail.

Statistical Analysis

When baking a cake, the average homemaker does not understand the chemical effects of the ingredients she uses. However, if she is careful and follows directions, the product is quite gratifying. Somewhat similar application of this principle will yield excellent results in manipulation

33

of statistical formulas. In other words, it is not necessary to be as concerned with the derivation of the formulas as with their application to practical testing problems. It is our purpose, then, to present some simple statistical techniques that will give useful answers to the questions listed above.

The sample problem.   A motor fitness test was administered to fifty pupils in junior high school; one of the items was a series of two-minute sit-ups. The following test scores were chosen to illustrate the application of selected statistical techniques in finding answers to the five questions posed.

48	32	18	28	28
39	30	30	27	41
42	31	31	33	39
43	32	32	30	38
45	33	33	31	35
22	12	33	32	37
23	15	26	33	35
24	16	26	29	34
25	19	27	29	36
23	20	28	27	36

Frequency table.   A large number of test scores can be more efficiently handled if the scores are grouped than if they are considered individually. Grouping is accomplished by constructing a frequency table (see Table 1). Proceed as follows:

1. Find the range of scores by subtracting the lowest score from the highest.

2. Select a step interval (sometimes called a class interval and abbreviated S.I. or i) that will result in not more than twenty or less than ten intervals. For a large number of test scores the number of step intervals

TABLE 1.   *Tabulation of Two-Minute Sit-up Scores Made by Fifty Junior High School Pupils*

Mid-points	Step Intervals	Tallies	Frequency
47.5	45.5—49.4	1	1
43.5	41.5—45.4	111	3
39.5	37.5—41.4	1111	4
35.5	33.5—37.4	┼┼┼ 1	6
31.5	29.5—33.4	┼┼┼ ┼┼┼ ┼┼┼	15
27.5	25.5—29.4	┼┼┼ ┼┼┼	10
23.5	21.5—25.4	┼┼┼	5
19.5	17.5—21.4	111	3
15.5	13.5—17.4	11	2
11.5	9.5—13.4	1	1
			N = 50

should approach ten, whereas in a small number of cases the step intervals should be nearer 20. In the sample problem, with fifty cases, the total step intervals should be nearer to ten; therefore, the range of 36 is divided by ten, giving 3.6. Rounding this figure off gives a step interval of four.

3. Begin constructing the frequency table by selecting a starting point that will include the lowest test score in the first step interval. In the sample problem we could use either nine or ten. As ten seems to be a more convenient number to start with, we will use it. Table 1 contains the frequency table with ten step intervals.

4. Tally the test scores in their proper classes as illustrated in the table. The column adjacent to the tally column is labeled "frequency" (often designated as f), representing the frequency of scores occurring in the various intervals.

5. When interpreting the distance of a step interval, we must keep in mind that a given score also falls within a range. For example, 5 may be interpreted as anything from 4.5 up to and including 5.4. We apply this reasoning when discussing the range of a step interval. In Table 1 the range of the first step interval is from 9.5 up to, and including, 13.4. That is, all scores from 9.5 to 13.4, inclusive, would be tallied in this interval. The lower limit of the next step interval is 13.5, and the upper limit is 17.4.

The mean or average.   It is important to know the one best score that is most representative of the group. The mean or average is the measure of *central tendency* most commonly used. It may be computed through adding up the scores and dividing by the number of scores added together. However, once the data are grouped as in Table 1, the simplest method is to proceed as follows:

1. Select the step interval in which you guess the mean will fall (in most instances it will be the interval containing the greatest number of frequencies) and draw two parallel lines across the paper as in Table 2.

2. Alongside the f (frequency) column, make a d (deviation) column. This column is filled in by counting the *deviations* that each step interval is removed from the interval in which you have guessed the mean to fall. The deviations above the mean are assigned positive values, while those below it are given negative ones.

3. Next to the d column construct an fd column. The figures for this column are obtained by multiplying the values in the f column by those in the corresponding d column.

4. Add the f column; the total should be that of the number (N) of pupils tested.

5. Compute the sum of the fd column by adding up the positive and negative values separately. Determine the difference between these two scores. If the sum of the scores on the negative side of the mean is larger than the sum of the positive scores, assign this difference a negative sign; whereas, if the positive is larger, assign the difference a positive

TABLE 2. *Calculation of Mean from Two-Minute Sit-up Data Grouped in a Frequency Table*

Step Intervals	f	d	fd
45.5–49.4	1	4	4
41.5–45.4	3	3	9
37.5–41.4	4	2	8
33.5–37.4	6	1	6
29.5–33.4	15		27 ⟋ −42
25.5–29.4	10	−1	−10
21.5–25.4	5	−2	−10
17.5–21.4	3	−3	−9
13.5–17.4	2	−4	−8
9.5–13.4	1	−5	−5
	N = 50		Σ = −15

$$M. = G.M. + \left(\frac{\Sigma\, fd}{N} \times S.I. \right) \qquad M = 31.5 + \left(\frac{-15}{50} \times 4 \right)$$

G.M. = 31.5   M = 30.3
Σ fd = −15
S.I. = 4

value. In Table 2 the negative is the larger; therefore the difference is assigned a negative value.

6. The formula for computing the mean is:

$$M = G.M. + \left(\frac{\Sigma\, fd}{N} \times S.I. \right)$$

M = mean
G.M. = guessed mean, or mid-point of the step interval in which the mean was selected. It is computed by dividing the step interval by two and adding this to the lower limit of the step interval in which the mean was guessed. (For illustrative purposes, Table 1 contains the midpoints of each of the ten step intervals.)
Σ = summation of scores
Σ fd = total of the fd column
S.I. = step interval.

Table 2 shows the computation of the mean for the sample problem.

When interpreting the mean it should be remembered that this measure of central tendency is affected by extreme scores. In some instances this may result in erroneous conclusions about the data. For example, a person may say, "The average salary of the residents on my street is $10,000." This may be true, but perhaps 99 per cent of the families have an average income amounting to $5,000, whereas 1 per cent receive an extremely high wage. This, of course, unduly affects the mean, hence giving an incorrect picture of the situation.

Actually, the average or mean may be compared to the fulcrum on a teeter board when the board is in perfect equilibrium. If we place an exceptionally heavy person on one end and a very light person on the other, the fulcrum will have to be placed closer to the heavy person in order to balance the teeter board. So too, in a distribution of scores, the mean will fall at the point where the data on either side of this central point are in balance: one extremely low score will pull the mean toward it, and an exceptionally high score will do likewise.

Median. In most situations, the mean is used as the score which best represents how well a group performed on a test. However, there are conditions in which extreme scores as already mentioned may affect the mean so that it becomes an unreliable measure of central tendency. The median, or the point above and below which one half or 50 per cent of the scores fall (also a measure of central tendency), is unaffected by extreme scores. The median can be computed for ungrouped data when N is odd or even as well as for grouped data. Scores are always arranged in order of magnitude.

Ungrouped data, N odd: 7, 11, 15, 19, 22. The median is 15, the point above and below which 50 per cent of the scores fall.

Ungrouped data, N even: 4, 5, 7, 11, 15, 18, 19, 21. Eleven and 15 are the two middle scores; hence it becomes necessary to determine the midpoint between 11 and 15, which is 13; that is, the lower limit of 11 plus one half the difference between 10.5 and 15.5, or 10.5 + 2.5.

To compute the median when data are grouped, turn to page 48 under percentiles, for the median, fiftieth percentile, and second quartile (Q_2) are one and the same.

The following is an example of when the physical educator might choose the median in preference to the mean in representing the most reliable measure of central tendency. Suppose that the principal of your school wishes to know the average fitness score in a remedial class. There are ten pupils in the class who have been working very hard throughout the year; one youngster has not been applying himself. The 11 scores are as follows:

    36   71   72   73   75   78   80   81   85   85   86

In this case the mean equals 75 (74.72), whereas the median, obviously a much more representative score for the majority of the class, equals 78, a difference of three points. The score of 36 resulted in a low and unreliable representation of class performance. From this example one can see how the expression "figures lie" evolved. In a distribution which is symmetrical, or normal, the mean and the median would be equal.

Standard deviation.   The mean, or average, is referred to as a measure of central tendency; that is, the score that best represents how the pupils as a group stand. To determine how the scores cluster about the mean, it becomes necessary to know the measure of variability of the data. This statistic is referred to as the standard deviation, and may be defined as that measure which indicates the scatter or spread of the middle 68.26 per cent of the scores about the mean. For example, a mean of 50 with a standard deviation of 5 would be interpreted as: approximately 68 per cent of the students scored between 50 ± 5, or from 45 to 55 (normal distribution).

The standard deviation (written as σ, the Greek letter sigma) is computed in the following way (Table 3):

$$\sigma = \text{S.I.} \sqrt{\frac{\Sigma\, fd^2}{N} - \left(\frac{\Sigma\, fd}{N}\right)^2} \qquad \sigma = 4 \sqrt{\frac{179}{50} - \left(\frac{-15}{50}\right)^2}$$

$$\text{S.I.} = 4$$
$$\Sigma\, fd^2 = 179$$
$$N - 50$$
$$\Sigma\, fd = -15$$

TABLE 3.   *Calculation of Standard Deviation from Two-Minute Sit-up Data Grouped in a Frequency Table*

Step Intervals	f	d	fd	fd²
45.5–49.4	1	4	4	16
41.5–45.4	3	3	9	27
37.5–41.4	4	2	8	16
33.5–37.4	6	1	6	6
29.5–33.4	15		27 / −42	
25.5–29.4	10	−1	−10	10
21.5–25.4	5	−2	−10	20
17.5–21.4	3	−3	−9	27
13.5–17.4	2	−4	−8	32
9.5–13.4	1	−5	−5	25
	N = 50		Σ = −15	Σ = 179

1. Construct an fd^2 column alongside the fd column. The figures for this column are obtained by multiplying the scores in the fd column by

the corresponding score in the d column. It should be recognized that all the scores in this column will be positive, for a negative multiplied by a negative yields a positive, as is the case for those scores falling below the mean. (See Table 3).

2. Add the scores in the fd^2 column and insert the value in the following formula:

$$\sigma = \text{S.I.} \sqrt{\frac{\Sigma\, fd^2}{N} - \left(\frac{\Sigma\, fd}{N}\right)^2}$$

$\sigma =$ standard deviation
$\Sigma\, fd^2 =$ total of the fd^2 column
$N =$ number of cases
$\Sigma\, fd =$ sum of the fd column
S.I. $=$ step interval.

Table 3 gives the solution for the problem of determination of the standard deviation for the sample analysis. Appendix A contains square root tables to help in making these computations.

The standard deviation of the scores should always be given when reporting the mean. This statistic tells how well the major portion of the pupils scored about the mean. A large standard deviation indicates that the data are variable and hence heterogeneous, whereas a small deviation shows that the group is quite homogeneous. For example, if in a fitness test administered to 100 pupils the mean was found to be 65 and the standard deviation 10, we would know that 68 per cent of the youngsters scored between 55 and 75, a very homogeneous group. On the other hand, if merely the mean were reported, this would actually tell us very little. Possibly two or three extreme scores occurred, which caused the mean to be significantly shifted toward either the low or high end of the scale. The standard deviation, also being affected by extreme scores, immediately tips us off as to the homegeneity of the data.

One way in which to obtain an estimate of whether our standard deviation is unusually large or small is to remember that there should be about six standard deviations between our lowest and highest scores. For example, in a distribution with a low score of 30 and a high score of 120, the range would equal 90. The standard deviation should approximate 15, or one-sixth of the range, provided the distribution is normal. This simple calculation results in a measure that serves as a reference point in helping us to evaluate the size of the standard deviation.

If we have only a few cases (when N is less than 30) and it is not feasible to group the data, the standard deviation for ungrouped data can be computed in the following manner:

TABLE 4.   *Computing Standard Deviation When N is Small (30 or less)*

X	d	d²
5	0	0
4	−1	1
6	1	1
3	−2	4
7	2	4
25		10

Computing the mean:

$$M = \frac{25}{5} = 5$$

Computing the standard deviation:

$$\sigma = \sqrt{\frac{\Sigma\, d^2}{N-1}}$$

where:

σ = standard deviation
d = deviation of each score from mean (X — M)
$\Sigma\, d^2$ = sum of squared deviations of each score about the mean
N = number of scores.

then:

$$\sigma = \sqrt{\frac{10}{5-1}} = \sqrt{2.5}$$

$$\sigma = 1.58$$

The normal curve.   The normal curve is a graph very similar to that representing the probability of what would occur if the combination of heads and tails resulting from one flip of ten coins were plotted on graph paper. Table 5 illustrates the various combinations resulting from such an experiment. Figure 2 is a graph of these theoretical results, while the smoothed line superimposed on the graphed combinations represents a normal curve.

This type of curve is also referred to as a probability curve, because chance happenings, such as rolling dice, flipping coins, and most all occurrences depending on a large number of chance happenings, will result in such a graph. The normal curve is selected for study because frequently the data found in educational testing follow the properties of the normal curve. For example, scores resulting from measuring a large group in spelling, in arithmetic, for IQ, or for fitness, height, weight, and skills ability will be distributed in accordance with properties of the normal curve.

Figure 3 illustrates the normal curve divided into three parts on either

TABLE 5. *Possible Combinations Resulting from Tossing Ten Coins Simultaneously**

		Probability Ratio
1 H10	1 chance in 1024 of 10 heads	$\dfrac{1}{1024}$
10 H9 T1	10 chances in 1024 of 9 heads and 1 tail	$\dfrac{10}{1024}$
45 H8 T2	45 chances in 1024 of 8 heads and 2 tails	$\dfrac{45}{1024}$
120 H7 T3	120 chances in 1024 of 7 heads and 3 tails	$\dfrac{120}{1024}$
210 H6 T4	210 chances in 1024 of 6 heads and 4 tails	$\dfrac{210}{1024}$
252 H5 T5	252 chances in 1024 of 5 heads and 5 tails	$\dfrac{252}{1024}$
210 H4 T6	210 chances in 1024 of 4 heads and 6 tails	$\dfrac{210}{1024}$
120 H3 T7	120 chances in 1024 of 3 heads and 7 tails	$\dfrac{120}{1024}$
45 H2 T8	45 chances in 1024 of 2 heads and 8 tails	$\dfrac{45}{1024}$
10 H1 T9	10 chances in 1024 of 1 head and 9 tails	$\dfrac{10}{1024}$
1 T10	1 chance in 1024 of 10 tails	$\dfrac{1}{1024}$

1024

* Adapted from Garrett, Henry E.: Statistics in Psychology and Education. 6th ed. New York, Longmans, Green & Co., Inc., 1970, p. 92.

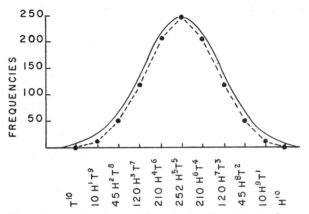

Figure 2. Theoretical results obtained from tossing ten coins simultaneously. (Garrett, Henry E.: Statistics in Psychology and Education. New York, Longmans, Green & Co., 1953, p. 91.)

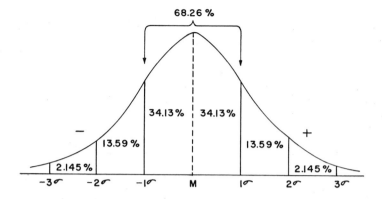

Figure 3. Division of normal curve into standard deviation units.

side of a center line that in turn bisects the curve. The middle line represents the mean of the scores. The three lines on either side of the mean are equidistant along the base line and are referred to as standard deviation units. The right side of the mean is positive, indicating the direction toward the high scores of the distribution, while the left side is negative, or toward the lower scores of the distribution. Thus the normal curve is divided into six standard deviations, three on each side of the mean.

By methods employed in calculus, it is possible to compute the area under each segment of the curve. It so happens that, in a normal curve or distribution, one standard deviation above the mean contains 34.13 per cent of the scores; between one and two standard deviations 13.59 per cent of the scores fall; and between two and three standard deviations lie 2.145 per cent of the scores. As the normal curve is bilateral, the same percentages apply to the negative side of the curve.

In adding up the percentages, the sum comes to 99.73 per cent, which means that 0.27 per cent of the scores are not included. Obviously, to include more cases we would have to embrace more standard deviations on either side of the mean. However, for most purposes, six standard deviations will satisfactorily serve our needs, as very few test scores fall outside of these limits.

Table 6 has been prepared for our convenience when referring to the fractional parts of a standard deviation under the normal curve. For example, what per cent of the cases fall 1.8 standard deviations above the mean (positive side of the curve)? In the extreme left-hand column of Table 6 we locate 1.8; in the adjacent column we find that 46.41 per cent of the cases fall between the mean and 1.8 standard deviations. What per cent fall 1.86 standard deviations above the mean? The same procedure is followed with the exception that we must look across the top of the table for the .06 column; down this column opposite the 1.8 we note that 46.86 per cent of the cases fall between the mean and 1.86 standard deviations.

Use of the normal curve in interpretation of data.   Usually, when we have administered a test in physical education, we may safely assume that the data will distribute themselves in a normal manner, that is, will follow the properties of the normal curve. Going on this assumption, we then can use the normal probability table for determining what percentage of our students scored at various standard deviation distances from the mean. As an illustration, in the sample problem the mean was 30.3 and one standard deviation is equal to 7.5. According to our normal curve table, a range of one standard deviation either side of the mean contains 68.26 per cent of the cases. In the sample problem, one standard deviation equals 7.5 and, when added to and subtracted from the mean, results in a range of about 23 to 38. Thus we may say that approximately 68 per cent of our pupils scored within this range. If we had 100 pupils, close to 68 of them would have a score not lower than 23 or higher than 38.

Standard scores.   In order to interpret a test score to a pupil, we should have a basis for comparison. Merely telling Johnny that he scored 60 on a test does not divulge much information. However, if we quote the percentage of pupils scoring above and below the score of 60, Johnny immediately will comprehend his relative position in the group. Converting the distance a given score is removed from the mean into standard deviation units enables one to refer to the table of the normal curve and read the percentage of scores falling within this area. To illustrate, let us say that the mean is 50 and the standard deviation is 8. If a pupil scores 54 on the test, what percentage of the pupils scored above and below this point? In this case the pupil scored a distance of 4 points above the mean. Dividing 4 by the standard deviation of 8 equals the 0.5 standard deviation unit that this score of 54 is above the mean. Referring to Table 6, we note that 19.15 per cent of the cases fall between the mean and 0.5 standard deviation. Thus, approximately 69 per cent (50% + 19%) of the pupils scored below 54, while 31 per cent scored above 54. The number of deviation units by which a test score is removed from the mean is referred to as a standard score. The formula for its computation may be written:

$$\text{Standard score} = \frac{X - M}{\sigma}$$

X = any test score
M = mean
σ = standard deviation of data.

TABLE 6. *Percentage Parts of the Total Area under the Normal Probability Curve Corresponding to Distances on the Base Line between the Mean and Successive Points from the Mean in Units of Standard Deviation**

Example: Between the mean and a point 1.57 sigma is found 44.18 per cent of the entire area under the curve.

Units	.00	.01	.02	.03	.04	.05	.06	.07	.08	.09
0.0	00.00	00.40	00.80	01.20	01.60	01.99	02.39	02.79	03.19	03.59
0.1	03.98	04.38	04.78	05.17	05.57	05.96	06.36	06.75	07.14	07.53
0.2	07.93	08.32	08.71	09.10	09.48	09.87	10.26	10.64	11.03	11.41
0.3	11.79	12.17	12.55	12.93	13.31	13.68	14.06	14.43	14.80	15.17
0.4	15.54	15.91	16.28	16.64	17.00	17.36	17.72	18.08	18.44	18.79
0.5	19.15	19.50	19.85	20.19	20.54	20.88	21.23	21.57	21.90	22.24
0.6	22.57	22.91	23.24	23.57	23.89	24.22	24.54	24.86	25.17	25.49
0.7	25.80	26.11	26.42	26.73	27.04	27.34	27.64	27.94	28.23	28.52
0.8	28.81	29.10	29.39	29.67	29.95	30.23	30.51	30.78	31.06	31.33
0.9	31.59	31.86	32.12	32.38	32.64	32.90	33.15	33.40	33.65	33.89
1.0	34.13	34.38	34.61	34.85	35.08	35.31	35.54	35.77	35.99	36.21
1.1	36.43	36.65	36.86	37.08	37.29	37.49	37.70	37.90	38.10	38.30
1.2	38.49	38.69	38.88	39.07	39.25	39.44	39.62	39.80	39.97	40.15
1.3	40.32	40.49	40.66	40.82	40.99	41.15	41.31	41.47	41.62	41.77
1.4	41.92	42.07	42.22	42.36	42.51	42.65	42.79	42.92	43.06	43.19
1.5	43.32	43.45	43.57	43.70	43.83	43.94	44.06	44.18	44.29	44.41
1.6	44.52	44.63	44.74	44.84	44.95	45.05	45.15	45.25	45.35	45.45
1.7	45.54	45.64	45.73	45.82	45.91	45.99	46.08	46.16	46.25	46.33
1.8	46.41	46.49	46.56	46.64	46.71	46.78	46.86	46.93	46.99	47.06
1.9	47.13	47.19	47.26	47.32	47.38	47.44	47.50	47.56	47.61	47.67
2.0	47.72	47.78	47.83	47.88	47.93	47.98	48.03	48.08	48.12	48.17
2.1	48.21	48.26	48.30	48.34	48.38	48.42	48.46	48.50	48.54	48.57
2.2	48.61	48.64	48.68	48.71	48.75	48.78	48.81	48.84	48.87	48.90
2.3	48.93	48.96	48.98	49.01	49.04	49.06	49.09	49.11	49.13	49.16
2.4	49.18	49.20	49.22	49.25	49.27	49.29	49.31	49.32	49.34	49.36

As another example, let us say that Johnny scored 38 sit-ups in the sample problem. What percentage of the pupils scored above and below him? The problem is solved in the following manner:

$$X = 38$$
$$M = 30$$
$$\sigma = 7.5$$

$$\text{Standard score} = \frac{38 - 30}{7.5} = 1.07 \ \sigma \text{ units}$$

TABLE 6. (Continued)

Units	.00	.01	.02	.03	.04	.05	.06	.07	.08	.09
2.5	49.38	49.40	49.41	49.43	49.45	49.46	49.48	49.49	49.51	49.52
2.6	49.53	49.55	49.56	49.57	49.59	49.60	49.61	49.62	49.63	49.64
2.7	49.65	49.66	49.67	49.68	49.69	49.70	49.71	49.72	49.73	49.74
2.8	49.74	49.75	49.76	49.77	49.77	49.78	49.79	49.79	49.80	49.81
2.9	49.81	49.82	49.82	49.83	49.84	49.84	49.85	49.85	49.86	49.86
3.0	49.865									
3.1	49.903									
3.2	49.93129									
3.3	49.95166									
3.4	49.96631									
3.5	49.97674									
3.6	49.98409									
3.7	49.98922									
3.8	49.99277									
3.9	49.99519									

* Adapted from: Biometrika Tables for Statisticians, Vol. 1, 1954. Edited by E. S. Pearson and H. O. Hartley.

The standard deviation unit that the score of 38 is removed from the mean is 1.07. As shown in Table 6, 1.07 standard deviations from the mean include 35.77 per cent of the cases. Thus we may say that approximately 86 per cent of the pupils scored below Johnny, while only 14 per cent of them scored above him.

Scales and percentile tables. Scales provide a means for placing various test scores on a common table from 0 to 100. Scaling data enables one to:

1. Compare and average unlike scores, e.g., data obtained from track events, skill testing, fitness testing, and swimming results may be averaged, thus providing a general index.

2. Group or classify pupils.

3. Interpret individual standings against the group.

4. Make norms from test data.

Three scales—Sigma, Hull, and T—and the percentile table will be discussed in this section. All that one needs for constructing the three scales is the mean and the standard deviation of the data. The only difference in these three scales is the number of standard deviations contained in each. The Sigma scale includes 3 standard deviations on either side of the mean; the Hull scale, 3.5 standard deviations; while the T-scale is made up of 5 standard deviations on either side of the mean.

The percentile table consists of points along the 0 to 100 table where a certain percentage of scores lie above and below. It is calculated directly from the frequency table.

Sigma scale (Table 7).   The Sigma scale is calculated as follows:

1. Compute the mean and standard deviation as described.

2. Place the numbers 1 to 100 in a column, and opposite 50 place the mean of the data.

TABLE 7.   *Calculation of Sigma, Hull, and T-Scales for Two-Minute Sit-ups**

Scale Score	Sigma Scale		Hull Scale		T-Scale	
	Computed	Rounded Off	Computed	Rounded Off	Computed	Rounded Off
100	52.8	53	56.8	57	67.8	68
90	48.3	48	51.5	52	60.3	60
80	43.8	44	46.2	46	52.8	53
70	39.3	39	40.9	41	45.3	45
60	34.8	35	35.6	36	37.8	38
50	30.3	30	30.3	30	30.3	30
40	25.8	26	25.0	25	22.8	23
30	21.3	21	19.7	20	15.3	15
20	16.8	17	14.4	14	7.8	7
10	12.3	12	9.1	9	—	—
0	7.8	8	3.8	4	—	—

Sigma Scale	Hull Scale	T-Scale
$M \pm \dfrac{3\sigma}{5}$	$M \pm \dfrac{3.5\sigma}{5}$	$M \pm \dfrac{5\sigma}{5}$
Rate $= 30.3 \pm \dfrac{(3)\ (7.5)}{5}$	Rate $= 30.3 \pm \dfrac{(3.5)\ (7.5)}{5}$	Rate $= 30.3 \pm \dfrac{(5)\ (7.5)}{5}$
Rate $= 30.3 \pm 4.5$	Rate $= 30.3 \pm 5.3$	Rate $= 30.3 \pm 7.5$

* Note: For convenience of presenting the scales, the column 0 to 100 has been divided into tenths rather than hundredths. In this case the denominators of the formulas become 5 rather than 50.

3. Multiply the standard deviation by 3 and divide this by 50.

4. Consecutively add this number to the mean for determining points 51 to 100 on the 0 to 100 scale; and consecutively subtract this number from the mean for determining assigned values from 49 to 0. Note that in Table 7 the scales are computed in tenths, rather than hundredths, for ease of presentation. Hence the rate is computed by dividing by 5 rather than by 50.

Hull scale.   The same procedure for constructing the Sigma scale is used here, with the exception of step 3. Multiply the standard deviation by 3.5, divide by 50, and serially add to and subtract from the mean this result, as was done in step 4 above, for determining the values to assign on the 0 to 100 scale.

T-scale. Once again, the only difference is step 3. Multiply the standard deviation by 5, divide by 50, and consecutively add to and subtract from the mean this result. Table 7 contains the three scales constructed from the data obtained in the two-minute sit-up test.

Choice of three scales. The customary argument against use of the Sigma scale is that not a sufficient number of scores are contained within six standard deviations. For example, if a youngster scored only 5 or 6 sit-ups he would not be included on the lower end of the scale, as illustrated in Table 7. This same type of reasoning could be applied to the upper end of the scale. Too frequently there would be pupils obtaining scores which would not be on either end of the Sigma scale.

By the same token, the T-scale may be criticized for just the opposite effect. From our data in Table 7, we cannot use the lower end of the scale, as it is impossible to score a negative number of sit-ups. Likewise a junior high school pupil would find it extremely difficult to score 68 sit-ups in two minutes, which is necessary to earn 100 points on the T-scale. Although the Hull scale appears to reach a happy medium, it is more difficult to interpret. Because of this, the T and sigma scales are most commonly employed.

Percentiles and quartiles. A *percentile* indicates that point at which a certain percentage of scores lies above and a certain percentage falls below. The interpretation of the percentile is somewhat similar to that of the standard score in that both percentile and standard score indicate the percentages falling above and below a given score. The difference between the two is that the percentile table does not take into consideration the mean and variability of the scores. The percentile table *does not have equal scale units of uniform length.* It may be effectively used as a method to show relative standing of individuals in terms of rank. The percentile, by definition, represents the point at which a certain percentage of subjects scored above and below, regardless of the distribution of scores. The advantage of using percentiles as a norm or standard is ease of interpretation by both pupil and teacher. For example, a youngster receiving a percentile score of 70 on a particular test can readily understand that 30 per cent of his classmates scored above him and 70 per cent scored below him. This ease of understanding was one reason that the norms for the AAHPER Youth Fitness Test were stated in terms of percentiles.

The three percentiles that divide the table into quarters are called *quartiles.* The first quartile, Q_1, is the twenty-fifth percentile and is the point at which 25 per cent of the scores fall below and 75 per cent above. Specifically, from Table 8, Q_1 for the two-minute sit-ups equals 26.

TABLE 8.   *Computation of Percentiles for Two-Minute Sit-ups*

Step Intervals	f	cf		
45.5–49.4	1	50	P100	48
41.5–45.4	3	49	P90	41
37.5–41.4	4	46	P80	36
33.5–37.4	6	42	P70	33
29.5–33.4	15	36	P60	32
25.5–29.4	10	21	P50	31
21.5–25.4	5	11	P40	29
17.5–21.4	3	6	P30	27
13.5–17.4	2	3	P20	25
9.5–13.4	1	1	P10	20
	N = 50		P0	12

P10

$$50$$
$$.10$$
$$\overline{5.0}$$

$$17.5 + \left(\frac{2}{3} \times 4 \right) = 20.2$$

P20

$$50$$
$$.20$$
$$\overline{10.0}$$

$$21.5 + \left(\frac{4}{5} \times 4 \right) = 24.7$$

P30

$$50$$
$$.30$$
$$\overline{15.0}$$

$$25.5 + \left(\frac{4}{10} \times 4 \right) = 27.1$$

P40

$$50$$
$$.40$$
$$\overline{20.0}$$

$$25.5 + \left(\frac{9}{10} \times 4 \right) = 29.1$$

P50

$$50$$
$$.50$$
$$\overline{25.0}$$

$$29.5 + \left(\frac{4}{15} \times 4 \right) = 30.6$$

P60

$$50$$
$$.60$$
$$\overline{30.0}$$

$$29.5 + \left(\frac{9}{15} \times 4 \right) = 31.9$$

P70

$$50$$
$$.70$$
$$\overline{35.0}$$

$$29.5 + \left(\frac{14}{15} \times 4 \right) = 33.2$$

P80

$$50$$
$$.80$$
$$\overline{40.0}$$

$$33.5 + \left(\frac{4}{6} \times 4 \right) = 36.2$$

P90

$$50$$
$$.90$$
$$\overline{45.0}$$

$$37.5 + \left(\frac{3}{4} \times 4 \right) = 40.5$$

P0 = Lowest score
P100 = Highest score

TABLE 8. *(Continued)*

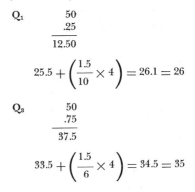

$$Q_1 \quad \frac{\begin{array}{r}50\\.25\end{array}}{12.50}$$

$$25.5 + \left(\frac{1.5}{10} \times 4\right) = 26.1 = 26$$

$$Q_3 \quad \frac{\begin{array}{r}50\\.75\end{array}}{37.5}$$

$$33.5 + \left(\frac{1.5}{6} \times 4\right) = 34.5 = 35$$

Hence, 75 per cent of the pupils did more than 26 sit-ups, while 25 per cent did less than 26 sit-ups. The second quartile, Q_2, is the fiftieth percentile and indicates the point at which half the scores lie above and half below. Q_2 is also a measure of central tendency similar to the mean, and is referred to as the median. Unlike the mean, the median is not affected by extreme scores. If, for example, a child scored an exceptionally large or small number of sit-ups, the mean would be pulled toward this extreme score, but the median would not. Regardless of the distribution of scores, the median indicates the point at which half of the test scores will fall above and half below. Because of this factor the median at times becomes a more reliable measure of central tendency than does the mean. On the normal curve, both the mean and median occupy the identical position.

The third quartile, Q_3, is the seventy-fifth percentile and indicates the point where 25 per cent of the scores fall above and 75 per cent lie below.

Using the data for two-minute sit-ups, percentiles are computed in the following manner (Table 8):

1. Construct a cumulative frequency column *(cf)* as shown in Table 8. This is done by serially adding the frequency column.

2. Multiply the desired percentile by the number of cases. For example, in computing the tenth percentile (P10) as illustrated in Table 8, multiply 10 per cent times 50, which equals 5.

3. Follow up the cumulative frequency column and observe that the 5 falls between 3 and 6.

4. Write down the lower step interval in which 5 falls, or 17.5.

5. Subtract 3 in the cumulative frequency column from 5, which equals 2.

6. There are 3 frequencies in the step interval 17.5 to 21.4; hence we must go two-thirds of this distance. This is then multiplied by the step interval, and the result is added to 17.5, the lower limit of the step interval, for the final result.

Product-moment correlation coefficient. On page 27 we learned why the correlation coefficient is an extremely important statistic when it comes to selecting a test for use in the program. As we have previously noted, the correlation coefficient basically indicates the degree of association btween two variables. Those who are interested in actually computing a correlation coefficient will find it both interesting and not too difficult.

Computing correlation coefficient using a scatter diagram. There is only one new mathematical step to be learned in order to compute a correlation coefficient. Its calculation can best be demonstrated by means of a scatter diagram, which is illustrated in Figure 4. Table 9 contains two sets of hypothetical scores obtained from the administration of a badminton skill test to a group of senior high school girls on two successive days. As you perhaps have surmised already, the problem at hand is to determine the reliability of this test—or how closely the sets of measures agree. This is the basic experimental design employed in determining the reliability of a skill test by what is referred to as the test-retest method of measuring reliability. The same would be true for determining objectivity, if *two* or more examiners were involved in gathering the data.

1. Our first endeavor will be to establish two frequency tables in the same manner as outlined on page 34.

X VARIABLE (FIRST TRIAL)

Y VARIABLE (SECOND TRIAL)	10–12.4	13–15.4	16–18.4	19–21.4	22–24.4	25–27.4	28–30.4	31–33.4	34–36.4	37–39.4	40–42.4	43–45.4	46–48.4	f_y	d_y	fd_y	fd_y^2	X'–	Y'+
45–47.4													(35)	1	5	5	25		35
42–44.4											(20)			1	4	4	16		20
39–41.4				(3)		(6)					(30)			5	3	15	45	3	36
36–38.4							(12)	(16)	(10)					5	2	10	20		38
33–35.4						(2)		(9)	(8)					6	1	6	6		19
30–32.4			/		///	///	THL							12	40/47				
27–29.4			/	(2)		/ (4)	////	/ (2)						7	-1	-7	7	6	2
24–26.4					////	(4)								6	-2	-12	24	4	
21–23.4					(6)	/								3	-3	-9	27		6
18–20.4			(12)		(4)									2	-4	-8	32		16
15–17.4			(15)											1	-5	-5	25		15
12–14.4		(24)												1	-6	-6	36		24
f_x	0	1	2	2	4	9	11	7	5	4	4	0	1	N=50	Σ=-7	Σ=263	Σ=198		
d_x	-5	-4	-3	-2	-1		1	2	3	4	5	6	7						
fd_x	-0	-4	-6	-4	-4	-18/83	11	14	15	16	20	0	7	Σ=65					
fd_x^2	0	16	18	8	4		11	28	45	64	100	0	49	Σ=343					

Figure 4. Scatter diagram method of computing correlation coefficient.

TABLE 9. *Data from Badminton Skill Test Administered on Successive Days to Determine Test Reliability*

First Trial (x)	Second Trial (y)	First Trial (x)	Second Trial (y)
47	45	25	30
41	43	26	31
42	39	26	30
40	41	21	30
30	39	33	29
29	40	30	27
23	39	29	29
40	37	25	27
39	36	28	27
37	38	28	29
35	36	21	27
36	38	30	25
39	33	29	26
37	35	27	24
34	33	25	24
35	35	26	26
34	33	25	25
31	33	25	21
31	30	24	21
31	30	22	23
33	32	24	20
32	31	18	20
33	31	18	17
28	30	13	12
28	31	30	32

2. Commencing at the upper left hand corner of the scatter diagram, write in each step interval, beginning with the lowest at the left for the first set of test scores. Do likewise with the second set of data, placing the highest step interval in the upper left hand corner. For example the first two scores [47 and 45] are plotted in the most upper right hand square of the scattergram (47 of first trial falls in step interval 46 to 48.4 and 45 of second trial falls in interval 45 to 47.4).

Formula: Where:

$$r = \frac{\dfrac{\Sigma\, x'y'}{N} - (C_x \cdot C_y)}{\sigma_x \cdot \sigma_y}$$

r = correlation coefficient

$\Sigma\, x'y'$ = summation of cross-products

N = number of pairs of cases

C_y = correction factor for y, or $\dfrac{\Sigma\, fd_y}{N}$

3. Plot the scores. From Table 9 the first pair of scores is 47 and 45. Under X variable (first trial on scatter diagram) find interval 46–48.4, follow down the column to the opposite step interval 45–47.4 (second trial), and place one tally. Do likewise for the second pair of scores; i.e., 41 is located in step interval 40–42.4 (first trial) and 43 in interval 42–44.4. Place a tally at this intersect. Continue for the remaining pairs.

$$C_x = \text{correction factor for x, or } \frac{\Sigma\, fd_x}{N}$$

$$\sigma_y = \text{standard deviation for Y scores}$$

$$\sigma_x = \text{standard deviation for X scores.}$$

Computations:

$$\Sigma\, x'y' = 198$$

$$N = 50$$

$$C_y = \frac{\Sigma\, fd_y}{N} = \frac{-7}{50} = -0.14$$

$$C_x = \frac{\Sigma\, fd_x}{N} = \frac{65}{50} = 1.30$$

$$\sigma_y = \sqrt{\frac{\Sigma\, fd_y{}^2}{N} - C_y{}^2} = \sqrt{\frac{263}{50} - 0.02} = 2.29$$

$$\sigma_x = \sqrt{\frac{\Sigma\, fd_x{}^2}{N} - C_x{}^2} = \sqrt{\frac{343}{50} - 1.69} = 2.27$$

$$r = \frac{\dfrac{198}{50} - (-0.14 \times 1.30)}{(2.29)\,(2.27)}$$

$$r = 0.80$$

4. Indicate the assumed means for each variable by drawing lines through the step intervals containing greatest number of frequencies.

5. Fill in *f, d, fd,* and *fd²* columns and rows respectively for the first set of data on the X axis, and for the second set of scores on the Y axis.

6. The X'Y' column contains the cross-products of the deviations of each score from its mean. It is computed by counting the squares from each mean, multiplying them and in turn multiplying this product times the total number of frequencies in that particular square.

7. Under the column labeled X'Y', the cross-products in each row are summed. The total of the cross-products in the rows of the upper right hand and lower left hand quadrants of the scatter diagram are recorded under the plus column. The totals for the upper left and lower

right quadrants are placed in the negative column. The summation of the positive and negative columns is done algebraically.

The scatter diagram method of computing r loses some accuracy when N is less than 50 and when there are fewer than twelve step intervals. It is very useful in demonstrating graphically the degree of relationship between the two variables in question. The scatter diagram also permits computation of the mean, standard deviation, and correlation coefficient in a single operation. One must not forget, if the standard deviation is calculated from the scatter diagram to be used in describing the mean, that it must first be multiplied by the step interval. Attention is brought to the fact that this was not necessary in computing r on the scatter diagram, as all numbers were in graphic units and hence comparable.

Regression lines. It might be worthwhile at this time to define and illustrate the working of regression lines, in order to give a clearer conception of the nature of the correlation coefficient now that the method of its computation has been explained. Figure 5 is a graph of the means of the data for the lateral rows (X variable) and the vertical columns (Y variable) from Figure 4. The lines have been drawn to represent the best fit line for the means of the columns and the means of the rows. The angle formed by the two regression lines represents the coefficient

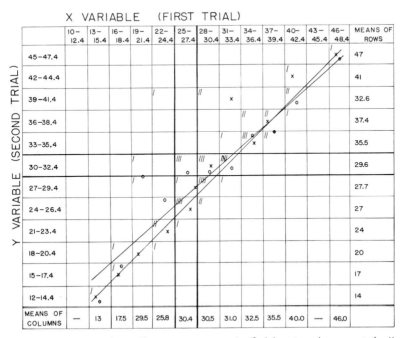

Figure 5. Regression lines. The row means are signified by x's and represent the X variable, or first trial. The column means represent the second trial and are indicated by small o's.

of correlation. The means for the rows are found simply by considering each score as if it were equal to the midpoint of the step interval in which it occurs. For example, the only score found in the first row from the top is in the step interval 45.5–48.4; hence the mean for that row equals 47, the midpoint of the step interval. The third row from the top contains five scores, and by averaging the midpoints of the intervals in which each of these scores fall, the resulting mean for that row is found to equal 32.6.

Figure 6 consists of six correlation coefficient scatter diagrams that have been simplified to show the relationship between the angle of the regression lines and the various values of r, ranging from $+1$ to -1. Diagram A in Figure 6 shows two regression lines lying one on top of the other, which results in a correlation of $+1$. Diagram F illustrates a perfect negative relationship: as in diagram A, its lines of best fit lie on top of one another; but here they run in opposite directions. Diagram D indicates a zero correlation, as the two lines are perpendicular to each other. There

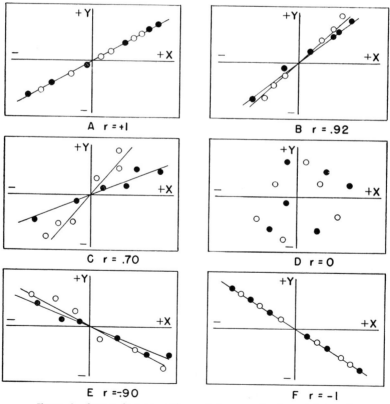

Figure 6. Scatter diagrams with correlations ranging from $+1$ to -1.

is no relationship whatsoever between these two variables, whatever they may be.

It may be stated, then, that the smaller the angle between the lines of best fit, the higher the value of the correlation coefficient. When the angle between the two lines of best fit approaches 0, the correlation nears 1. By the same token, as the angle approaches 90 degrees, the correlation approximates 0.

Diagram *E* in Figure 6 illustrates the position of two lines of best fit when a negative correlation exists. The computer *r* between the two variables is approximately −.90. The negative sign is affixed to indicate that as one variable increases, the other decreases, as would be the case in a correlation of time in running the 100 yard dash against leg strength, assuming that the faster one runs the stronger his legs must be.

Correlation when N is small.   Computing a correlation coefficient with a small number of cases is done in the following manner:

1. Arrange the data as shown in Table 10. The first and second columns of figures the paired test scores.

TABLE 10.   *Calculation of the Correlation Coefficient Using Sum of Squares Method With Raw Data*

X	Y	x $(X-M)$	y $(Y-M)$	x^2	y^2	xy
20	13	8	6	64	36	48
18	9	6	2	36	4	12
14	8	2	1	4	1	2
11	6	−1	−1	1	1	1
9	5	−3	−2	9	4	6
7	5	−5	−2	25	4	10
5	3	−7	−4	49	16	28
Σ 84	49	0	0	188	66	107
$M = 12$ $M = 7$						

2. Compute the mean for each column by obtaining the total of each and dividing that sum by the number of cases in the column.

3. The figures in the third column are obtained by subtracting the mean of column 1 from each score in it. Similarly, the figures in the fourth column are obtained by subtracting the mean of column 2 from each score in column 2.

4. The fifth and sixth columns are obtained by finding the square of the values in the third and fourth columns respectively.

5. The figures in the seventh column are obtained by multiplying each value in column 3 by the corresponding value in column 4.

6. Columns 5, 6, and 7 are individually summed.

The formula for computing r by what is called the sum of the squares method is as follows:

$$r_{xy} = \frac{\Sigma\, xy}{\sqrt{\Sigma\, x^2 \cdot \Sigma\, y^2}}$$

Where:

r_{xy} = correlation of X on Y
$\Sigma\, xy$ = summation of cross-products
$\Sigma\, x^2$ = sum of squares for x
$\Sigma\, y^2$ = sum of squares for y.

$$r_{xy} = \frac{\Sigma\, xy}{\sqrt{\Sigma\, x^2 \cdot \Sigma\, y^2}}$$

$$r_{xy} = \frac{107}{\sqrt{(188)\,(66)}} = \frac{107}{\sqrt{12,408}}$$

$$r_{xy} = \frac{107}{111.39}$$

$$r_{xy} = 0.96$$

Rank-difference correlation. The rank-difference correlational method, referred to as Rho (ρ) and symbolized by that Greek letter, sometimes is used in validating skill tests. It is a method whereby scores are merely arranged in serial order or rank. For example, if we wished to correlate standings in a round-robin tournament with scores on a skill test, which would give us an indication of the validity of the test, we might proceed as follows:

1. Arrange the skill test scores in order from highest to lowest, as depicted in Table 11.

2. Assign each test score a rank; notice that test scores 3 and 4 are identical and have each been assigned a median rank. The same is true for scores 8 and 9.

3. List alongside this rank column the standings of each subject in the round-robin tournament.

4. Subtract the rank number of each pupil's test score from the number of his standing in the round-robin, and enter the results in a difference column (D) (i.e., subtract standing in round-robin column scores from rank column scores).

5. Square each entry in the D column, to eliminate negative values, and arrange the results in a difference squared column (D^2).

6. The rank-difference correlation coefficient is computed by totaling the values in the D^2 column and inserting all the problem data into the formula. The coefficient of .96 indicates that the results of this hypothetical badminton test are in close agreement with the standings in the round-

$$\rho = 1 - \frac{6 \Sigma D^2}{N(N^2 - 1)}$$

Where:

ρ = rank difference correlation coefficient
D^2 = difference between paired ranks squared
N = number of pairs.

Therefore:

$$\rho = 1 - \frac{6(7)}{10(10^2 - 1)}$$

$$\rho = 1 - \frac{42}{990}$$

$$\rho = 0.96$$

TABLE 11.   *Ranks Assigned on Badminton Skill Test and Round-Robin Tournament*

Subjects	Skill Test Scores	Rank	Standing in Round-Robin	D	D²
1	38	1	1	0	0
2	37	2	3	—1	1
3	36	3.5	2	1.5	2.25
4	36	3.5	4	—0.5	0.25
5	32	5	5	0	0
6	29	6	6	0	0
7	28	7	8	—1	1
8	27	8.5	7	1.5	2.25
9	27	8.5	9	—0.5	0.25
10	24	10	10	0	0
					$\Sigma = 7.00$

robin tournament. Hence, for this particular case, we would conclude that the badminton test is valid.

The rank-difference method can be used in measuring such associations as subjective judgments of participants' performances in team activities and skill tests as, for example, between a subjective ranking of volley ball, soccer, football, and basketball players and the scores made on the particular skill tests designed for these activities.

Interpreting the correlation. On page 28 we described a standard for evaluating the size of the correlation so that we could interpret how reliable, objective, or valid a test might be. Ignoring the size of the sample, a very neat and more precise manner of ascertaining the amount of relationship in a correlation is to square the r. This r^2 is called the *coefficient of determination*. It tells us the proportion of the variance in one variable that is associated with the variance in the other variable. For example, if X correlated with Y so that the r were to equal .90, the $(.90)^2$ times 100 would tell us that 81 per cent of the variance in X can be accounted for by the variance in Y. Nineteen per cent of the variance is unaccounted for in this correlation. Thus we have a measure showing specifically the amount of relationship in a correlation coefficient of any given size. For a correlation of 1, which of course is perfect, 100 per cent of the X variance would be accounted for in the variance of Y.

Reliability of Statistics

Provided we wish to pursue our statistical knowledge further, it is necessary to determine the confidence, faith or trust we might place in the scores or data we have gathered. This area of statistical study is called *reliability*, and it forms the structure upon which all experimental studies are based. We are going to introduce you to three measures of statistical reliability, which are easily computed and which will allow you to solve some experimental problems which may arise in the gymnasium or classroom.

Definition of terms. Before we commence, it is necessary to learn the definitions for *sample, population, statistic,* and *parameter.* A *sample* is a small, representative part of the population. A *population* is all the people related to the particular variable you wish to measure. For example, if we wished to know the average number of sit-ups eighth-grade girls in the Los Angeles school system could perform, we could do one of two things: (1) measure *all* the children in the system; or (2) measure a small representative number of girls.

All girls in the school system would constitute the *population,* whereas a representative group from the population would be referred to as a *sample.* To be sure, it would be much easier to measure a sample (from three to four hundred, for example) rather than measuring the entire population, which might comprise thirty to forty thousand scores. In selecting our sample we must make certain that it is a random selection (i.e., each individual in the population had an equal chance to be chosen) and that the sample is sufficiently large to allow valid representation.

If we were to measure the population (all girls in the system) and compute the mean, this average would be referred to as a *parameter,* while the mean computed from the sample would be a *statistic.* As one graduate student has suggested, "a statistic is to the sample as a parameter is to the population." In other words, the parameter is the true value, while the statistic is, hopefully, a reliable representation of the parameter. *Reliability,* then, is that portion of statistics which allows us to represent in a valid manner the true measure of a population without testing all of the individuals comprising the population. The reliability of several statistics will be our immediate concern.

Standard error of the mean (σ_M). This measure of reliability reveals the proximity of a statistical mean to the population mean (parameter); its size depends upon the variability of the scores about the statistical mean (σ) and upon the number of cases (N) in the sample. The formula reads as follows:

$$\sigma_M = \frac{\sigma}{\sqrt{N}}$$

Where:

σ = estimate of the population standard deviation

You will insert the standard deviation you computed from your sample as this estimate.

N = the number of cases in your sample

In situations where N is less than 30 it is customary to compute the standard deviation by subtracting 1 from the number of cases:

$$\sigma = \sqrt{\frac{\Sigma\, d^2}{N-1}}$$

rather than:

$$\sigma = \sqrt{\frac{\Sigma\, d^2}{N}}$$

The reason for this is that the standard deviation computed from a random sample is slightly less than the population sigma. Therefore, when a small number (less than 30) of cases occurs in a sample, an adjustment is necessary.

Interpreting σ_M. As previously mentioned, the standard error of the mean allows us to determine the amount of confidence we might place in the statistical mean; or just how well our sample mean represents the true mean of the population.

Hypothetically, suppose we were to randomly select 100 samples (N = 30) from a population. We then administer a sit-up test to each of the sample groups. Do you believe, upon computing a mean for each of the 100 samples, that all would be identical? Of course not. However, provided our samples were truly random, the means would be close, the small differences being attributed to *sampling error.* Then if we were to compute the mean of our 100 sample means, it should represent the true or population mean. If we then computed the standard deviation of these means, the resulting statistic would represent the standard error of our mean. In other words, the means computed from *these* samples would distribute themselves in a normal probability curve as depicted in Figure 7.

Note the similarity between this distribution and Figure 3 which appears on page 42. The latter represents actual scores, whereas Figure 7 reflects a *hypothetical* distribution of means as we suggested in the above example.

Value of σ_M. Of what value is the standard error of the mean? It tells us how reliable our sample mean is in relationship to the true mean. For example, in Figure 7, our standard error of the mean added to and subtracted from our computed mean gives us the range in which we would expect our mean to fall 68 times out of 100. Or, looking at it in another way, suppose we were to draw 100 successive samples from the population; it would be valid to state that 68 of those means would lie within ± 1 standard error of the mean.

Let us compute and interpret the standard error of the mean from the following data which were obtained by administering 2-minute sit-up tests to senior high school boys:

$$\sigma = 12$$
$$M = 40$$
$$N = 36$$
$$\sigma_M = \frac{\sigma}{\sqrt{N}}$$
$$\sigma_M = \frac{12}{\sqrt{36}} = 2$$

Range.   To determine the range in which we would expect our mean to fall 68 times out of 100, we would multiply the standard error of the

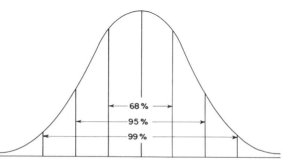

Figure 7.   Hypothetical distribution of means obtained by drawing successive samples from the population. The sample means are distributed equally on both sides of the population mean.

mean by 1 (1 standard error) and then add and subtract this quantity to and from the mean:

$$M = 40$$
$$\sigma_M = 2$$
$$M \pm (1 \times \sigma_M)$$
$$40 \pm (1 \times 2) = 38 - 42$$
$$\text{(range)}$$

Sixty-eight times out of 100 we would expect the true mean to fall between 38 and 42; in other words, if we repeated the sit-up test on one hundred samples, we would then expect that, 68 times out of 100, the means would fall between 38 and 42. Thirty-two times out of 100 the means would fall above and below the range (16 of the means below 38 and 16 above 42).

Supposing we extended our range to include two standard errors of the mean, what might we infer?

$$M \pm 2 \, \sigma_M$$

or:

$$40 \pm (2 \times 2) = 36 - 44$$
$$\text{(range)}$$

From Table 6 we find that two standard errors include 95.44 per cent of the distribution (2×47.72). Consequently, we can state that 95.44 times out of a 100 our true mean will fall within the range 36 to 44; or, if we repeated the testing by drawing 100 samples, 95.44 times out of 100 the means would lie within this range. Actually, what we have covered so far is not very different from the concepts learned while studying the standard deviation earlier in this chapter.

Confidence intervals. When dealing with the standard error of the mean, usually two ranges, or confidence intervals, as they are more appropriately called, are reported in research literature. These are the limits covering 95 and 99 per cent of the distribution of hypothetical means. If you look at Table 6 you will observe that 1.96 standard errors include exactly 95 per cent of the distribution (2×47.50), while 2.58 standard errors include 99 per cent of the distribution (2×49.51). The statistician refers to these as the .05 and .01 levels of confidence respectively. This is true because in the former, one would expect the true mean to fall within the interval 95 times out of 100 and in the latter situation, 99 times out of 100. Briefly summarizing, then:

$M \pm 1.96 \, \sigma_M = .05$ level of confidence.
   (5/100 the true mean would fall outside the interval)
$M \pm 2.58 \, \sigma_M = .01$ level of confidence.
   (1/100 the true mean would fall outside the interval)

On this basis let us determine the .05 and .01 confidence intervals for the following problem:

Given:

$$M = 40$$
$$\sigma_M = 2$$

Determine:

(A) the .05; and
(B) the .01 levels of confidence.

Solution:

A. $40 \pm 1.96 \times 2 = 40 \pm 3.92$
B. $40 \pm 2.58 \times 2 = 40 \pm 5.16$

In problem (A) we would expect the true mean to fall within the interval 36.08 to 43.92 in 95 times out of 100, while in problem (B) the true mean would lie within the range 34.84 to 45.16 in 99 times out of 100.

The standard error of the mean gives us insight regarding the reliability of our computed statistic, without requiring us to (1) measure the entire population or (2) draw a hundred or so successive samples in order to estimate the accuracy of a single sample mean. If you were commissioned to determine the average speed with which Little League pitchers could throw, the knowledge you have gained thus far could prove extremely worthwhile. As there are over a million children scattered around the globe playing ball, it would obviously be quite impractical and perhaps impossible to measure the entire population of pitchers. Rather, we would obtain a random sample with an adequate number of youngsters, then compute the mean and its standard error to establish our confidence intervals.

Significance of the difference between two means. There might be an occasion when you would like to compare the performance of two different schools on a particular test. For example, let us pose the following question: "Are the boys in East High School potentially better basketball players than those at Central?" Following administration of a basketball skill test such as the Knox test (p. 213) to both schools, we would compute the two means in ascertaining if one school were better than the other. The difference which might occur between the two means would have to be tested to determine whether it was a true difference or was due to sampling error. By computing the standard error of the difference (σ_{diff}) we can determine whether or not a real difference exists between our two sample means, just as we did in computing the standard error of the mean in order to ascertain the reliability of our sample mean.

If we find the mean difference to occur at least 95 times out of 100 (.05 level of confidence) or even better, 99 times out of 100 (.01 level of confidence) we would conclude that the difference between our two means did not occur through chance. On the other hand, if the difference occurred less than 95 times out of 100, we would assume the difference between the two means to be a chance difference.

The null hypothesis. The null hypothesis is used in testing differences that occur between means. It states that since both samples came from the same population, the difference which does occur between the means came about through chance alone. We accept this hypothesis when differences occur less than 95 times out of 100 (less than .05 level of confidence); we reject the null hypothesis when differences occur 95 or more times out of 100 (.05 and/or .01 levels of confidence). There is a simple statistical formula that allows us to determine whether or not the difference between two means occurred through chance or in fact is a real or true difference; it is called the *t* test or *t* ratio.

The t test. The ratio of the difference between two means to the standard error of the difference (σ_{diff}) is called the *t* test and is written in the following manner:

$$t = \frac{M_1 - M_2}{\sigma_{\text{diff}}}$$

Depending upon whether our two samples are correlated or not, the formula for the standard error of the difference takes two forms:

1. When the means are uncorrelated (independent), that is, when they come from different samples as in the basketball problem mentioned above, the formula for the standard error of the difference may be written:

$$\sigma_{\text{diff}} = \sqrt{\sigma_{M_1}{}^2 + \sigma_{M_2}{}^2}$$

2. When the means are correlated, that is, when they come from the same group tested before and after; or in situations in which two groups are equated on a test, then:

$$\sigma_{\text{diff}} = \sqrt{\sigma_{M_1}{}^2 + \sigma_{M_2}{}^2 - 2\,r_{12}\,\sigma_{M_1}{}^2\,\sigma_{M_2}{}^2}$$

in which r_{12} is the correlation between the two sets of data or scores.

t test for uncorrelated observations. To demonstrate the calculation of *t* for *uncorrelated* groups, we shall state the above proposition in the following problem: It is our consideration that, owing to better instruction, the boys at Central High are potentially better basketball players than the boys at East High. The null hypothesis in this instance would state: there is not a true difference between the two groups; a difference may occur between the two means because of chance alone. We shall now proceed to determine whether or not we accept or reject the null hypothesis.

Given:

	N	M	σ	σ_M
East High School	100	42 sec.	5	.5
Central High School	100	38 sec.	5	.5

$$t = \frac{M_1 - M_2}{\sigma_{diff}}$$

$$\sigma_{diff} = \sqrt{\sigma_{M_1}^2 + \sigma_{M_2}^2} = \sqrt{.25 + .25} = .71$$

$$t = \frac{42 - 38}{.71} = \frac{4}{.71} = 5.63$$

The t of 5.63 indicates that the difference of four between M_1 and M_2 lies 5.63 standard error of the differences beyond the average or mean difference(s). In a distribution of differences taken for the same population, the mean difference would equal zero, as depicted in Figure 8.

When using the t test the required level of significance is dependent upon the number of cases in our sample. From Table 12 we enter with $N - 1$ degrees of freedom (df) which equals $100 - 1$ or 99. To be significant at or beyond the .05 level of confidence, we need a t of at least 1.98 and for significance at the .01 level the t must equal 2.63. Consequently, we would reject the null hypothesis, as our t of 5.63 far exceeds 2.63. The difference existing between our two means is a true difference. The boys at Central have superior potential as basketball players because their average time in performing the Knox test is *faster* (smaller mean) than the participants at East High School, who are significantly slower in their performance.

Recall the standard score formula appearing on p. 43. The formula for the t test is quite similar. We are merely converting the difference between the two means to standard scores and through the use of Table 12

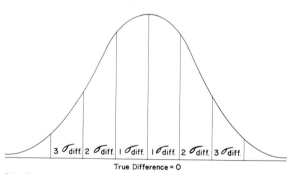

Figure 8. Distribution of differences obtained by drawing successive pairs of samples from the same population, computing the means, and plotting the differences between the means.

determining how far away from the mean difference (0) our difference lies. The mean difference of the distribution in Figure 8 equals zero because it is based on the sample mean differences computed from the identical population. Therefore, errors in sampling which overestimate the difference would cancel out the effects of those errors underestimating the difference. The net result would be a mean difference equal to zero.

t *test for correlated observations.* When two groups are equated or paired, we must take into consideration this dependency or correlation in computing the σ_{diff}. Also, in experiments where a single group is administered a pre-test and a post-test, the same consideration applies.

Let us pose a simple problem to illustrate the computation of t for correlated or dependent groups. As a result of a 10-week isometric strengthening program, will eighth grade girls increase their ability to perform 2-minute sit-ups? The raw data appear in Table 13. It will be necessary to compute the following statistics in which X represents scores before the exercise program and Y those scores following the program.

$$M_x = \frac{\Sigma_x}{N}$$

$$M_x = \frac{201}{10} = 20.1$$

$$\sigma_x = \sqrt{\frac{\Sigma d^2}{N-1}}$$

$$\sigma_x = \sqrt{\frac{468.9}{9}} = \sqrt{52.10}$$

$$\sigma_x = 7.22$$

$$\sigma_{M_x} = \frac{\sigma_x}{\sqrt{N}} = \frac{7.22}{3.16}$$

$$\sigma_{M_x} = 2.28$$

$$M_y = \frac{\Sigma_y}{N}$$

$$M_y = \frac{205}{10} = 20.5$$

$$\sigma_y = \sqrt{\frac{\Sigma d^2}{N-1}}$$

$$\sigma_y = \sqrt{\frac{398.5}{9}} = \sqrt{44.28}$$

$$\sigma_y = 6.65$$

$$\sigma_{M_y} = \frac{\sigma_y}{\sqrt{N}} = \frac{6.65}{3.16}$$

$$\sigma_{M_y} = 2.10$$

r_{xy} = correlation between X and Y. The computation was done as outlined on page 56. The r in this case was computed to equal .977.

$$\sigma_{diff} = \sqrt{\sigma_{M_x}^2 + \sigma_{M_y}^2 - 2\, r_{xy}\, \sigma_{M_x}\, \sigma_{M_y}}$$

$$\sigma_{diff} = \sqrt{2.28^2 + 2.10^2 - (2)\,(.977)\,(2.28)\,(2.10)}$$

$$\sigma_{diff} = \sqrt{9.61 - 9.36}$$

$$\sigma_{diff} = \sqrt{.25} = .50$$

$$t = \frac{M_x - M_y}{\sigma_{diff}} = \frac{20.1 - 20.5}{.50} = .80$$

Table 12.   t *Values Used in Determining Statistical Significance of the Difference between Two Means.*

Example: Twenty degrees of freedom (df) and a t value equal to 2.09 infers that 5 times in 100 trials one would expect a mean difference of this magnitude.

Degrees of Freedom	Probability			
	0.10	*0.05*	*0.02*	*0.01*
1	$t = 6.34$	$t = 12.71$	$t = 31.82$	$t = 63.66$
2	2.92	4.30	6.96	9.92
3	2.35	3.18	4.54	5.84
4	2.13	2.78	3.75	4.60
5	2.02	2.57	3.36	4.03
6	1.94	2.45	3.14	3.71
7	1.90	2.36	3.00	3.50
8	1.86	2.31	2.90	3.36
9	1.83	2.26	2.82	3.25
10	1.81	2.23	2.76	3.17
11	1.80	2.20	2.72	3.11
12	1.78	2.18	2.68	3.06
13	1.77	2.16	2.65	3.01
14	1.76	2.14	2.62	2.98
15	1.75	2.13	2.60	2.95
16	1.75	2.12	2.58	2.92
17	1.74	2.11	2.57	2.90
18	1.73	2.10	2.55	2.88
19	1.73	2.09	2.54	2.86
20	1.72	2.09	2.53	2.84
21	1.72	2.08	2.52	2.83
22	1.72	2.07	2.51	2.82
23	1.71	2.07	2.50	2.81
24	1.71	2.06	2.49	2.80
25	1.71	2.06	2.48	2.79
26	1.71	2.06	2.48	2.78
27	1.70	2.05	2.47	2.77
28	1.70	2.05	2.47	2.76
29	1.70	2.04	2.46	2.76
30	1.70	2.04	2.46	2.75
35	1.69	2.03	2.44	2.72
40	1.68	2.02	2.42	2.71
45	1.68	2.02	2.41	2.69
50	1.68	2.01	2.40	2.68
60	1.67	2.00	2.39	2.66
70	1.67	2.00	2.38	2.65
80	1.66	1.99	2.38	2.64
90	1.66	1.99	2.37	2.63
100	1.66	1.98	2.36	2.63
125	1.66	1.98	2.36	2.62
150	1.66	1.98	2.35	2.61

TABLE 12. *(Continued)*

Degrees of Freedom	Probability			
	0.10	0.05	0.02	0.01
200	1.65	1.97	2.35	2.60
300	1.65	1.97	2.34	2.59
400	1.65	1.97	2.34	2.59
500	1.65	1.96	2.33	2.59
1000	1.65	1.96	2.33	2.58
∞	1.65	1.96	2.33	2.58

TABLE 13. *Two-Minute Sit-up Scores, Before and Following a 10-week Isometric Exercise Program for Eighth Grade Girls (N = 10).*

Subject	Before Exercise X	After Exercise Y
1	12	14
2	10	9
3	23	24
4	25	24
5	29	30
6	32	29
7	14	15
8	17	18
9	19	21
10	20	21
N = 10	= 201	= 205

Entering Table 12 with 9 degrees of freedom (N — 1), the difference of .4 must be as large as 2.26 to be significant at the .05 level; for significance at the .01 level, the t must equal 3.25. Since our t equals .80, we must accept the null hypothesis, and conclude that the difference of .4 between the two means was a chance occurrence. Apparently, for some reason, the isometric exercise program failed to cause improvement in the two-minute sit-up test.

Short method for computing t, dependent sample. Providing one does *not* need the correlation coefficient between the two sets of scores, there is a shorter way to compute t; this method still considers the correlation between the two sets of dependent samples, but employs a simpler mathematical identity. The procedure is outlined in Table 14. Observe that the two methods agree as to the final t ratio.

TABLE 14.   *Short Method for Computing* t *(Dependent Sample)*

N	Before Exercise	After Exercise	D	D²
1	12	14	2	4
2	10	9	−1	1
3	23	24	1	1
4	25	24	−1	1
5	29	30	1	1
6	32	29	−3	9
7	14	15	1	1
8	17	18	1	1
9	19	21	2	4
10	20	21	1	1
	201	205	4	24

$$\Sigma d^2 = \Sigma D^2 - \frac{(\Sigma D)^2}{N}$$

$$\Sigma d^2 = 24 - \frac{(4)^2}{10}$$

$$\Sigma d^2 = 24 - 1.6 = 22.4$$

$$\sigma_D = \sqrt{\frac{\Sigma d^2}{N-1}}$$

$$\sigma_D = \sqrt{\frac{22.4}{9}} = \sqrt{2.49} = 1.58$$

$$\sigma_{diff} = \frac{\sigma_D}{\sqrt{N}}$$

$$\sigma_{diff} = \frac{1.58}{\sqrt{10}} = .50$$

$$t = \frac{M_1 - M_2}{\sigma_{diff}}$$

$$t = \frac{20.1 - 20.5}{.50} = .80$$

Summary and Conclusions

A few statistical procedures quite essential for analyzing test scores in physical education have been demonstrated. To be sure, there are many other techniques that could be applied in analyzing the data; however, we did start out in this chapter to answer five basic questions. Let us review these questions to see whether or not the answers are apparent.

1. How did the group as a whole do on the test? In order to answer

this question we need to know the measure of central tendency, or mean, that is indicative of the score most representative of the group. It is also necessary to know the measure of variability that tells us within what range the middle 68 per cent of the pupils scored. Thus the mean and standard deviation inform us as to the standing of the group as a whole.

2. How does each individual stand in relation to the group? On the basis of the information presented in this chapter, we have two possible answers to this question. In order of reliability, the standard score should be our first choice, because the measure of central tendency and variability of the group have both been taken into consideration in the computation of this score. The second choice is the percentile table, which may be used when we are dealing with a small group and a somewhat crude measure only is desired.

3. How can we homogeneously group the pupils? There are two plausible answers to this question. The most reliable method would be on the basis of the normal curve. As an illustration, let us asume that we wish to group our pupils in terms of general athletic ability. After the test is administered, the mean and standard deviation must be calculated. On the assumption that our group was normally distributed, we would split the six standard deviations into as many groups as we desired. Figure 7 illustrates the normal curve separated into five groups. This division was obtained by dividing 5, the desired number of classes, into 6 standard deviations. Applying this division of the normal curve to our two-minute sit-up data, we would proceed as follows: From Figure 7 we can see that between plus and minus .6 of standard deviation 45 per cent of the cases fall. We have designated this as the C group. To compute the limits, multiply .6 by the obtained standard deviation of 7.5, which equals 4.5. This number when added to and subtracted from the mean of 30.3 gives a range of 25.8 to 34.8. Hence all scores falling within these limits would constitute the C group. In like manner, the ranges between the remaining groups may be determined and all scores falling within these respective limits would be classified as indicated in Figure 9. The

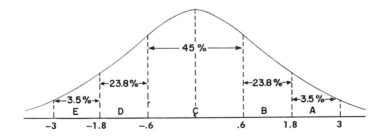

Figure 9. Normal curve divided into five parts for purposes of marking.

following are results obtained from the computations:

LETTER MARKS AND EQUIVALENT SCORES

$$43.9 - \uparrow \quad A$$
$$34.9 - 43.8 \quad B$$
$$25.8 - 34.8 \quad C$$
$$16.8 - 25.7 \quad D$$
$$16.7 - \downarrow \quad E$$

Homogeneity within a class may also be obtained through use of the percentile table. Once again, the same argument applies here as above, in that the measures of central tendency and variability are not taken into consideration. However, for use within a class, the percentiles are quickly computed and are satisfactory, when a small group is being classified according to merit. If four groups are desired, the three quartiles could be computed and the classifications assigned as follows:

$$0 \; \dfrac{\longleftarrow D \longrightarrow \; | \; \longleftarrow C \longrightarrow \; | \; \longleftarrow B \longrightarrow \; | \; \longleftarrow A \longrightarrow}{Q_1 \qquad\qquad Q_2 \qquad\qquad Q_3} \; 100$$

4. How can we use these scores for grading purposes? Scales, particularly the Hull scale, are the answer to this question. Actually any statistical method that is used in classifying or grouping test scores would also be applicable to grading, for marking is merely dividing the distribution of scores into classes or groups. The individual instructor must determine his percentage of A's, B's, C's, D's, and E's. After this decision is made, the scaled scores may be divided into four or five sections. By looking at Figure 9, one can see how this was accomplished when five-letter grades are desired.

5. How do we construct norms? The T-scale, sigma scale, percentiles, or Hull scale may be used in establishing norms. After the test scores have been scaled, you actually have a norm or standard. It should be remembered that a large number of cases, i.e., 500 or more, yields a more reliable norm than does a small number, say 50 cases. Few tests in physical education have norms, and most teachers, when first starting, lack equipment for testing. Items requiring little equipment, such as the standing broad jump, dashes, pull-ups, and sit-ups, can be effectively used for evaluating certain aspects of fitness. It is most desirable to construct your own norms for these types of tests. In those schools having a small number of pupils, scores collected over a period of two or three years may be combined, resulting in a larger number and thus creating more reliable standards.

6. Finally, understanding the reliability of statistics allows us to objectively determine the amount of confidence or faith we can place in our obtained data. Such statistics as the standard error of the mean,

standard error of the difference between means, and the *t*-test between correlated and uncorrelated means permit us to study many problems peculiar to the physical education program, as well as aiding us to understand our research literature.

BIBLIOGRAPHY

1. Edwards, Allen: Statistical Analysis. Revised ed. New York, Holt, Rinehart & Winston, 1964.
2. Garrett, Henry E.: Statistics in Psychology and Education. 6th ed. New York, Longmans, Green & Co., 1970.
3. Snedecor, George W., and Cochran, William G.: Statistical Methods. 6th ed. Ames, Iowa, The Iowa State University Press, 1967.
4. Weber, J. C., and Lamb, David R.: Statistics and Research in Physical Education. St. Louis, C. V. Mosby Co., 1970.

chapter 4

measuring strength

Reasons for Measuring Strength

Whether using dynamometers or subjective appraisal, there are four good reasons that show why evaluating the strength of pupils could be vitally important to the physical educator, to his program, and to his pupils: (1) strength is necessary for good appearance; (2) strength is basic to good performance in skills; (3) strength is valued highly as a measure of physical fitness; and (4) maintenance of strength may serve as a prophylaxis against certain orthopedic deficiencies.

Strength and appearance. A girl wants to be beautiful; a boy desires to be strong, with a nice-looking physique. These are natural desires—they are ranked at the top of the list as highly valued possessions by youth themselves. Providing that no pathologic condition is involved, a strong physique *can* be obtained in a comparatively short period of time. Masculine bodies can be made strong and flexible in a matter of months; Atlas does it. Girls' appearances *can* be improved both in body form and in basic movements of standing, walking, and sitting; modeling schools do it.

Through the cooperation of the physical education and the home economics departments, public schools usually have professional personnel trained for development and maintenance of beautiful physiques for both boys and girls. Guidance in grooming and nutrition coupled with proper body building programs, as determined from testing results, can be one of the most worthwhile endeavors in our entire education regimen. We *must* take advantage of this know-how if physical education as a profession is to achieve its greatest potential.

Strength as basic to good performance in skills. Strength is basic to performance in activities. By measuring we can determine the status of our pupils and hence construct a more effective program to meet pupil needs. By first assaying muscular development, it can be determined whether pupils are ready for instruction in sports skills. A pupil will not be able to hold the tennis racket as instructed if he has not sufficient strength. How can a pupil learn to pole vault if he cannot hold his own weight? Moreover, lack of sufficient strength results in rapid muscular fatigue, which limits the amount of practice time available for learning skills.

Proper muscular development helps to prevent muscular imbalances that may result in compensating movements when a child is attempting to learn new skills. We have all seen injured people favoring their good (strong) sides. A similar compensating mechanism may result if a youngster does not have sufficient strength to hold the tennis racket as instructed. In order to hold the racket he will compensate by calling into play more muscles than would properly be necessary. These compensating mechanisms may result in imbalances which, if not corrected, become progressively more difficult to rectify.

Strength as a measure of physical fitness. Probably nowhere in physical education is there a greater controversy than in the area of fitness. The discussion of physical fitness in Chapter 1 gave an idea of the difficulty involved in defining this condition. Until the time comes when the definition of fitness is agreed upon and we have the instruments for objectively measuring it, there will continue to be confusion as to what is the best evaluative approach to this problem. By no means does this imply that we should delete appraisal of fitness from the program because the experts fail to agree. On the contrary, we must employ the best and most practical tests available in order to learn more and more about the appraisal of general fitness. We should definitely consider any disagreements in this vital area as challenges rather than inhibitions, and take it upon ourselves to use, study, evaluate, and improve our testing procedures. No one will deny that our present measuring instruments in the area of fitness are far superior to no measurement at all.

There are numerous types of tests used in the evaluation of fitness. Although it is impossible to classify them, Karpovich[11] has suggested that the majority fall into three groups: muscular performance, organic function, and a combination of the two.

Muscular performance tests are tests of activities involving the large muscles of the body, such as running, pull-ups, dips, squat jumps, and broad jump. Examples of organic function tests include such items as pulse rate, pulse pressure, standing and sitting blood pressures, and energy cost of exercise. The third type includes tests in which the effects of a specific exercise are recorded in terms of pulse rate, pulse pressure, and blood pressure, usually both before and after exercise.

Strength tests are one of the most practical measures to evaluate fitness of youngsters in schools. They have been used quite successfully since around 1930. Today more and more emphasis seems to be placed on this type of test as a reflector of total fitness for the following reasons:

(1) strength is a highly objective measure; (2) strength is affected by disease processes such as infected tonsils, cancers, ulcers, abscesses, and colds, which produce a systemic reaction; and (3) strength is affected by emotional problems.

Objectivity of strength testing.   Strength is a highly objective measure, as day-to-day measurements indicate that consistent results can be obtained with a small margin of error. Metheny[16] reports objectivity coefficients for right grip strength of .957 and .953 for boys and girls, respectively, between the ages of two years-six months and six years-five months. From her study, Metheny concluded that reliable results may be obtained from tests of grip strength given over six days to children from two and one-half to six and one-half years of age, and that such results are no less reliable than those obtained when the test is administered to older children.

To further substantiate these findings, Metheny[16] quotes several studies in which objectivity coefficients for grip strength range from .82 to .94. The age range of the subjects in these studies was from four years to high school age. Clarke[5] reports objectivity coefficients for thirty-eight cable-tension strength tests ranging from .74 to .99. Thirty-three of the coefficients are between .90 and .99; three range between .82 and .89, while two are in the seventies.

Strength as affected by organic problems.   Numerous case studies have been reported in the literature to bear out the relationship between decline in strength and organic drains on the system. At the onset of infection there is a noticeable loss in strength; and, with recovery, strength returns to its original level. A few examples are cited below:

> A Lynbrook high school pupil's strength scores consistently dropped over a three-year period. The boy was finally sent to an orthopedic physician who diagnosed the condition as syringomyelia (development of cavities within the spinal cord).[2]
>
> When first tested a girl had an extremely low strength score. Referral to her family physician resulted in a diagnosis of malnutrition and goiter. Treatment by physician resulted in a 200 per cent increase in test score from September to May.[2]
>
> A New England high school football player had an exceptionally low score as contrasted to what should be expected from an athlete in training. The score was such a surprise to the physical educator that the boy was again measured, with the identical results. This boy finally admitted for the first time to a kidney injury sustained during football.[2]
>
> A boy's grip strength dropped from 125 to 119 in three weeks. The subject was hospitalized. A diagnosis of intestinal parasitism was made and a 7-foot tapeworm was removed. In the next eight weeks the boy's grip strength rose to 145 pounds.[5]

Strength as affected by emotional problems.   Strength is affected by emotional stress. Tensed or keyed-up individuals usually obtain exceptionally high or low strength scores. Once the condition is properly diagnosed and steps are taken to ameliorate the cause or causes, a return to normal is noted. The following studies serve as examples:

> A youngster received a low score on a fitness test which was administered in October of the school year. He was described as noncooperative, nervous, a constant talker and a wise guy. By March, after a regulated *individual* program was initiated, the youngster had increased his fitness by 150 per cent! Accompanying this increase in fitness were other notable improvements such as improved social adjustment, a more healthy appearance, and significant scholastic gains.[19]
>
> One youngster, selected because of low score, was given the title of "a probable delinquent" by his teacher. After consultation and establishment of a program, this lad by mid-year was a member of the YMCA. His reasons for joining? He wanted to become an athlete. The boy was reported to show vast improvement by April of the school year.[19]
>
> In a written report by a homeroom teacher the following appeared: Fall of the school year: infantile, pouting, tantrums, poor coordination, unpopular, poor work habits, cannot control talking in class, slovenly, cry baby, teases." By April with an accompanying increase in fitness scores, a significant change in social adjustment was noted.[19]

Occasionally, in administering fitness tests you will observe youngsters displaying maladjustment tendencies in their attitude toward taking the test. As examples the following are cited:

> In a girl who was proved to have a psychiatric disorder and whose history indicated that she was boss of the family at the age of twelve years, complete interpretation of strength scores was impossible because the youngster complained of spraining her back whenever she lifted. Further follow-up revealed serious behavior problems. Referral was made to a psychiatrist who treated the child.[2]
>
> The author has had several disheartening experiences while administering a simple strength test for research purposes to a group of eight- to twelve-year-old boys. In one instance a nice-looking youngster while standing in line experienced a complete emotional breakdown. I reported the incident to the homeroom teacher and the principal. They gave this information: The boy was overly protected; his mother did not want him to play with other children. He remained in the classroom during recess (the school had no physical education) to read or play by himself. As the boy's father was abroad this youngster missed much needed companionship, a situation which possibly could be helped by a good physical educator.

These case studies are but a few of the many that lend validity to strength testing as a means of reflecting general physical fitness. With this type of measurement program, the deficient pupils are located and the necessary steps may be taken to ameliorate the causes of their problems.

Strength testing can form a valuable and integral part of the professional physical education program.

Strength as prophylaxis.   Lack of minimal muscular strength may lead to certain chronic illnesses. Kraus and his co-workers[15] state that "lack of sufficient muscular activity not only means insufficient emotional release, but at the same time it decreases muscular strength." They claim that muscle disuse is a predisposing factor to general and local tension. Over 4000 cases of low back pain were studied by Kraus and associates, the patients being from private practice, from the Columbia Medical Center Low Back Clinic, and from the Low Back Service of the Institute of Physical Medicine and Rehabilitation of New York University's Bellevue Center. It was reported that approximately 80 per cent of the patients, after thorough examination by a team of specialists, were found to be free from organic disease; when treated with systematic exercise, they improved as their strength and flexibility increased. In follow-up studies, it was found that these patients lost ground as their physical activities were reduced or given up. Kraus and associates further reported that, of the number treated, relief of pain also paralleled improved muscle status.

Both Crile[7] and Cannon[2] bring our attention to the possible physiological imbalance resulting from overstimulation by the adrenal gland. This gland normally secretes a hormone that internally excites the body for activity. The activity that follows burns up the secretion, and thus the body is allowed to relax or function in a normal manner. The stimulation to the adrenal may also be caused by anxiety and worry. Without physical activity as a release, the hormone leaves the body tense and keyed up. This has been suggested as one of the causes for the increasing number of emotional disturbances in our population. Increased mechanization, spectator activities, and lack of interest in fitness present a tremendous challenge to the physical educator for developing fitness *and* teaching youngsters the values of *maintaining* physical fitness.

Muscular efficiency.   Physiologically, a muscle working near its maximum capacity works with less efficiency than does a muscle sufficiently strengthened to perform the task. For example, if one were putting the shot, the primary muscles involved would work much more efficiently if they possessed more than the minimal amount of strength necessary to perform the activity. The application of this principle prevails in any activity requiring strength.

Thus a muscle group working near its maximum capacity may easily become chronically fatigued, resulting in lowered vitality of the body and less proficiency in execution of skills. In addition, this is a contributing factor to accident proneness.

Hypokinetics (role of inactivity in production of disease).   In recent years there has been a growing interest in the role of inactivity as a cause of disease. Although conclusions are not definite and a great deal of research needs to be done, students of physical education should recognize the potential in this broad field. Kraus and his co-workers, in a report from the Institute of Physical Medicine and Rehabilitation, New York University, review some of the pertinent literature in the field of hypokinetic disease.[15]

The report states that the mechanized life in America leads to physical inactivity. This in turn is a large factor in a number of orthopedic, internal, and psychosomatic disease entities. The report further states that muscle tests may be used as a means of predicting the incidence of this disease group (hypokinetic disease) in a statistical population, and that study, treatment, and prevention of physical inactivity as an important etiologic factor of many disabling diseases is imperative for the national welfare.

The results of studies supporting the above statement, as reported by Kraus and associates, are as follows:

1. Coronary disease is twice as frequent in groups of sedentary persons as in the active.

2. Diabetes, duodenal ulcer, and a number of other conditions, internal, surgical, or both, are more frequent in the sedentary than in the active.

3. Electromyographic activity of tense muscle is highly increased and goes hand in hand with increase of pain after irritating interview. The tension syndrome produced by insufficient outlet for fight and flight response provides the basis for a large number of orthopedic difficulties, including stiff neck and painful back. Tension headaches also belong in this group.

4. Lack of physical fitness parallels emotional difficulties.

5. Incidence of dental caries is in inverse proportion to weakness of bite force.

More research is needed in this area to gain greater insight to the cause and effect of muscular deficiencies as they contribute to disease. Owing to the increasing population, to crowded metropolitan areas, and to more push buttons for performing physical labor, a rich new field has appeared to challenge physical educators everywhere.

Instruments for Measuring Strength

Back and leg dynamometer (Figs. 16 and 17).   The dynamometer is a scale mounted on a stall bar bench or wooden platform. The chain and the handle attached to it provide for adjustment according to the size of the subject. The scale measures from 0 to 2500 pounds and is divided into units of 10 pounds. In addition to the dial hand there is a maximum indicator that remains in place after maximum effort by the subject.

Manuometer (Fig. 10).   The manuometer is used to record strength of the grip (finger flexors). It consists of two heavy springs mounted between steel bars. The bars are curved to "fit the grip." The scale is from

0 to 200 pounds. The dial hand is returned to the zero point manually. Figure 10 illustrates the manuometer with a push-and-pull attachment that enables one to measure the strength of the pectoral muscles and the shoulder retractors.

Tensiometer (Fig. 11).   The tensiometer* measures the pulling force

*Manufactured by the Pacific Scientific Co., Inc., 1430 Grande Vista Avenue, Los Angeles, Calif.

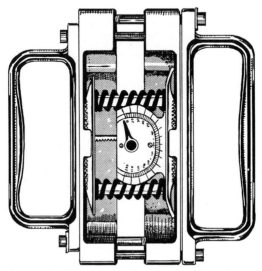

Figure 10.   Manuometer with push-and-pull attachment.

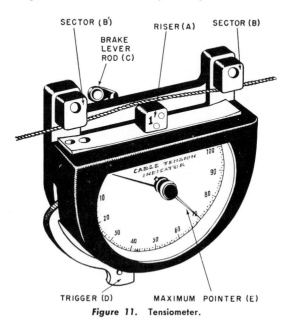

Figure 11.   Tensiometer.

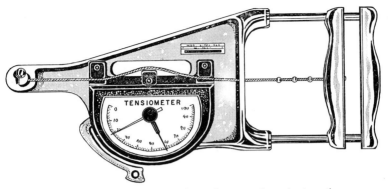

Figure 12. Tensiometer attachment for measuring grip strength.

on a cable. As the force on the cable increases, the riser on the tensiometer over which the cable passes is depressed. There is a maximum pointer to facilitate reading the subject's score. Two tensiometers are needed for most testing situations—one that registers to 100 pounds and another that will record up to 400 pounds. The lower end of the 400-pound instrument is not accurate (below 30 pounds), while the 100-pound instrument does not allow testing of stronger muscle groups (e.g., knee extensors).

Figure 12 represents an attachment to the tensiometer that permits the measurement of grip strength.

Strength Tests

Strength Index (SI). The Strength Index is the gross score obtained from lung capacity and the following six strength tests: right grip, left grip, back lift, leg lift, pull-ups, and push-ups (the latter two tests combined in a formula provide an arm strength score). The SI is proposed in physical education as a measure of general athletic ability. There is considerable statistical evidence to support this contention. Satisfactory validity has been obtained against such criteria as: earning letters on major sports high school athletic teams, batteries of track and field athletic events, and the equation of participants on various sports teams.

Physical Fitness Index (PFI). The Physical Fitness Index is a score derived from comparing an achieved Strength Index with a norm based upon the individual's sex, weight, and age. A PFI of 100 is considered average. This test is proposed as a measure of physical fitness, indicating the immediate ability of the individual for physical activity. The validity of this assumption is based on such evidence as: a theoretical relationship between strength and proficiency for physical activity; the resultant defections accompanying a loss of strength; case studies revealing the effect of organic conditions upon loss in strength, resulting in a lowered PFI; and the relationship between the PFI and physicians' judgments of fitness status.

ADMINISTRATION AND EVALUATION OF THE PFI

Sequence of test items   (Figure 13, Conventional PFI Score Card).
1. Age recorded in years and months.
2. Height to nearest half inch; subject in stocking feet.
3. Weight to nearest half pound; subject in gym clothes and stocking feet.
4. Lung capacity, using wet spirometer; recorded in cubic inches.
5. Grip strength using manuometer; recorded to nearest pound.
6. Back lift using dynamometer; recorded in pounds.
7. Leg lift using dynamometer; recorded in pounds.

PFI Score Card

Name (Print)								
	Last		First					
Grade								
Date	First Test		Second Test		Third Test		Fourth Test	
Age	Yrs.	Mos.	Yrs.	Mos.	Yrs.	Mos.	Yrs.	Mos.
Weight		Lbs.		Lbs.		Lbs.		Lbs.
Height		Ins.		Ins.		Ins.		Ins.
Multiplier								
Pull-ups								
Push-ups								
Arm Strength								
Leg Lift								
Back Lift								
Left Grip								
Right Grip								
Lung Capacity								
Strength Index								
Normal SI								
PFI								

Figure 13. Score card for PFI test.

8. Pull-ups: *boys*. Horizontal bars with attached rings; record maximum number.

Pull-ups: *girls*. Rings attached to adjustable horizontal bar. Body at right angles to bar with heels under bar resting on floor. Record maximum number.

9. Dips: *boys*. Performed on parallel bars. Record maximum number. Push-ups: *girls*. Performed on stall bar bench. Record maximum number.

Administration of test items *Lung capacity* (Fig. 14). This is the amount of air that can be expired after the deepest possible inspiration. Lung capacity, sometimes called vital capacity, is related to one's size and, to a lesser extent, the strength of one's respiratory muscles.

1. The spirometer should be placed at a height that allows the subject to stand erect at the beginning of the test.

2. The subject should then forcefully inhale and exhale twice before taking the test (hyperventilate).

3. The subject should be cautioned not to allow air to escape through his nose or around the mouthpiece.

4. As the subject nears completion of the effort he should bend slightly forward to get as much air as possible into the spirometer.

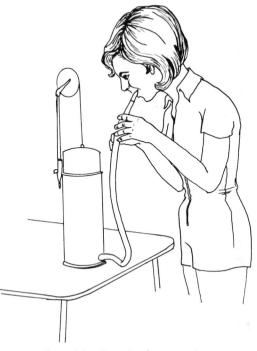

Figure 14. Measuring lung capacity.

5. The tester should watch the needle to obtain the maximum reading.

Grip strength (Fig. 15):

1. The subject's hands should be first chalked. Place the concave edge of the manuometer between the first and second joints of the fingers, with the dial toward the palm.

2. The subject is allowed any movement while squeezing his instrument, *provided* he does not hit any object with his fist. The most common movement is the upper cut.

3. The right grip is tested first.

Back lift (Fig. 16):

1. The subject stands on the dynamometer base, with feet parallel and about 6 inches apart. The malleoli of the ankle joint should be as nearly opposite the attachment of the dynamometer to its base as possible.

2. The subject stands with head erect, back straight, and chalked fingers extending down the thighs. The examiner holds the bar at the

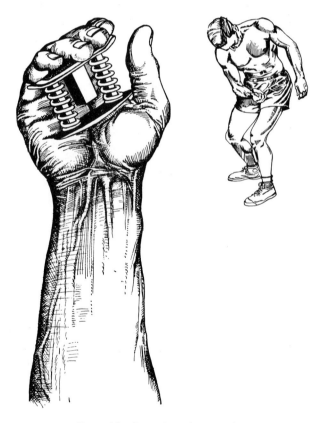

Figure 15. Measuring grip strength.

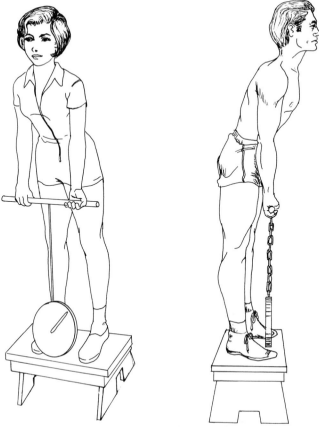

Figure 16. Measuring back lift.

tips of subject's fingers to obtain proper adjustment. The bar is then connected to the chain.

3. The subject bends slightly forward, with knees straight, and grasps the bar near either end. The grip is mixed, one hand forward and one backward.

4. The subject is asked to lift straight up while the examiner spots by placing his hands over the subject's to prevent the latter's hands from slipping.

Leg lift (Fig. 17).   This is the most difficult test to administer.

1. The subject assumes the same position as in the back lift. A belt is used around the subject's hips to stabilize the bar, as the lifting force of the legs is much too great to be held by the hands.

2. The subject holds the center of the bar, palms down, at the level of the pubic bone.

3. As the tester faces the subject, the belt loop is attached to the left

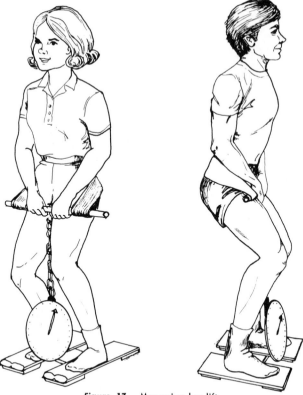

Figure 17. Measuring leg lift.

end of the bar. The belt is then brought around the lower portion of the sacrum to be attached to the right end of the handle as seen in Figure 18.

4. To make the attachment to the right side of the bar, proceed as follows: Form a loop in the belt by folding it back. The loop should be just opposite the end of the handle. Holding the loop in the left hand, reach down between the belt and subject to grasp the end of the belt in the right hand. Slide the loop over the bar and pull the end of the belt up against the subject's hip. With the belt in this position, the pulling

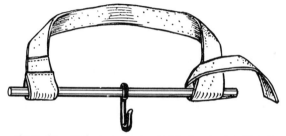

Figure 18. Method of securing belt to bar for leg lift test.

force of the bar will hold the tail end of the belt against the subject's body, preventing the bar from sliding—similar to a timber hitch.

5. The subject, with head up and back straight, bends at the knees. The handle is hooked onto the chain so that the subject's knees are flexed between 115 and 125 degrees.

6. The bar will be on the subject's thighs during the lift. The subject may place his hands either in the middle or at the ends of the bar.

7. The subject is asked to lift straight up. At the completion of the lift the subject's knee joints should be almost completely extended to insure maximum effort.

Pull-ups: boys (Fig. 19).   The subject starts from complete extension.* Count one for each pull-up. The examiner should spot to prevent swaying.

---

*Note: If rings are not available, the subject should perform the pull-ups with "palms-toward-body" grip.

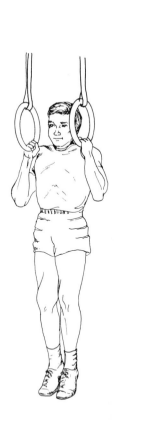
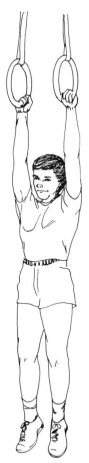

Figure 19. Pull-ups: boys.

Up to four half-counts are allowed for either: (1) kipping, (2) lack of complete flexion (chin should be even with hands), or (3) lack of complete extension (arms straight).

Pull-ups: girls (Fig. 20).   The rings are attached to a horizontal bar so that they are even with subject's sternal apex. A mat should be placed under the bar to prevent slipping of feet.*

The body is at right angles to the rings. Count one for each complete pull-up. Up to four half-counts are allowed for sagging, pumping, or knee bending. The Gay apparatus, or an adaptation of it like that in Figure 19, facilitates this testing procedure.

Dips: boys (Fig. 22).   Parallel bars or wall parallel bars are used; the former have an advantage in that they may be adjusted to height. The bars should be shoulder high.

Count one for mounting the bars. The subject dips to the point where

---

*Note: If rings are not available, the subjects should perform the pull-ups with "palms-toward-body" grip.

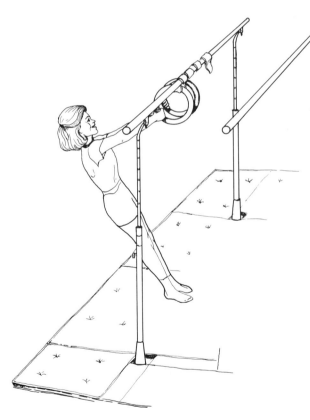
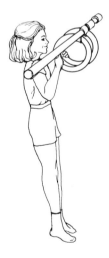

Figure 20. Pull-ups: girls.

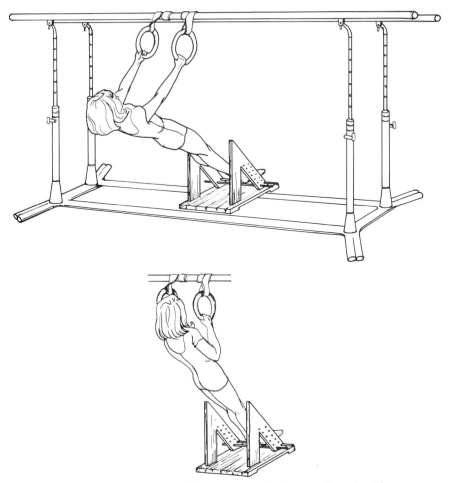

Figure 21. Adaptation of Gay apparatus for testing pull-ups for girls.

the elbow forms a right angle. The examiner notes this place with his fist, which the subject touches each time he comes down. Up to four half-counts are allowed for incomplete push-ups, kicking, or kipping.

Push-ups: girls (Fig. 23). A stall bar bench is used. The subject assumes the front leaning rest position, with arms straight, on a bench 13 inches high.

1. With head up and back straight the subject lowers her body so that her chest touches, or nearly touches, the bench.

2. Each push-up counts one. Up to four half-counts are allowed for arching, swaying, or incomplete movements.

Scoring the PFI. Figure 13 shows the most common type of score card used in the PFI testing.

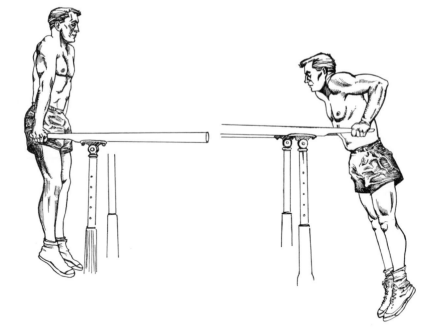

Figure 22. Dips: boys.

Arm strength. Arm strength for both girls and boys is computed by the following formula:

$$(\text{Dips} + \text{Pull-ups}) \left(\frac{W}{10} + H - 60 \right)$$

W = weight in pounds
H = height in inches (disregard H − 60 if height is less than 60 inches).

Example:

Subject's weight = 150 pounds
Subject's height = 65 inches
Pull-ups   =   4
Push-ups or dips =   6

Inserting in the formula:

$$\text{Arm strength} = (4 + 6)\left(\frac{150}{10} + 65 - 60 \right) = (10)\ (20)$$

$$\text{Arm strength} = 200$$

Computing the SI. To the arm strength is added the lung capacity, back and leg strength, and grip strength. The total score is the Achieved or Obtained Strength Index.

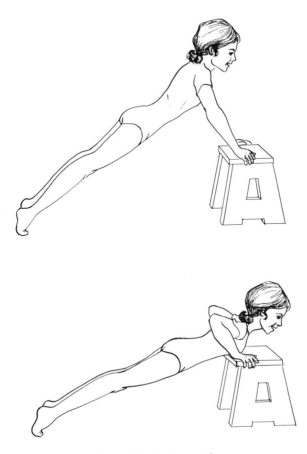

Figure 23. Push-ups: girls.

Computing the PFI.   To obtain the PFI the following formula is used:

$$\text{PFI} = \frac{\text{Achieved SI}}{\text{Norm}} \times 100$$

The norm is obtained from Tables 15 and 16, which have been constructed on the basis of sex, age, and weight of the subject. (Norms for men and women [ages 19 to 38 years] as well as the ones reproduced here are available from the Medart Company in St. Louis.) For example: A boy's weight is 150 pounds; his age is fifteen years; his obtained SI is 2200; his norm SI (from Table 16) is 2188. Thus, 2200 divided by 2188, times 100, equals a PFI of 101.

The validity of Rogers' PFI norms has been questioned, chiefly in that

Table 15. *Strength Index Norms for Girls (Belt)**

AGE

Weight	8	8-6	9	9-6	10	10-6	11	11-6	12	12-6	13	13-6	14	14-6	15	15-6	16	16-6	17	17-6	18	Weight
180															2840	2933	2990	2984	2960	2912	2835	180
178														2721	2796	2885	2940	2934	2912	2865	2790	178
176													2598	2681	2752	2837	2890	2884	2863	2819	2745	176
174												2192	2560	2610	2707	2789	2840	2835	2815	2772	2700	174
172											2364	2137	2523	2600	2663	2741	2790	2785	2766	2726	2655	172
170										2350	2332	2122	2186	2559	2619	2693	2740	2735	2718	2679	2610	170
168										2220	2300	2387	2449	2518	2575	2615	2690	2685	2670	2632	2565	168
166									2085	2190	2268	2352	2412	2478	2531	2597	2640	2635	2621	2586	2520	166
164									2058	2160	2236	2318	2374	2437	2486	2519	2590	2586	2573	2539	2475	164
162									1923	2030	2130	2201	2283	2337	2397	2412	2510	2586	2521	2493	2430	162
160							1818	1897	2002	2100	2172	2218	2300	2356	2398	2153	2190	2486	2176	2146	2385	160
158							1793	1871	1974	2070	2140	2213	2263	2313	2354	2105	2410	2436	2428	2399	2340	158
156						1736	1769	1815	1946	2010	2108	2178	2226	2275	2310	2337	2390	2386	2379	2353	2295	156
154						1711	1744	1818	1919	2010	2076	2144	2188	2234	2265	2309	2310	2337	2331	2306	2250	154
152					1681	1687	1720	1792	1891	1980	2044	2109	2151	2194	2221	2261	2290	2287	2282	2260	2205	152
150				1625	1657	1663	1695	1766	1863	1950	2012	2074	2114	2153	2177	2213	2210	2237	2234	2213	2160	150
148			1524	1602	1633	1639	1670	1740	1835	1920	1980	2039	2077	2112	2133	2165	2190	2187	2186	2166	2115	148
146			1502	1578	1609	1615	1646	1714	1807	1890	1918	2001	2010	2072	2089	2117	2110	2137	2137	2120	2070	146
144		1419	1479	1555	1584	1590	1621	1687	1780	1860	1916	1970	2002	2031	2044	2069	2090	2088	2089	2073	2025	144
142	1310	1398	1457	1531	1560	1566	1597	1661	1752	1830	1881	1915	1965	1991	2000	2021	2010	2038	2010	2027	1980	142
140	1319	1376	1435	1508	1536	1542	1572	1635	1724	1800	1852	1900	1928	1950	1956	1973	1990	1988	1992	1980	1935	140
138	1298	1354	1113	1485	1512	1518	1547	1609	1696	1770	1820	1865	1891	1909	1912	1925	1940	1938	1944	1933	1890	138
136	1278	1333	1391	1461	1188	1491	1523	1583	1668	1740	1788	1830	1854	1869	1868	1877	1890	1888	1895	1887	1845	136
134	1257	1311	1368	1438	1163	1469	1498	1556	1641	1710	1756	1796	1816	1828	1823	1829	1810	1839	1847	1840	1800	134
132	1237	1290	1316	1111	1139	1445	1474	1530	1613	1680	1724	1761	1779	1788	1779	1781	1790	1789	1798	1794	1755	132
130	1216	1268	1324	1391	1415	1121	1419	1504	1585	1650	1692	1726	1742	1747	1735	1733	1740	1739	1750	1747	1710	130
128	1195	1246	1302	1368	1391	1397	1124	1178	1557	1620	1660	1691	1705	1706	1691	1685	1690	1689	1702	1700	1665	128
126	1175	1225	1280	1344	1367	1373	1100	1152	1529	1590	1628	1656	1668	1666	1647	1637	1610	1639	1653	1654	1620	126
124	1154	1203	1257	1321	1312	1318	1375	1125	1502	1560	1596	1622	1630	1625	1602	1589	1590	1590	1605	1607	1575	124
122	1134	1182	1235	1297	1318	1324	1351	1399	1474	1530	1564	1587	1593	1585	1558	1541	1540	1540	1556	1561	1530	122
120	1113	1160	1213	1274	1294	1300	1326	1373	1446	1500	1532	1552	1556	1544	1514	1493	1490	1490	1508	1514	1485	120
118	1092	1138	1191	1251	1270	1276	1301	1317	1418	1470	1500	1517	1519	1503	1470	1445	1440	1440	1460	1467	1440	118
116	1072	1117	1169	1227	1246	1252	1277	1321	1390	1440	1468	1482	1482	1463	1426	1397	1390	1390	1411	1421	1395	116
114	1051	1095	1146	1204	1221	1227	1252	1294	1363	1410	1436	1448	1444	1422	1381	1349	1340	1341	1363	1374	1350	114
112	1031	1074	1124	1180	1197	1203	1228	1268	1335	1380	1404	1413	1407	1382	1337	1305	1290	1291	1314	1328	1305	112
110	1010	1052	1102	1157	1173	1179	1203	1242	1307	1350	1372	1378	1370	1341	1293	1253	1210	1241	1266	1281	1260	110
108	989	1030	1080	1134	1149	1155	1178	1216	1279	1320	1340	1313	1333	1300	1249	1205	1190	1191	1218	1234	1215	108
106	969	1009	1058	1110	1125	1131	1154	1190	1251	1290	1308	1308	1296	1260	1205	1157	1140	1141	1169	1188	1170	106
104	948	987	1035	1087	1100	1106	1129	1163	1224	1260	1276	1274	1258	1219	1160	1109	1090	1092	1121	1141	1125	104
102	928	966	1013	1063	1076	1082	1105	1137	1196	1230	1244	1239	1221	1179	1116	1061	1040	1012	1072	1095	1080	102
100	907	944	991	1040	1052	1058	1080	1111	1168	1200	1212	1204	1184	1138	1072	1013	990	992	1024	1048	1035	100
98	886	922	969	1017	1028	1034	1055	1085	1140	1170	1180	1169	1147	1097	1028	965	940	942	976	1001	990	98
96	866	901	917	993	1004	1010	1031	1059	1112	1140	1148	1134	1110	1057	984	917	890	892	927	955	945	96
94	845	879	924	970	979	985	1006	1032	1085	1110	1116	1100	1072	1016	939	869	840	843	879	908	900	94
92	825	858	902	946	955	961	982	1006	1057	1080	1084	1065	1035	976	895	821	790	793	830	862	855	92
90	804	836	880	923	931	937	957	980	1029	1050	1052	1030	998	935	851	773	740	743	782	815	810	90
88	783	814	858	900	907	913	932	954	1001	1020	1020	995	961	894	807	725	690	693	734	768	765	88
86	763	793	836	876	883	889	908	940	973	990	988	960	921	854	763	677	640	643	685	722	720	86
84	742	771	813	853	858	864	883	901	946	960	956	926	886	813	718	629	590	594	637	675	675	84
82	722	750	791	829	831	810	839	875	918	930	921	891	819	773	671	581	540	541	588	629	630	82
80	701	728	769	806	810	816	834	819	890	900	892	856	812	732	630	533	490	494	540	582	585	80
78	680	706	717	783	786	792	809	823	862	870	860	821	775	691	586	485	410	444	492	535		78
76	660	685	725	759	762	768	785	797	834	840	828	786	738	651	542	437	390	394	443	489		76
74	639	663	702	736	737	743	760	770	807	810	796	752	700	610	497	389	340	345	395			74
72	619	642	680	712	713	719	736	744	779	780	764	717	663	570	453	341	290	295	346			72
70	598	620	658	689	689	695	711	718	731	750	732	682	626	529	409	293	240	245				70
68	577	598	636	666	665	671	686	692	723	720	700	647	589	488	365	245	190					68
66	557	577	614	642	641	647	662	666	695	690	668	612	552	448	321	197	140					66
64	536	555	591	619	616	622	637	639	668	660	636	578	514	407	276	149						64
62	516	534	569	595	592	598	613	613	640	630	604	543	477	367	232							62
60	495	512	547	572	568	574	588	587	612	600	572	508	440	326								60
58	474	490	525	549	544	550	563	561	584	570	540	473	403									58
56	454	469	503	525	520	526	539	535	556	540	508	438										56
54	433	447	480	502	495	501	514	508	529	510	476											54
52	413	426	458	478	471	477	490	482	501	480												52
50	392	404	436	455	447	453	465	456	473													50
	8	8-6	9	9-6	10	10-6	11	11-6	12	12-6	13	13-6	14	14-6	15	15-6	16	16-6	17	17-6	18	
**	10.3	10.8	11.1	11.7	12.1	12.1	12.3	13.1	13.9	15	16	17.4	18.6	20.3	22.1	24	25	24.9	24.2	23.3	22.5	

*Reproduced with permission of Frederick Rand Rogers.
**Weight Deviation Multiplier.

Norms for individuals whose weights are above limits for which norms are included are calculated by adding to the norm for any chosen weight the pound difference that weight and the individual's weight times the Weight Deviation Multiplier.

Table 16. *Strength Index Norms for Boys (Belt)**

AGE

Weight	8	8-6	9	9-6	10	10-6	11	11-6	12	12-6	13	13-6	14	14-6	15	15-6	16	16-6	17	17-6	18	Weight
180															2664	2813	2917	2993	3056	3105	3159	180
178															2632	2778	2880	2954	3016	3064	3118	178
176															2601	2743	2843	2916	2976	3023	3077	176
174														2363	2569	2708	2805	2877	2936	2983	3035	174
172														2336	2537	2674	2768	2838	2896	2942	2994	172
170														2308	2505	2639	2731	2799	2856	2901	2953	170
168														2280	2474	2604	2694	2761	2816	2860	2911	168
166													2067	2253	2442	2569	2657	2722	2776	2819	2870	166
164													2043	2225	2410	2534	2620	2683	2736	2779	2829	164
162													2020	2198	2378	2499	2583	2645	2696	2738	2787	162
160												1848	1996	2170	2316	2465	2546	2606	2656	2697	2746	160
158												1827	1972	2142	2315	2430	2509	2567	2616	2636	2704	158
156											1718	1807	1949	2115	2283	2395	2472	2528	2576	2615	2663	156
154											1699	1786	1925	2087	2251	2360	2435	2490	2536	2575	2622	154
152											1680	1766	1902	2060	2219	2325	2398	2451	2496	2534	2580	152
150										1610	1661	1745	1878	2032	2188	2291	2361	2412	2456	2493	2539	150
148										1591	1642	1724	1854	2001	2156	2256	2324	2373	2416	2452	2498	148
146										1573	1623	1704	1831	1977	2124	2221	2287	2335	2376	2411	2456	146
144									1525	1554	1604	1683	1807	1949	2092	2186	2250	2296	2336	2371	2415	144
142									1506	1536	1585	1663	1784	1922	2060	2151	2213	2257	2296	2330	2374	142
140								1470	1487	1517	1566	1642	1760	1894	2029	2116	2176	2219	2256	2289	2332	140
138								1451	1468	1498	1547	1621	1736	1866	1997	2082	2139	2180	2216	2218	2291	138
136							1401	1431	1449	1480	1528	1601	1713	1839	1965	2047	2102	2141	2176	2207	2249	136
134							1382	1412	1430	1461	1509	1580	1689	1811	1933	2012	2065	2102	2136	2167	2208	134
132							1362	1392	1411	1443	1490	1560	1666	1784	1901	1977	2028	2064	2096	2126	2167	132
130						1318	1343	1372	1392	1424	1471	1539	1642	1756	1870	1942	1991	2025	2056	2085	2125	130
128					1273	1299	1324	1353	1373	1405	1452	1518	1618	1728	1838	1907	1954	1986	2016	2044	2084	128
126				1227	1255	1280	1304	1333	1354	1387	1433	1498	1595	1701	1806	1873	1917	1948	1976	2003	2043	126
124			1185	1209	1236	1261	1285	1314	1334	1368	1414	1477	1571	1673	1774	1838	1879	1909	1936	1963	2001	124
122		1146	1169	1192	1218	1242	1266	1294	1315	1350	1395	1457	1548	1646	1743	1803	1842	1870	1896	1922	1960	122
120		1130	1152	1174	1199	1223	1246	1275	1296	1331	1376	1436	1524	1618	1711	1768	1805	1831	1856	1881	1919	120
118	1092	1114	1135	1156	1181	1204	1227	1255	1277	1312	1357	1415	1500	1590	1679	1733	1768	1793	1816	1840	1877	118
116	1077	1098	1119	1139	1162	1185	1208	1235	1258	1294	1338	1395	1477	1563	1647	1699	1731	1754	1776	1799	1836	116
114	1061	1082	1102	1121	1144	1166	1188	1216	1239	1275	1319	1374	1453	1535	1615	1664	1694	1715	1736	1759	1795	114
112	1046	1066	1085	1104	1125	1146	1169	1196	1220	1257	1300	1354	1430	1508	1584	1629	1657	1677	1696	1718	1753	112
110	1030	1050	1069	1086	1107	1127	1150	1177	1201	1238	1281	1333	1406	1480	1552	1594	1620	1638	1656	1677	1712	110
108	1014	1034	1052	1068	1088	1108	1130	1157	1182	1219	1262	1312	1382	1452	1520	1559	1583	1599	1616	1636	1670	108
106	999	1018	1035	1051	1070	1089	1111	1138	1163	1201	1243	1292	1359	1425	1488	1524	1546	1560	1575	1595	1629	106
104	983	1002	1018	1033	1051	1070	1092	1118	1144	1182	1224	1271	1335	1397	1457	1490	1509	1522	1536	1555	1588	104
102	968	986	1002	1016	1033	1051	1072	1099	1125	1164	1205	1251	1312	1370	1425	1455	1472	1483	1496	1514	1546	102
100	952	970	985	998	1014	1032	1053	1079	1106	1145	1186	1230	1288	1342	1393	1420	1435	1444	1456	1473	1505	100
98	936	954	968	980	995	1013	1034	1059	1087	1126	1167	1209	1264	1314	1361	1385	1398	1405	1416	1432	1464	98
96	921	938	952	963	977	994	1014	1040	1068	1108	1148	1189	1241	1287	1329	1350	1361	1367	1376	1391	1422	96
94	905	922	935	945	958	975	995	1020	1049	1089	1129	1168	1217	1259	1298	1316	1324	1328	1336	1351		94
92	890	906	918	928	940	956	976	1001	1030	1071	1110	1148	1194	1232	1266	1281	1287	1289	1296	1310		92
90	874	890	902	910	921	937	956	981	1011	1052	1091	1127	1170	1204	1234	1246	1250	1251	1256			90
88	858	874	885	892	903	918	937	962	992	1033	1072	1106	1146	1176	1202	1211	1213	1212	1216			88
86	843	858	868	875	884	898	918	942	973	1015	1053	1086	1123	1149	1171	1176	1173	1176				86
84	827	842	851	857	866	879	898	923	954	996	1034	1065	1099	1121	1139	1141	1139	1134	1136			84
82	812	826	835	840	847	860	879	903	935	978	1015	1045	1076	1094	1107	1107	1102	1096				82
80	796	810	818	822	829	841	860	883	916	959	996	1024	1052	1066	1075	1072	1065	1057				80
78	780	794	801	804	810	822	840	864	897	940	977	1003	1028	1038	1043	1037	1028	1018				78
76	765	778	785	787	792	803	821	844	878	922	958	983	1005	1011	1012	1002	991					76
74	749	762	768	769	773	784	802	825	858	903	939	962	981	983	980	967	953					74
72	734	746	751	752	755	765	782	805	839	885	920	942	958	956	948	933						72
70	718	730	735	734	736	746	763	786	820	866	901	921	934	928	916	898						70
68	702	714	718	716	718	727	744	766	801	847	882	900	910	900	885							68
66	687	698	701	699	699	708	724	746	782	829	863	880	887	873								66
64	671	682	684	681	681	689	705	727	763	810	844	859	863	845								64
62	656	666	668	664	662	669	686	707	744	792	825	839	840									62
60	640	650	651	646	644	650	666	688	725	773	806	818										60
58	624	634	634	628	625	631	647	668	706	754	787	797										58
56	609	618	618	611	607	612	628	649	687	736	768											56
54	593	602	601	593	588	593	608	629	668	717	749											54
52	578	586	584	576	570	574	589	610	649	699												52
50	562	570	568	558	551	555	570	590	630	680												50
	8	8-6	9	9-6	10	10-6	11	11-6	12	12-6	13	13-6	14	14-6	15	15-6	16	16-6	17	17-6	18	
**	7.80	8.00	8.35	8.80	9.26	9.54	9.67	9.78	9.52	9.30	9.50	10.30	11.80	13.80	15.89	17.41	18.52	19.36	20	20.40	20.68	

*Reproduced with permission of Frederick Rand Rogers.
**Weight Deviation Multiplier.

the standards are too high. Appendix C shows the experience of the New Britain, Connecticut, public school system in using the PFI for eight years; it gives norms as well as the general modus operandi of the program.

Interpreting the PFI.   On the norm chart the first quartile is equal to a PFI of 85, which tells us that 25 per cent of the children score below 85 while 75 per cent score above; the median is 100, the point at which half of the children score above and half below; and the third quartile equals 115, the point at which 25 per cent of the children score above and 75 per cent below. It is advisable to retest youngsters scoring 85 and under to make certain that the score is correct. If it is correct, they should be interviewed, a health habit questionnaire (p. 399), and a case study form (p. 397), or similar record should be completed to help ascertain the cause or causes of low fitness. On the basis of this information an individual program should be prescribed.

Precautions in PFI testing.   The following is a list of precautions that should be recognized as essential to PFI testing:

1. *Equipment*
   a. *Spirometer:* Make certain that the water is at the proper level before and at intervals during the testing. Check to be sure that no water is in the hose. On occasion, during the testing, if the collected air is too rapidly forced from the spirometer, water is spilled. If a bubbling noise occurs while a subject is being tested, the water level is too low. Air may escape at the attachment of the hose to the spirometer and at the place where collected air is released. A piece of shiny metal or a small mirror held near these points serves as a good check.
   b. *Dynamometer:* The greatest problem is calibration of this instrument. One method is to hang weights from the dynamometer. The difficulty here is that sufficient weights usually are not available to check the entire range of the instrument. For example, a weight of 150 pounds would tell you only the accuracy of the instrument at the lower end of the scale. The most satisfactory method is to send the instrument back to the factory every two years for calibration.
2. *Subjects*
   a. All subjects should have a medical examination and be completely free from ruptures or muscular weaknesses that might be aggravated by the test.
   b. The subjects should have experienced taking the test at least once before the test results can be considered reliable.
   c. A few seconds of alternate toe touching and bobbing should precede the back lift test. Two or three deep knee bends should precede the leg lift test.
   d. In administering the back and leg lift tests, select an object across

the room, about eye level, for the subjects to watch. This helps to insure that the head will be up and back straight.

e. In administering the leg lift tests to a subject for the first time, instruct him to practice the movement a couple of times before hooking the bar to the dynamometer. This will give him the feel of what is desired. While the subject is lifting, the tester should place his hands on the side of the subject's thighs. In this way the examiner can aid in preventing the subject from swaying either backward or forward. At the same time it will give the subject a feeling of security.

f. When hooking the bar to the chain for either back or leg lifts, make sure that there are no kinks that would allow a sudden jolt while the subject is pulling. Kinks frequently occur at the point where the chain is connected to the dynamometer. Taping this connection prevents the last link from slipping down toward the scale and becoming kinked.

g. Tape an angle of 120 degrees on the wall where the leg lift is being administered, for convenience in estimating the angle.

h. Allow a five-minute rest between pull-ups and push-ups.

Simplification of PFI.   Clarke and Carter[6] at Oregon and Seymour[20] at Springfield College found that the Strength Index could be simplified considerably by using fewer items. The regression equations, which all correlate at least .977 with the Strength Index, are as follows:

Upper elementary school boys
$$SI = 1.05 \text{ (leg lift)} + 1.35 \text{ (back lift)} + 10.92 \text{ (dips)} + 133$$

Junior high school boys
$$SI = 1.33 \text{ (leg lift)} + 1.20 \text{ (arm strength)} + 286$$

Senior high school boys
$$SI = 1.22 \text{ (leg lift)} + 1.23 \text{ (arm strength)} + 499$$

Evaluation of the PFI.   In Chapter 2 the criteria of scientific authenticity for selecting a test were discussed. Included among the criteria were: reliability, objectivity, validity, and administrative feasibility. Let us evaluate the PFI and SI against these criteria.

Reliability and objectivity.   In 1925, Rogers[18] obtained reliability and objectivity coefficients for the PFI test items ranging from .86 (leg strength) to .97 (lung capacity) for the seven items. The objectivity of the Strength Index was found to be .94.

Validity.   Rogers defines the fitness that the PFI measures as the status of general health. He states that it is a positive measure indicating relative amounts of power for activity. Chamberlain and Smiley,[3] in one study, and Hernlund,[10] in another, demonstrated that physicians' judgments of health status and PFI scores resulted in a correlation of .60.

CABLE-TENSION STRENGTH TESTS

Clarke,[4] over a period of ten years, has developed tests for measuring strength of thirty-eight muscle groups using a tensiometer. These tests were constructed originally with the idea in mind for use with orthopedic disabilities in hospitals and Veterans Administration centers. However, application of these tests has been made in numerous research studies, particularly at Springfield College.

The tests have been used with children as well as with adults.[5] Although the greatest application of these tests is being made in research, it seems logical that once norms are established the tests will form a valuable adjunct to the measurement program in public schools. The equipment is economical and the techniques of administration are easily acquired.

Equipment.   In addition to the tensiometer (Fig. 11), the equipment used for the majority of the cable-tension strength tests is illustrated in Figure 24.

Chain and Cable.   Twelve to eighteen inches of $\frac{1}{16}$-inch extra flexible 7x7 cable are attached by tying, or preferably by using a No. 14-6 solderless lug (used in electrical fittings), to a link chain about 3 feet long. The chain should be able to withstand a pulling force of 700 pounds. At the other end of the cable, another solderless lug is used, which permits attachment to the regulation strap.

Regulation strap.   This strap consists of a double-thickness piece of parachute webbing, 2½ feet in length. The material is stitched firmly around a D-ring, which may be purchased from a harness shop. A keeper, from the same webbing, is made of double thickness to give stiffness.

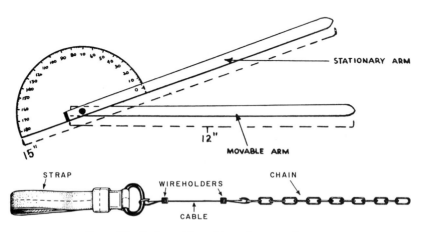

Figure 24. Equipment for cable-tension strength testing.

Goniometer.   This instrument is used for measuring the joint angles. It consists of a 180-degree protractor made from Plexiglas. (The 6-inch protractor is most practical.) Attached to the protractor are two arms, 15 inches long. One of these arms is stationary, extended along the zero line; the other should be permitted to rotate through 180 degrees. The use of a winged nut and bolt placed through an eyelet at the point of rotation of the movable arm helps in maintaining set angles during testing procedures.

A series of No. "0" wall hooks is spaced 6 inches apart from the floor to the ceiling, over which the chain on the pulling strap is attached, depending upon the test. This arrangement permits placing the chain over the proper hook, which will allow the force of the pull to be directed at right angles, regardless of the position of the joint.

In addition to the regulation strap, cable, and chain, Clarke has developed a trunk harness, trunk strap, and finger strap. A description of these materials and of the administration of the thirty-eight strength tests appears in the manual, "Cable-Tension Strength Tests," published by Brown-Murphy Company, Chicopee, Massachusetts.

Elbow flexion and ankle plantar flexion tests.   Figure 25 illustrates the elbow flexion (*A*) and ankle plantar flexion (*B*) cable-tension strength tests. Directions for administration of these two sample tests follow.

Elbow flexion (Fig. 25, *A*):

Starting position:

1. Subject in supine position, hips and knees flexed, feet resting on table; free hand resting on chest.

2. Subject's upper arm on the side tested is adducted and extended at the shoulder to 180 degrees; elbow in 115 degree flexion; forearm in mid-prone position.

Attachments:

1. Regulation strap around forearm midway between wrist and elbow joints.

2. Pulling assembly hooked to wall at subject's feet.

Precautions:

1. Prevent raising elbow and abducting upper arm by bracing at elbow.

Objectivity coefficient is .95.

Ankle plantar flexion (Fig. 25, *B*):

Starting position:

1. Subject in supine position; hips in 180-degree extension and adduction; knees in 180-degree extension; arms folded on chest.

2. Ankle on side tested in 90-degree plantar flexion; mid-position of inversion and eversion.

Attachments:

1. Regulation strap around foot, above metatarsal-phalangeal joint.

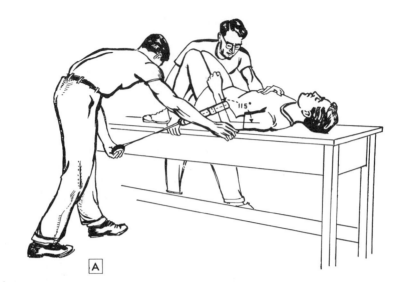

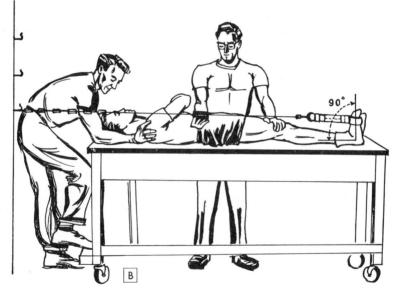

Figure 25. A, Elbow flexion strength test. B, Ankle plantar flexion strength test.

2. Pulling assembly is attached to wall at subject's head.
Precautions:
1. Prevent inversion or eversion at ankle joint, and raising of leg.
2. Brace behind shoulders to stabilize subject.
Objectivity coefficient is .93.

KRAUS-WEBER STRENGTH TESTS

Recognizing that the number of patients with low back disorders was increasing and that, as demonstrated through clinical experience, the majority of the disorders might have been prevented by maintaining a certain level of fitness, Kraus and Hirschland[14] examined 4458 American school children on a battery of six muscular strength tests. These tests, according to Kraus and Hirschland, represented minimum-fitness tests; that is, they were tests that indicated a level of strength and flexibility in certain key muscular groups below which functioning of the whole body as a healthy organism seemed endangered. Kraus and Hirschland noted that the patients whose physical fitness level fell below these minimum requirements appeared to be "sick people," individuals who bore all the earmarks of "constant strain," and who frequently manifested signs of emotional instability.

The Kraus-Weber tests were constructed over a period of eighteen years from clinical experience. The six tests selected for administration to the school children are purportedly the most valid out of a larger battery administered in clinical situations.

Administration.   There should not be any warm-up prior to taking the tests.

In the description of the six tests which follows the words "upper" and "lower" are used to indicate test movements rather than any specific areas.

Test 1 (Fig. 26).   In this test the strength of the abdominal and psoas muscles is determined.

Designation.   "Abdominals plus psoas" or A+.

Position of person being tested.   The subject is supine, with hands behind neck; the examiner holds the subject's feet down on the table.

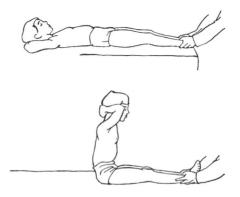

Figure 26. Strength test: abdominal and psoas muscles.

Command. "Keep your hands behind your neck and *try to roll up* into a sitting position."

Precautions. If the person being tested is unable to perform this movement at first try, it may be because he has not understood the directions. Help him a little and then let him try again. Watch for a "stiff back sit-up." This may indicate that either the subject has not understood you and needs a further explanation with emphasis on "rolling up," or that he has *very* poor abdominals and is doing most of the work with his psoas.

Watch also for a twist of the upper body as the subject sits up. If one is noted it may be due to unequal development of the back muscles.

Marking. If the person being tested cannot raise his shoulders from the table the mark is 0. If, unaided, he is able to reach a sitting position the mark is 10. If the examiner must help half-way to the sitting position the mark would be 5. The distance from supine to sitting is marked from 0 to 10.

Test 2 (Fig. 27)   This is a further test for abdominal muscles.

Designation. "Abdominals minus psoas" or A−.

Position of person being tested. The subject is supine, with hands behind neck and knees bent. The examiner holds the subject's feet down on the table.

Command. "Keep your hands behind your neck and *try to roll up* into a sitting position."

Precautions. The precautions are the same as for Test 1, but as Test 2 is usually more difficult the tendency toward "stiff back sit-up" will be even more pronounced and to it is added the tendency to help with one or the other elbow.

Marking. Same as Test 1.

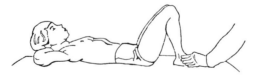

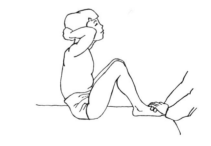

Figure 27. Strength test: abdominal minus psoas muscles.

Test 3 (Fig. 28).   This tests the strength of the psoas, and lower abdominals.

Designation.   "Psoas" or P.

Position of person being tested.   The subject is supine with hands behind neck and legs extended.

Command.   "Keep your knees straight and lift your feet 10 inches off the table. Keep them there while I count." The count is ten seconds. (Adding any three-syllable word after each number makes the count fairly reliable as to time. For example. "One chimpanzee, two chimpanzee, three chimpanzee," and so on.)

Precautions.   If the person tested has not understood your command, he may try to raise his chest when he raises his feet and will need further explanation. Watch for an extremely arched back, which may indicate very weak abdominal muscles or poor postural habits, contributing to sway back or lordosis.

Marking.   Holding for ten full seconds is passing and is marked as 10. Anything less is recorded as that part of the ten seconds that was held: 4 for four seconds, 7 for seven seconds, etc.

Test 4 (Fig. 29)   This tests the strength of the upper back muscles.

Designation.   "Upper back" or UB.

Position of person being tested.   The subject is prone with a pillow under his abdomen, but far enough down to give the body the feeling of being a seesaw, one end of which could be held in the air if the other

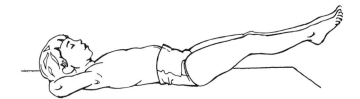

Figure 28.   Strength test: psoas and lower abdominal muscles.

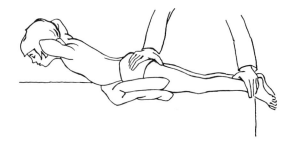

Figure 29.   Strength test: upper back muscle.

end were weighted. The commands will aid in getting the subject in the proper position.

Commands. "Roll over onto your stomach and lift up the middle so that I can slide this pillow under you." (Be sure the pillow is large enough to really support the subject.) "Now I am going to hold down your feet while you put your hands behind your neck and raise up your chest, head, and shoulders. Hold them up while I count." The count is ten seconds.

Precautions. Do not let the person being tested drop his chest onto the table or rest his elbows. Watch for pronounced muscular development on one side of the spine. If this condition is present, the back should be checked from time to time to guard against scoliosis (curvature of the spine).

Marking. Holding for ten full seconds is passing and is marked as 10. Anything less than ten seconds is recorded as that part of ten seconds that was held. For example, a person staying up for four seconds would get a mark of 4.

Test 5 (Fig. 30).   This tests the strength of the lower back.

Designation. "Lower back" or LB.

Position of person being tested. The subject remains prone over the pillow, but removes his hands from behind his neck, places them down on the table, and rests his head on them.

Commands. "I am going to hold your chest down on the table; try to lift your legs up, but do not bend your knees." There may be a tendency to bend the knees or even to support the legs by keeping the toes on the table. It may be necessary to assist the subject to the required position. "Now, hold this position while I count." The count is ten.

Marking. Holding for ten full seconds is passing and is marked as 10. Anything less is recorded as that part of the ten seconds that was held; for example, four seconds would be scored as 4.

Test 6 (Fig. 31).   This tests the length of back and hamstring muscles.

Designation. "Back and hamstrings" or BH.

Position of person being tested. The subject stands erect in stocking or bare feet, with hands at his sides.

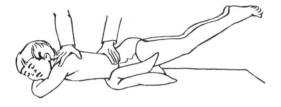

Figure 30. Strength test: lower back muscle.

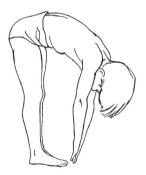

Figure 31. Strength test: hamstring muscles and length of back muscles.

Commands. "Put your feet together, keep your knees straight; now lean down slowly and see how close you can come to touching the floor with your fingertips. Stay down as far as you can for a count of three. *Do not bounce.*"

Precaution. Watch out for bouncing. The furthest point reached without bouncing and held for three counts is the marking point. The examiner should hold the knees of the person being tested in order to prevent any bend.

Marking. Touch is designated by T. *Touch* is only given when the floor-touch is held for three counts. Less than *touch* is marked by the distance in inches between the floor and the fingertips. For example, a person unable to touch the floor by 2 inches would be marked "−2."

Results. Owing to the large number of American failures, Kraus and Hirschland[13] examined 2870 European children for purposes of comparison. Table 17 contains the results of this study.

TABLE 17. *Comparison of Results in Administering the Kraus-Weber Tests to American and European Children (6-16)*

	Austrian	Italian	Swiss	American
Number tested	678	1036	1156	4264
Failure	9.5%	8.0%	8.8%	57.9%
Incidence of failure	9.7%	8.5%	8.9%	80.0%

Kraus, Hans, and Hirschland, Ruth P.: Minimum Muscular Fitness Tests in School Children. Research Quart., 25: 183, 1954.

Kraus and Hirschland state that the children (ages of 6 and 16 years) were from public school systems in suburban and small urban communities. The sizes of these cities, both European and American, were comparable.

Figure 32 contains four graphs with a breakdown of flexibility failures, weakness failures, children failing at least one test, and total number of

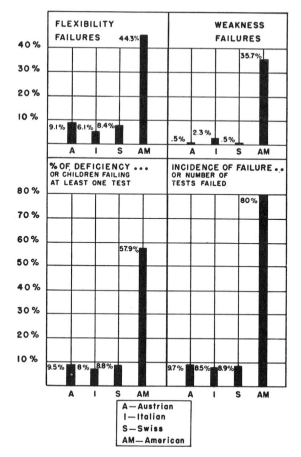

Figure 32. Minimum muscular fitness tests in school children. (Kraus, Hans, and Hirschland, Ruth P.: Research Quart., 25: 184, 1954.)

tests failed. These data reveal that American children certainly are below par as compared with their European contemporaries. Muscular flexibility tests resulted in by far the highest percentage of failures (44.3 per cent), while muscular weakness constituted 35.7 per cent of American failures.

President's commission.   Since the publication of these data, the problem of physical fitness has received national attention. In fact, President Eisenhower in 1956 established a Fitness Commission, appointing Vice-President Nixon as Chairman.

The first meeting of the President's Commission was held in Annapolis, Maryland, where educators met to discuss the issue. As a result of the fitness conference, President Eisenhower, in hopes of mitigating the problem of low fitness among American children, created:[8]

1. A Council on Youth Fitness at the Cabinet level to give top priority

to this field and to coordinate better the activities of some thirty-five federal agencies.

2. A Citizens' Advisory Committee on the Fitness of American Youth, composed of key citizens in fields appropriate to fitness, to examine and explore the facts and thereafter alert America on what can and should be done.

Other studies. The Kraus-Weber findings have led to further studies by physical educators to gain additional information in regard to the fitness of youth in America. For example, a study by Fox and Atwood,[9] in which 575 Iowa City school children in grades one through six were tested on the Kraus-Weber test, revealed the following facts:

1. In one or more of the tests, 66.1 per cent failed.

2. There were 56.9 per cent flexibility failures.

3. There were 34.8 per cent muscular weakness failures.

4. Of the six-year-olds, 42 per cent failed the abdominal tests; there was a progressive decrease to a low of 4 per cent of twelve-year-olds failing.

5. As abdominals increased in strength with increase in age, an increase in failure was noted on the psoas test.

6. Boys failed flexibility at a greater rate than girls.

7. The school with the better physical education program had fewer failures.

A list of behavior traits from Bakwin and Bakwin were given to the classroom teachers. Six per cent of the group checked by the teachers as showing some consistent form of emotional disturbance failed three tests; or 25 per cent of those failing three tests showed some evidence of maladjustment.

In another study, by Phillips and associates, the Kraus-Weber test of muscular fitness was administered to 1456 elementary school children from an Indiana city.[17] In order to determine the reliability of the test items, 215 of the children were tested twice. Also 126 of the children were tested for grip strength of the preferred hand to determine the relationship between grip strength and success on the Kraus-Weber test. The following results were obtained:

1. The reliability for the total Kraus-Weber battery and four of the individual test items resulted in coefficients exceeding .950 in all cases.

2. No relationship was established between grip strength and the Kraus-Weber tests.

3. The Indiana group was found to be somewhat superior to the Kraus sample in all failure comparisons.

4. Girls were more successful on the flexibility test than boys.

5. For both sexes, lack of flexibility increased with age.

6. For both sexes there was a decided decrease in strength item failure as age increased. At eleven years of age, failure on any strength item was less than 8 per cent.

7. Not more than six of the 1456 children failed each of the back strength items.

On the basis of this study the authors suggested that the back tests are not discriminatory and either should be eliminated or some other test submitted. They further recommended that flexibility figures and strength weakness figures be separated according to sex differences in interpreting or reporting the results. Their reasoning is that as flexibility decreases with age and strength increases, the total figures imply that no changes are occurring.

Among the most revealing fitness studies compiled recently is one by Campbell and Pohndorf dealing with a comparison of United States and British children. These examiners administered the AAHPER Physical Fitness Tests to over 10,000 British boys and girls. The results showed British youngsters far superior to the United States boys in all fitness tests except the softball throw. They have greater shoulder girdle strength, superior agility, and greater abdominal endurance, leg explosive power, and circulatory endurance. British girls also outdid their American counterparts. Furthermore, they showed superiority in performance over United States boys at ages 10 through 13 on their mean scores in five of the seven tests. These data are summarized in Figure 33.

Knuttgen[12] tested 319 male and 134 female Danish school children on the AAHPER test and compared his results with the American standards. He found that approximately 70 per cent of the boys' scores and 86 per cent of the girls' scores exceeded the corresponding American mean scores. The author suggests three general differences between the life of the Dane and that of the American. (1) There is, by necessity, more activity in the daily life of the Danish child, the bicycle being the principal means of transportation. Virtually no teen-agers or people in their twenties own automobiles because of the tremendous expense. The state-operated television operates only a few hours daily. (2) There is a distinct difference in school physical education programs, the Danish schools emphasizing soccer for boys and longball or handball (field-type with goals) for girls, with both sexes participating in gymnastics during the winter. The classes meet at least three times a week, with close supervision by the school administrators and by the Education Ministry personnel. (3) There appears to be a much higher interest in sports participation in Denmark, with about 45 per cent of the total population between the ages of 15 and 40 years participating in some form of sports activity.

Discussion of Kraus-Weber Test. Certain limitations of the Kraus-Weber tests have been suggested, as follows:

1. There are no allowances made for partial scores. The pupil either passes or fails the test item.

2. For the upper and lower back test these questions have been raised: How was the ten-second time duration determined? Should this

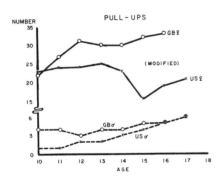

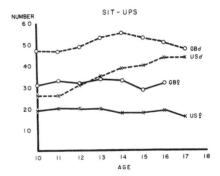

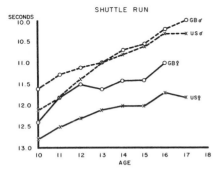

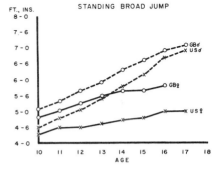

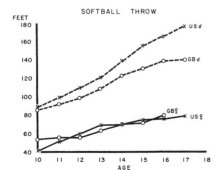

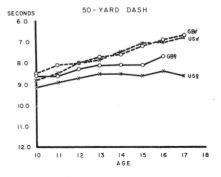

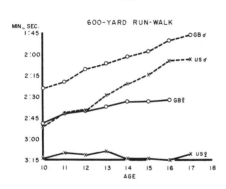

Figure 33. Comparison of boys and girls in the United States and Great Britain on AAHPER fitness test items (U.S. N = 8,500; G.B. N = 10,040). (Courtesy of Dr. R. H. Pohndorf, University of Ilinois.)

time interval vary with age level? Is the muscle sample adequate; that is, should shoulder girdle, legs, and feet be included?

Among the advantages of the Kraus-Weber test is its ease of administration. The only equipment needed is a table and a pillow or blanket. A pupil can be tested in two minutes. In addition to locating pupils with severe muscular weaknesses, the upper and lower back tests permit the trained eye of a physical educator to note muscular imbalances of the powerful back muscles. These lateral imbalances of muscular development should be noted as early as possible so that immediate steps can be taken for their correction. If left alone the strong muscle is apt to continue to get stronger, and a spinal curvature may result.

It may be worthwhile to note here that too frequently physical educators do not apply to best advantage their knowledge gained from kinesiology, physiology, body mechanics, and study of the atypical child. In the administration of such a test as the Kraus-Weber, the physical educator should approach the problem from a clinical standpoint. Through such clinical practice the examiner may become proficient in evaluating the general fitness characteristics of the child. For example, as the youngster is being examined, observe, in addition to muscular weaknesses, such characteristics as:

1. Signs of extreme tension.
2. Alertness of the child as commands are given.
3. Nutritional status.
4. Orthopedic deficiencies.
5. Muscle tonus.

It is here that information from background courses in the basic sciences, as mentioned above, is brought together and applied in a general fitness evaluation of the pupil. Through this type of approach a wealth of information may be gleaned from the examination, which can form the basis for follow-up work and program construction.

The approach to such evaluation requires skill that can be gained only through practice. Like the surgeon, the physician, and the therapist, the physical educator must train himself to be a craftsman in working with the human body. The Kraus-Weber test appears to be of value in this particular area of the testing program for use with elementary and junior high school children.

Summary and Conclusions

The use of strength tests in the public schools can form a valuable adjunct to the physical education program in terms of assaying general physical fitness. Measurement can be exciting in stimulating both you and your pupils to pass from low mediocrity to high excellence in terms of meeting the program objectives. Because of the stable nature of strength, the test results are reliable and objective. The fact that strength is related to ability in skills and is affected by organic drains and to some extent by emotional disturbances lends validity to these tests.

In almost any measuring instrument devised for use with human beings, shortcomings are always present. This is true with the strength tests that have been presented in this chapter. It would be foolhardy not to recognize the limitations accompanying each test. However, it is just as reckless not to measure at all, merely because a test is not perfect. Think, for example, of the skiers who will sit in front of the fire in the evening by the hour and argue over the advantages of various waxes and combinations that should be used, depending upon the snow conditions. Certainly, they all do not agree. However, by the same token, because of obvious shortcomings in certain waxing combinations, the skiers do not throw away the waxes and ski on bare boards. After all, the value of skiing goes beyond the type of wax used. So too, in physical education we should concern ourselves *more with the program that results from testing, and not so much with the test.*

BIBLIOGRAPHY

1. Amar, J.: The Human Motor. New York, E. P. Dutton & Co., 1920.
2. Cannon, W. B.: The Wisdom of the Body. Revised ed. New York, W. W. Norton & Co., Inc., 1939.
3. Chamberlain, C. G., and Smiley, D. F.: Functional Health and the Physical Fitness Index. Research Quart., Vol. 2, March, 1931.
4. Clarke, H. Harrison: A Manual: Cable-Tension Strength Tests. Chicopee, Massachusetts, Brown-Murphy Co., 1953.
5. Clarke, H. Harrison: Application of Measurement to Health and Physical Education. 4th ed. New York, Prentice-Hall, Inc., 1967, p. 171.
6. Clarke, H. Harrison, and Carter, Gavin H.: Oregon Simplification of the Strength and Physical Fitness Indices for Upper Elementary, Junior High, and Senior High School Boys. Research Quart., March, 1959.
7. Crile, G. W.: Man, an Adaptive Mechanism. New York, The Macmillan Co., 1916.
8. Fitness of American Youth. J. Am. A. Health, Physical Education, Recreation, September, 1956, p. 20.
9. Fox, Margaret G., and Atwood, Janet: Results of Testing Iowa School Children for Health and Fitness. J. Am. A. Health, Physical Education, Recreation, September, 1955, p. 20.
10. Hernlund, V. F.: The Selection of Physical Tests for Measuring Y.M.C.A. Secretaries. Supplement to Research Quart., March, 1935, pp. 235–241.
11. Karpovich, Peter V., and Sinning, Wayne E.: Physiology of Muscular Activity. 7th ed. Philadelphia, W. B. Saunders Company, 1971, p. 281.
12. Knuttgen, Howard G.: Comparison of Fitness of Danish and American School Children. Research Quart., 32:190–196, 1961.
13. Kraus, Hans, and Hirschland, Ruth P.: Minimum Muscular Fitness Tests in School Children. Research Quart., 25:177–188, 1954.
14. Kraus, Hans, and Hirschland, Ruth P.: Muscular Fitness and Orthopedic Disability. New York State J. Med. 54:212–215, 1954.
15. Kraus, Hans, Prudden, Bonnie, Weber, Sonja, and Hirscham, Kurt: Hypokinetic

Disease: Role of Inactivity in Production of Disease. Institute for Physical Medicine and Rehabilitation, New York University, Bellevue Medical Center, New York, 1955.

16. Metheny, Eleanor: Breathing Capacity and Grip Strength of Preschool Children. Iowa City, University of Iowa Studies in Child Welfare, Vol. 18, No. 2, 1940, pp. 114–115.

17. Phillips, Marjorie, et al.: Analysis of Results from the Kraus-Weber Test of Minimum Muscular Fitness in Children. Research Quart., 26:314–323, 1955.

18. Rogers, Frederick Rand: Physical Capacity Tests in the Administration of Physical Education. (Contributions to Education No. 173.) New York, Bureau of Publications, Teachers College, Columbia University, 1925.

19. Rogers, Frederick Rand: Reported in Physical Fitness News Letter, No. 6, May 20, 1955. Published by H. Harrison Clarke, University of Oregon, Eugene, Oregon.

20. Seymour, Emery W.: Follow-up Study on Simplifications of the Strength and Physical Fitness Indexes. Research Quart., May, 1960.

21. Zimmerli, Elizabeth: Case Studies of Unusual Physical Fitness Indices. Supplement to Research Quart., March, 1935.

chapter 5

motor fitness tests

The term "motor fitness" became popular during World War II. It may be defined as a limited phase of motor ability, emphasizing capacity for vigorous work. The aspects selected for emphasis are endurance, power, strength, agility, flexibility, and balance. More specifically, motor fitness might be referred to as efficient performance in such basic requirements as running, jumping, dodging, falling, climbing, swimming, lifting weights, carrying loads, and enduring sustained effort in a variety of situations. This type of measurement logically reflects the kind of fitness required of most military personnel. Numerous tests of motor fitness were devised and used in the various branches of the armed services.

The ease of administration, the small amount of training required for testing, and the economy of equipment involved contribute to the utility of these tests. The test results may be used to show the fitness status of the pupil, to measure improvement, and to serve as a basis for general ability classification in the physical education program. Although certain of the tests have norms constructed from a Sigma or T-scale, it is recommended that each teacher construct norms from his own pupils. He will then know that the scaled scores apply to his own group. Such factors as age, height, and weight of participants, and nature and intensity of the program will affect the norms.

Motor fitness tests are not beyond the reach of any school system desirous of initiating a measurement program. The tests are functional as well as objective in measuring a certain phase of fitness. It is possible to train student leaders to help in the administration of the test batteries. Because the tests are self-administered, the pupils may practice on their own to gain higher scores, at the same time increasing fitness.

It should be remembered that before data are collected for use in evaluation, as well as for constructing norms, the pupils should have sufficient experience with the test items. During the practice sessions the youngsters may become oriented as to the proper execution of the test as well as to the underlying reasons for the testing program. Brief discussions as to what the various items measure, as well as the need for maintenance of a certain degree of fitness, are vital adjuncts to the total program and should not be neglected.

It seems feasible at this time to mention a possible shortcoming of the sit-up test, which is included in a number of the motor fitness batteries contained in this chapter. The sit-up test, administered with the subject's knees straight, in most cases, is used to measure endurance and explosive power of the abdominal muscles. However, with the subject's legs straight, the primary muscle involved in executing this movement may be the iliopsoas, particularly if the back is arched. As this muscle is attached to the bodies of the lumbar vertebrae it may, in persons with weak abdominal muscles, cause serious strain at the lumbosacral joint. As a matter of fact, one of the important reasons Kraus gives for including this movement in his test battery (p. 97) is to observe whether or not there is an exaggerated lumbar curve as the child commences to sit up. If there is, the instructor is immediately warned that the child's abdominal muscles and perhaps the pelvic stabilizers are weak. In such instances as this it becomes obvious that the pull of the iliopsoas could cause low back strain, resulting in pain at the lumbosacral joint. In order to eliminate any possibility of injury it would be prudent to allow the subjects to perform sit-ups with hips and knees flexed (bent-knee sit-ups). This method minimizes the effectiveness of the iliopsoas muscle, and therefore a more pure abdominal action is involved.

Actually, there is very little reason for including the straight-leg sit-up movement in physical education programs. To strengthen the abdominal muscles, as in football, the bent-knee sit-up is a much better conditioner than is the straight-leg sit-up. To strengthen the iliopsoas, running exercises, which stress exaggerated raising of the knees, or jumping activities may be used. The iliopsoas muscle usually appears to be well developed in even the most emaciated cadavers, a further confirmation of the theory that the most efficient exercises for strengthening the abdominal muscles should leave the iliopsoas as nearly inactive as possible.

If you wish to use a motor fitness test containing the sit-up test with legs straight, you may substitute the bent-knee test, as long as any scoring tables that may accompany the test are not employed. If the sit-up test with knees straight is used, be alert for any exaggerated lumbar curves among the children.

AAHPER Youth Fitness Test

The American Association for Health, Physical Education and Recreation launched a Youth Fitness Project in 1957.[1] A national survey of

8500 boys and girls in the fifth through the twelfth grades was conducted to determine the general fitness level of these representative American youth. The battery of tests given them consisted of pull-ups, sit-ups, 40-yard shuttle run, 50-yard dash, 600-yard run-walk, standing broad jump, and a softball throw for distance.

In 1965 (under the Chairmanship of Dr. Paul Hunsicker, University of Michigan) some 9200 children from ten to seventeen years of age were tested and new norms were published.[1] The same test items were used with one exception: the flexed arm hang (Fig. 35) was substituted for modified pull-ups in the girls' test battery. There are two sets of percentile norms, one based on age and the other on the exponent Classification Index devised by Neilson and Cozens (p. 162). Norms based upon the Classification Index appear in Appendix D.

Administration of test items. In administering the tests it is suggested that the pull-up for boys, flexed arm hang for girls, sit-up, shuttle run, and standing broad jump all be given in one period; the 50-yard dash, softball throw for distance, and 600-yard run-walk may be given in a second period. Pupils should be given reasonable warm-up time prior to the testing.

Pull-ups: boys

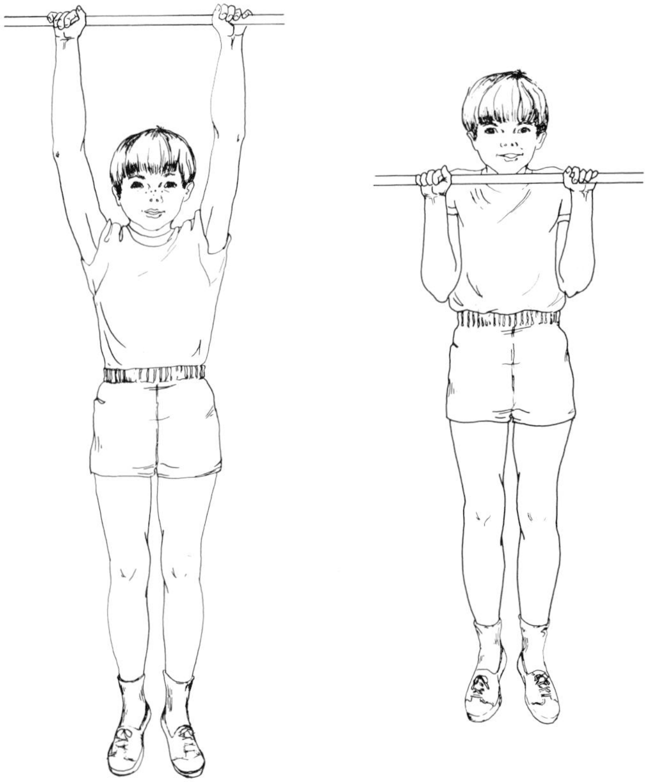

Figure 34. Pull-ups: boys.

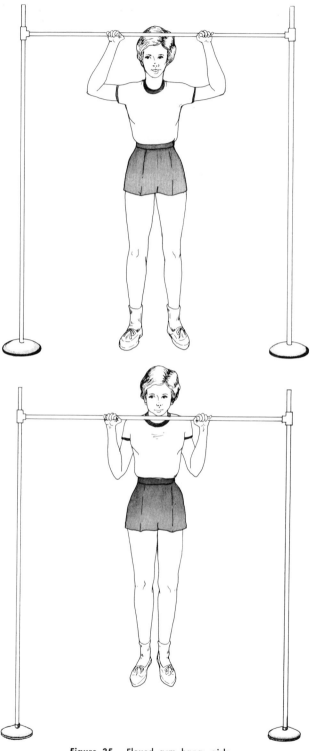

Figure 35. Flexed arm hang: girls.

Equipment.   A metal or wooden bar approximately 1½ inches in diameter is preferred. A doorway gym bar can be used, and, if no regular equipment is available, a piece of pipe or even the rungs of a ladder can also serve the purpose (Fig. 34).

Description.   The bar should be high enough so that the pupil can hang with his arms and legs fully extended and his feet free of the floor. He should use the overhand grasp (Fig. 34). After assuming the hanging position, the pupil raises his body by his arms until his chin can be placed over the bar and then lowers his body to a full hang as in the starting position. The exercise is repeated as many times as possible.

Rules

1. Allow one trial unless it is obvious that the pupil has not had a fair chance.

2. The body must not swing during the execution of the movement. The pull must in no way be a snap movement. If the pupil starts swinging, check this by holding your extended arm across the front of the thighs.

3. The knees must not be raised and kicking of the legs is not permitted.

Scoring.   Record the number of completed pull-ups to the nearest whole number.

Flexed arm hang: girls

Equipment.   A horizontal bar approximately 1½ inches in diameter is preferred. A doorway gym bar can be used; if no regular equipment is available, a piece of pipe can serve the purpose. A stop watch is needed.

Description.   The height of the bar should be adjusted so it is approximately equal to the pupil's standing height. The pupil should use an overhand grasp. With the assistance of two spotters, one in front and one in back of pupil, the pupil raises her body off the floor to a position where the chin is above the bar, the elbows are flexed, and the chest is close to the bar (Fig. 35). The pupil holds this position as long as possible.

Rules

1. The stop watch is started as soon as the subject takes the hanging position.

2. The watch is stopped when (a) pupil's chin touches the bar, (b) pupil's head tilts backwards to keep chin above the bar, (c) pupil's chin falls below the level of the bar.

Scoring.   Record in seconds to the nearest second the length of time the subject holds the hanging position.

Sit-ups: boys and girls

Equipment.   Mat or floor.

Description.   The pupil lies on his back, either on the floor or on a mat, with legs extended and feet about two feet apart. His hands are placed on the back of the neck with the fingers interlaced. Elbows are retracted. A partner holds the ankles down, the heels being in contact with the mat or floor at all times (Fig. 36). The pupil sits up, turning the trunk to the left and touching the right elbow to the left knee, returns to starting

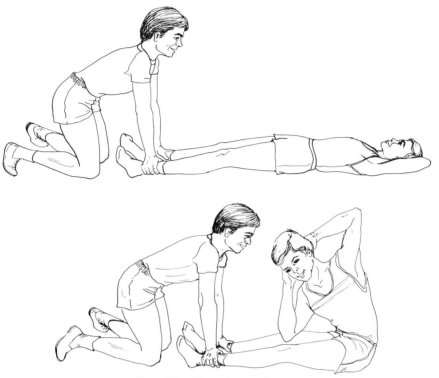

Figure 36. Sit-ups: boys and girls.

position, then sits up turning the trunk to the right and touching the left elbow to the right knee. The exercise is repeated, alternating sides.

Rules

1. The fingers must remain in contact behind the neck throughout the exercise.

2. The knees must be on the floor during the sit-up but may be slightly bent when touching elbow to knee.

3. The back should be rounded and the head and elbows brought forward when sitting up as a "curl"-up.

4. When returning to starting position, elbows must be flat on the mat before sitting up again.

Scoring. One point is given for each complete movement of touching elbow to knee. No score should be counted if the fingertips do not maintain contact behind the head, if knees are bent when the pupil lies on his back or when he begins to sit up, or if the pupil pushes up off the floor from an elbow. The maximum limit in terms of number of sit-ups shall be: 50 sit-ups for girls, 100 sit-ups for boys.

Shuttle run: boys and girls

Equipment.   Two blocks of wood, 2 inches × 2 inches × 4 inches, and stopwatch. Pupils should wear sneakers or run barefooted.

Description.   Two parallel lines are marked on the floor 30 feet apart. The width of a regulation volleyball court serves as a suitable area. Place the blocks of wood behind one of the lines as indicated in Figure 37. The pupil starts from behind the other line. On the signal "Ready? Go!"

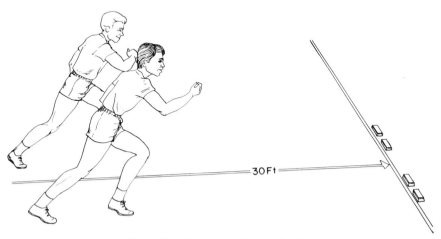

Figure 37.   Shuttle run: boys and girls.

the pupil runs to the blocks, picks one up, runs back to the starting line, and places the block behind the line; he then runs back and picks up the second block, which he carries back across the starting line. If the scorer has two stopwatches or one with a split-second timer, it is preferable to have two pupils running at the same time. To eliminate the necessity of returning the blocks after each race, start the races alternately, first from behind one line and then from behind the other.

Rules.   Allow two trials with some rest in between.

Scoring.   Record the time of the better of the two trials to the nearest tenth of a second.

Standing broad jump: boys and girls

Equipment.   Mat, floor, or outdoor jumping pit, and tape measure.

Description.   Pupil stands as indicated in Figure 38, with the feet several inches apart and the toes just behind the take-off line. Preparatory to jumping, the pupil swings the arms backward and bends the knees. The jump is accomplished by simultaneously extending the knees and swinging forward the arms.

Rules

1. Allow three trials.

2. Measure from the take-off line to the heel or other part of the body that touches the floor nearest the take-off line.

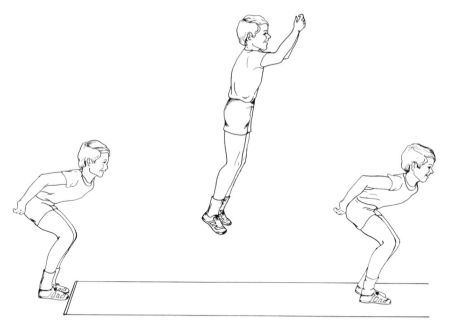

Figure 38. Standing broad jump: boys and girls.

3. When the test is given indoors, it is convenient to tape the tape measure to the floor at right angles to the take-off line and have the pupils jump along the tape. The scorer stands to the side and observes the mark to the nearest inch.

Scoring. Record the best of the three trials in feet and inches to the nearest inch.

50-yard dash: boys and girls

Equipment. Two stopwatches or one with a split-second timer.

Description. It is preferable to administer this test to two pupils at a time. Have both take positions behind the starting line. The starter will use the commands "Are you ready?" and "Go!" The latter will be accompanied by a downward sweep of the starter's arm to give a visual signal to the timer, who stands at the finish line (Fig. 39).

Rules. The score is the amount of time between the starter's signal and the instant the pupil crosses the finish line.

Scoring. Record in seconds to the nearest tenth of a second.

Softball throw for distance: boys and girls

Equipment. Softball (12-inch), small metal or wooden stakes, and tape measure.

Description. A football field marked in conventional fashion (five-yard intervals) makes an ideal area for this test. If this is not available, it is suggested that lines be drawn parallel to the restraining line, five yards apart. The pupil throws the ball while remaining within two parallel lines, six feet apart (Fig. 40). Mark the point of landing with one of the

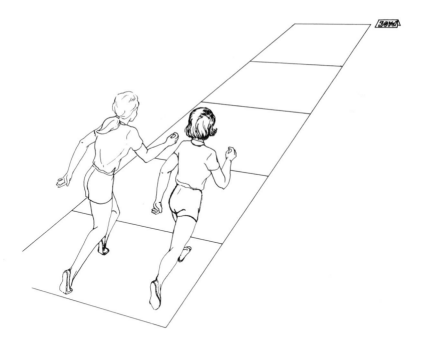

Figure 39. Fifty-yard dash: boys and girls.

small stakes. If his second or third throw is farther, move the stake accordingly so that, after three throws, the stake is at the point of the pupil's best throw. It was found expedient to have the pupil jog out to his stake and stand there; then, after five pupils have completed their throws, the measurements were taken. By having the pupil at his particular stake, there is little danger of recording the wrong score.

Rules

1. Only an overhand throw may be used.
2. Three throws are allowed.

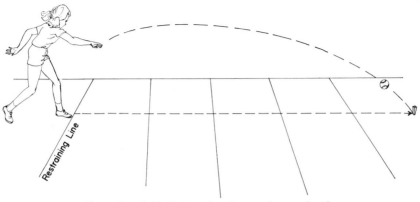

Figure 40:   Softball throw for distance: boys and girls.

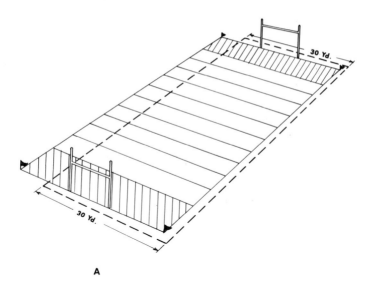

A

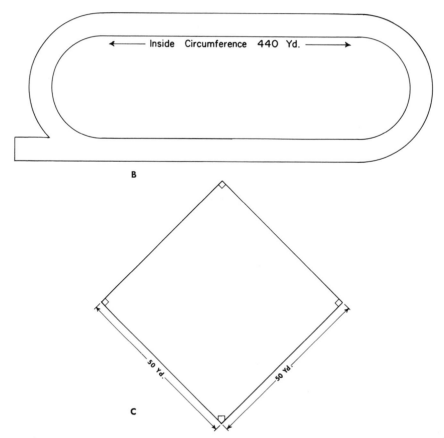

Figure 41. A, Football field for 600-yard run-walk. B, Inside track for 600-yard run-walk. C, Open area for 600-yard run-walk.

3. The distance recorded is the distance measured at right angles from the point of landing to the restraining line.

Scoring. Record the best of the three trials to the nearest foot.

600-yard run-walk: boys and girls

Equipment. Track or area marked according to Figures 41 *A, B,* and *C,* and stopwatch.

Description. Pupil uses a standing start. At the signal "Ready? Go!" the pupil starts running the 600-yard distance. The running may be interspersed with walking. It is possible to have a dozen pupils run at one time by having the pupils pair off before the start of the event. Then each pupil listens for and remembers his partner's time as the latter crosses the finish. The timer merely calls out the times as the pupils cross the finish.

Rules. Walking is permitted, but the object is to cover the distance in the shortest possible time.

Scoring. Record in minutes and seconds.

The Physical Performance Test for California (Revised)

During the school year 1969 to 1970, the Physical Performance Test for California was re-evaluated and new norms were established.[13] The events include standing long jump, bent-knee sit-up for time, side step, chair push-up, pull-up and jog-walk.

Administration of test items. It is recommended that the test be administered fall and spring to boys and girls, grades five through twelve. In schools in which classes meet only twenty minutes it is suggested that only one test event be administered per day; in class periods of thirty-five to forty minutes duration, two test events may be given.

Standing long jump (p. 116). Both feet must be on the take-off board when beginning the jump. Best of three trials is recorded to the nearest inch from the nearest point of body contact to the take-off line.

Bent-knee sit-ups. Subject supine on floor, heels not more than 12 inches from buttocks; angle of knees less than 90 degrees. Pupil places hands behind back of neck with fingers clasped and elbows squarely on mat. The pupil curls to a sitting position touching elbows to knees (Fig. 42). This completes one sit-up. The number of correctly executed sit-ups performed in a 60-second period shall constitute his score.

Side step (Fig. 43). Three parallel lines (1 inch wide) 5 feet long and 4 feet between each line are marked on the floor. The student begins by standing astride the center line with feet parallel. On command, the pupil slides or sidesteps to the left (crossing feet not permitted) until his left foot touches or crosses the line on the left. He has now scored one point. In the same manner the pupil rapidly sidesteps or slides back toward the right outside line. When the left foot touches area to right of center line, another point is scored. The pupil continues to move to the

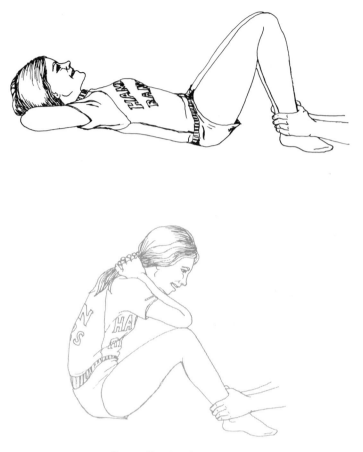

Figure 42. Bent-knee sit-up.

right and when right foot touches the right outside line another point is scored. Thus far the pupil would have a total of three points: one for touching or crossing the left outside line, one for crossing the center line with the left foot, and one for touching or crossing the outside right line with the right foot. The pupil now returns toward the left outside line and repeats this sliding or sidestepping from left line, across center to right line as many times as possible in 10 seconds. (The child's body should face forward, while the head turns toward the direction of movement; when touching an outside line both feet must be on that side of the center line.)

One trial is permitted after the pupil learns the skill. The score is the number of times the pupil crosses the center line with both feet and touches or crosses the outside left and right lines in ten seconds.

Chair push-ups (Fig. 44). Pupil grasps front corners of chair, assuming a front leaning rest position. Legs are together with both feet against the wall. The pupil's assistant holds the chair with both hands while bracing it with one foot. The body must be in a straight line and at right

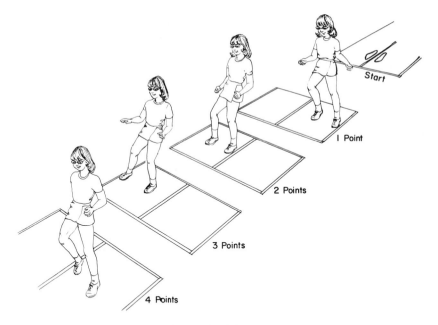

Figure 43. Side step.

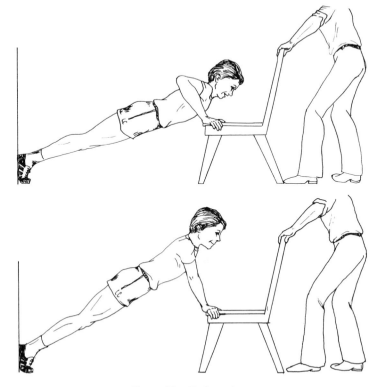

Figure 44. Chair push-up.

angles to the arms. The pupil lowers his body until the chest touches nearest edge of chair seat, which is the starting position. The chest touches at a point even with armpits or above nipple line.

Score is the number of push-ups completed. Those reaching 50 push-ups are stopped. No resting is permitted; the pupil must keep his body straight, touch his chest to edge of chair and push-up to full extension.

Pull-ups.   Bar should allow the pupil to hang at full extension with feet a few inches above ground. Using a forward grip, pupil raises body until chin is above bar and then returns to full extension. This completes one pull-up. Body must not swing during movement (partner may assist to prevent this) and no kicking is permitted. Score is the number of continuously executed pull-ups.

Jog-walk.   Duration is six minutes and score is the number of 110-yard segments the pupil covers in this period of time. The segment in which the individual finds himself at the end of the six minutes is also counted (Fig. 45).

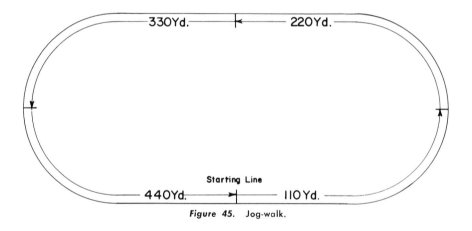

Figure 45.   Jog-walk.

Indiana Motor Fitness Test for High School and College Men

Using a twelve-item standard, involving at least two measures each of strength, velocity, motor ability, and endurance, Bookwalter has constructed a practical test of motor fitness.[2,3,15] The following four indices have been developed and validated for high school and college age men:

Motor Fitness Index I = (Chins + Push-ups) • (Vertical Jump)

Motor Fitness Index II = (Chins + Push-ups) • (Standing Broad Jump)

Motor Fitness Index III = (Straddle Chins + Push-ups) • (Vertical Jump)

Motor Fitness Index IV = (Straddle Chins + Push-ups) • (Standing Broad Jump)

The validities of the above indices with a twelve-item criterion are as follows: Index I, .859; Index II, .818; Index III, .841; and Index IV, .812. As these coefficients of validity are of approximate size, the instructor may select the index most applicable to his program and facilities. Indices I and III are preferable because of their higher validity coefficients.

Administration of test items (Fig. 46). *Chins.* The chins should be performed with either a palms-forward grip or palms-backward grip.

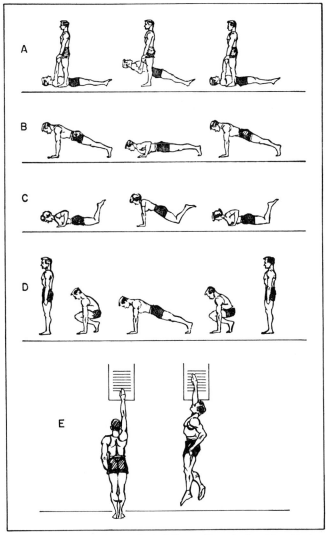

Figure 46. Test items for Indiana Physical Fitness Test. *A,* Straddle chinning. *B,* Push-ups (for boys). *C,* Push-ups (for girls). *D,* Squat thrusts (Burpee Test). *E,* Vertical jump (jump and reach). (Adapted from drawings by Henry Lohse, Department of Physical Education, Public Schools, Indianapolis, Indiana.)

Although the test directions allow the pupil to select any grip, the palms-backward method results on the average in two to two and one-half more chins. Whichever grip is selected, it should be consistent for all pupils.

When possible, the use of adjustable rings attached to the chinning bar may prove advantageous. Rings permit the wrists to rotate naturally in the execution of the chin, and they may be adjusted for convenience when measuring elementary and junior and senior high school pupils. Swinging or kicking is not permitted; the tester may and should steady the legs of the chinner. Half credits are not permitted, and the exercise should be continuous. It is prudent to place a mat beneath the rings or chinning bar.

Straddle chinning (Fig. 46, *A*). The class members should first be paired according to size and then counted off in groups of two. The number ones lie on their backs, arms sideward, with shoulders level on the floor. Upper arms are bent to vertical. Number twos stand astride and facing number ones, with feet outside and touching elbows of number ones. Partners clasp hands, bent-finger hold, and number ones chin upward as often as possible. The chest should meet firm resistance with partner's thighs each time. Both partners should keep legs and back straight. Arms of supporting partner are straight throughout. Partners may change places and repeat as before.

Push-ups (Fig. 46, *B, C*). These are executed from the floor. The chest must touch the floor each time and arms must be fully extended on the return. The back must be kept straight. No partial credit is allowed, and the exercise must be done continuously.

Vertical jump (Fig. 46, *E*). In the jump and reach test a blackened 1/4-inch plywood board, 5 feet long and 1 foot wide, may be used. The board is marked off in half inches and should be mounted on a basketball backstop, or if mounted on a wall it should be at least 6 inches out from the wall so that the subject will not scrape himself while executing the jump. The jumper toes a line, one foot in front of the board. The index fingers of both hands are chalked with magnesium. The subject reaches as high as possible with heels kept on the floor and makes a mark on the board with his chalked fingers. He next executes three jumps from a crouched position, making a mark each time on the board. The distance from the top of the reach mark to the top of the highest jump mark is recorded as his score. Measurement is taken to the nearest quarter inch. An assistant should stand on a table alongside the board so that the readings may be taken at eye level, insuring a greater degree of accuracy. The examiner should have a damp cloth to erase the chalk marks after each reading has been recorded.

Standing broad jump. The contestant toes a line 4 feet from the pit, or first 6-inch mark on a mat, and springs forward from both feet. The nearest point touched by any part of the body, at right angles to the take-off line, is his jump. Measurements are taken to the nearest inch.

If a mat is used, lines may be marked in 6-inch intervals and the nearest inches estimated. When performing this event in the gym, it is better if the subject jumps from the floor onto a well-secured mat.

Scoring the Indiana Motor Fitness Index. Table 18 contains norms established for 705 Indiana University men in a physical fitness program. The group was composed of both beginning and advanced students in about equal proportions, and should be fairly representative. The method for constructing these norms is simple and may be effectively used on data collected in your own school situation. Chapter 3 illustrates the method for constructing norms based upon a Sigma scale, which was applied in developing the Indiana norms.

As an illustration of the use of these norms, say a pupil scored six chins, eighteen push-ups, and jumped vertically 18.5 inches:

	RAW SCORE	SCALE SCORE (TABLE 18)
Chins	6	44
Push-ups	18	55
Vertical jump	18.50	37

Inserting the above data into Index I, which equals (chins + push-ups) times (vertical jump):

$$\text{Index I} = (44 + 55)\ (37) = 3663$$

This is divided by 100 (move decimal point two places to left), which equals 36.63 or 37, the Motor Fitness Index.

Norms for use in marking or classifying may be established from the Motor Fitness Index by computing the mean and standard deviation of the indices obtained from the local school population. As an example, say that 500 youngsters were tested. The first step would be to compute means and standard deviations for the three items: chins, push-ups, and vertical jumps. The raw scores would then be converted into scaled scores and the indices on the 500 pupils computed. The next step would be to determine the mean and standard deviation for all of the index scores. On the basis of these two statistics, mean and standard deviation, the norm could be constructed according to standard deviation units removed from the mean. If the mean for the index was computed to be 50 and the standard deviation 15, the divisions for classification into A, B, C, D, and F groups could be made. Figure 9 (p. 69) illustrates this procedure, in which the base line of the normal curve has been divided into the five classifications. That is, by dividing five (number of classifications) into six standard deviations, the distance along the base line to be allotted to each classification is determined. Thus, as seen in Figure 9, Group A covers the upper 1.2 σ; Group B the next 1.2 σ; Group C lies .6 σ to the right and left of the mean, while Groups D and E occupy the same relative

TABLE 18. *Scale Scores for Indiana Motor Fitness Index Items*

Scale score	Chins	Straddle chins	Push-ups	Vertical jump	Standing broad jump	Scale score
100	17	35	36	29.75	110	100
99				29.50		99
98				29.25		98
97		34	35	29.00	109	97
96	16				108	96
95			34	28.75		95
94		33		28.50	107	94
93						93
92		32	33	28.25	106	92
91	15			28.00		91
90			32		105	90
89		31		27.75		89
88				27.50	104	88
87			31	27.25		87
86	14	30				86
85			30	27.00	103	85
84				26.75		84
83		29			102	83
82			29	26.50		82
81	13	28		26.25	101	81
80			28			80
79				26.00	100	79
78		27		25.75		78
77			27	25.50	99	77
76						76
75	12	26	26	25.25	98	75
74				25.00		74
73		25			97	73
72			25	24.75		72
71				24.50	96	71
70	11	24	24	24.25		70
69					95	69
68				24.00		68
67		23	23	23.75	94	67
66						66
65	10	22	22	23.50	93	65
64				23.25		64
63					92	63
62		21	21	23.00		62
61				22.75	91	61
60	9		20	22.50		60
59		20			90	59
58				22.25		58
57		19	19	22.00	89	57
56						56
55			18	21.75	88	55
54	8	18		21.50		54
53					87	53
52			17	21.25		52
51		17		21.00	86	51
50			16	20.75		50
49	7	16			85	49
48				20.50		48
47			15	20.25	84	47
46		15				46
45			14	20.00	83	45
44	6			19.75		44
43		14		19.50	82	43
42			13			42
41		13		19.25	81	41
40			12	19.00		40
39	5				80	39
38		12		18.75		38
37			11	18.50	79	37
36						36
35		11	10	18.25	78	35
34	4			18.00		34
33		10		17.75	77	33
32			9			32
31				17.50	76	31
30		9	8	17.25		30
29						29
28	3			17.00	75	28
27		8	7	16.75		27
26				16.50	74	26
25		7	6			25
24				16.25	73	24
23	2			16.00		23
22		6	5		72	22
21				15.75		21
20			4	15.50	71	20
19		5				19
18	1			15.25	70	18
17		4	3	15.00		17
16				14.75	69	16
15			2			15
14		3		14.50	68	14
13				14.25		13
12			1		67	12

Table 18. (Continued)

11		2		14.00		11
10		1		13.75	66	10
9				13.50		9
8					65	8
7				13.25		7
6				13.00	64	6
5						5
4				12.75	63	4
3				12.50		3
2					62	2
1				12.25		1

Courtesy of Bookwalter, K. W.: Further Studies of Indiana Motor Fitness Index. Bulletin of the School of Education, Bureau of Cooperative Research and Field Service, Indiana University, Vol. 19, No. 5, September, 1943.

positions in the lower half of the curve as occupied by B and A in the upper half.

The computed values, where the mean equals 50 and the standard deviation equals 15, would be as follows:

LETTER MARKS AND EQUIVALENT SCORES

$$78 - \uparrow \; A$$
$$60 - 77 \; B$$
$$41 - 59 \; C$$
$$23 - 40 \; D$$
$$\downarrow \; - 22 \; E$$

The scores for the "C" range were computed by simply multiplying 0.6 by the standard deviation, 15, then adding and subtracting this product to the mean. The top of the "B" range was determined by multiplying 1.8 by 15 and adding it to the mean. The bottom of the "D" classification was obtained by subtracting the product of 1.8 times 15 from the mean. Obviously, all scores above the top of the "B" range and below "D" would be classified as "A" and "E" respectively.

On the basis of this classification system, the index score of 37, as computed in the example problem, would result in a "D" mark.

In addition to the method of scoring shown here, tables have been prepared which permit one to score any of the four indices by taking into account differences in body size. The tables and method of computing the scores appear in references 2, 3, and 15.

This test was constructed to measure the components of motor fitness, with particular consideration as to administrative feasibility.[15, 16] The validity of the test was established by correlating it against a criterion of twelve motor fitness items ($r = .767$). Figure 47 is the score card, containing the test items, developed by Bookwalter for use with this particular fitness test. The code for physical classification of girls as shown on the score card is as follows:

SS — Short slender	MS — Medium slender	TS — Tall slender
SM — Short medium	MM — Medium medium	TM — Tall medium
SH — Short heavy	MH — Medium heavy	TH — Tall heavy

INDIANA PHYSICAL FITNESS TEST FOR HIGH SCHOOL BOYS AND GIRLS

INDIANA PHYSICAL FITNESS TEST
PUPIL SCORE CARD

Name. MARY JONES ... Male...... Female. ✓... Grade. 10 ....

School............... City................ County................

Class (sect) .... Hour.............. Days per week..........

Encircle the classification group in which this individual falls.

Boys	Up to	675–	710–	745–	780–	815–	850–	885–	920 and
	674	709	744	779	814	849	884	919	up
Girls	SS	SM	(SH)	MS	MM	MH	TS	TM	TH

Item No.	Event	Grade 10			Grade 11			Grade 12		
		Test Period (Date each period when testing)								
		1	2	3	1	2	3	1	2	3
1. Age to last ½ year		14								
2. Height (last full inch)		4–10								
3. Weight in pounds		112								
4. Classification index										
5. Straddle chins		10								
6. Squat thrust (20")		7								
7. Push-ups (floor)		14								
8. Sum of scores on items 5, 6, 7		31								
9. Vertical jump to last ½ inch		14								
10. Ind. phy. fit. score (item 8 times item 9)		434								
11. Per cent of change (optional)										

Figure 47. Pupil score card for secondary grades, Indiana physical fitness test. (State of Indiana: Physical Fitness Manual for High School Girls. Bulletin No. 137 (Revised), Department of Public Instruction, Indiana, 1944.)

The instructions for obtaining the Indiana physical fitness score, using the data appearing on the sample card along with the necessary scoring tables, may be found in references 15 and 16.

Elementary School Motor Fitness Test

Franklin and Lehsten adapted the Indiana test for use in the elementary school program, for boys and girls in grades four through eight.[5] The

TABLE 19. *Indiana Physical Fitness State Norms for Elementary School Boys (Grades 4–8)*

	Scale Score	Up to 609	610-644	645-679	680-714	715-749	750 and over	Scale Score	
	100	109	124	124	140	145	159	100	
	99	108	122	122	138	144	158	99	
	98	106	121	121	136	142	156	98	
	97	105	119	119	135	140	154	97	
E	96	104	118	118	133	139	152	96	
X	95	102	116	116	132	137	151	95	
C	94	101	115	115	130	135	149	94	
E	93	100	113	113	128	134	147	93	
L	92	99	111	112	127	132	145	92	
L	91	97	110	111	125	130	144	91	
E	90	96	108	109	123	129	142	90	
N	89	95	107	108	122	127	140	89	
T	88	93	105	106	120	125	138	88	
	87	92	104	105	118	124	136	87	
	86	91	102	103	117	122	135	86	
	85	90	101	102	115	120	133	85	
	84	88	99	100	113	119	131	84	
	83	87	98	99	112	117	129	83	
	82	86	96	97	110	115	128	82	
	81	85	95	96	108	114	126	81	
	80	83	93	94	107	112	124	80	
	79	82	92	93	105	110	122	79	
	78	81	90	92	103	109	121	78	
G	77	79	89	90	102	107	119	77	
O	76	78	87	89	100	105	117	76	
O	75	77	86	87	99	104	115	75	
D	74	76	84	86	97	102	114	74	
	73	74	83	84	95	100	112	73	
	72	73	81	83	94	99	110	72	
	71	72	80	81	92	97	108	71	
	70	70	78	80	90	95	107	70	
	69	69	77	78	89	94	105	69	
	68	68	75	77	87	92	103	68	
	67	67	74	76	85	90	101	67	G
	66	65	72	74	84	89	100	66	O
	65	64	71	73	82	87	98	65	O
	64	63	69	71	80	85	96	64	D
	63	61	68	70	79	84	94	63	
	62	60	66	68	77	82	92	62	
	61	59	65	67	75	80	91	61	
	60	58	63	65	74	79	89	60	
	59	56	62	64	72	77	87	59	
	58	55	60	62	70	75	85	58	
	57	54	59	61	69	74	84	57	F
	56	53	57	59	67	72	82	56	A
	55	51	56	58	66	70	80	55	I
	54	50	54	57	64	69	78	54	R
	53	49	53	55	62	67	77	53	
	52	47	51	54	61	65	75	52	
	51	46	50	52	59	64	73	51	

TABLE 19. *(Continued)*

Scale Score	Up to 609	610-644	645-679	680-714	715-749	750 and over	Scale Score	
50	45	48	51	57	62	71	50	
49	44	47	49	56	60	70	49	
48	42	45	48	54	59	68	48	
47	41	44	46	52	57	66	47	F
46	40	42	45	51	55	64	46	A
45	38	41	43	49	54	63	45	I
44	37	39	42	47	52	61	44	R
43	36	38	40	46	50	59	43	
42	35	36	39	44	49	57	42	
41	33	34	38	42	45	54	41	
40	32	33	36	41	44	52	40	
39	31	31	35	39	42	50	39	
38	29	30	33	37	40	48	38	
37	28	28	32	36	39	47	37	
36	27	27	30	34	37	45	36	
35	26	25	29	33	35	43	35	
34	24	24	27	31	34	41	34	
33	23	22	26	29	32	40	33	P
32	22	21	24	28	30	38	32	O
31	21	19	23	26	29	36	31	O
30	19	18	21	24	27	34	30	R
29	18	16	20	23	25	33	29	
28	17	15	19	21	24	31	28	
27	15	13	17	19	22	29	27	
26	14	12	16	18	20	27	26	
25	13	10	14	16	19	26	25	
24	12	9	13	14	17	24	24	
23	10	7	11	13	15	22	23	
22	9	6	10	11	14	20	22	
21	8	4	8	9	12	19	21	
20	6	3	7	8	10	17	20	
19	5	1	5	6	9	15	19	
18	4		4	4	7	13	18	I
17	3		3	3	5	12	17	N
16	1		1	1	3	10	16	F
15					2	8	15	E
14					1	6	14	R
13						4	13	I
12						3	12	O
11						1	11	R
10							10	
9							9	
8							8	
7							7	
6							6	
5							5	
4							4	
3							3	
2							2	
1							1	

Courtesy of Franklin, C. C., and Lehsten, N. G.: Indiana Physical Fitness Tests for the Elementary Level (Grades 4-8). The Physical Educator, 5:38–45, May 1948.

TABLE 20. *Indiana Physical Fitness State Norms for Elementary School Girls (Grades 4-8)*

CLASSIFICATION INDEX GROUPINGS

	Scale Score	Up to 609	610-644	645-679	680-714	715-749	750 and over	Scale Score
	100	110	121	146	154	129	105	100
	99	109	119	144	152	128	104	99
	98	107	118	142	150	126	103	98
	97	106	116	141	148	124	102	97
	96	104	115	139	146	123	100	96
E	95	103	114	137	144	121	99	95
X	94	101	112	136	142	120	98	94
C	93	100	111	134	140	118	97	93
E	92	98	109	132	138	116	96	92
L	91	97	108	131	136	115	94	91
L	90	96	106	129	134	113	93	90
E	89	94	105	127	132	112	92	89
N	88	93	103	126	130	110	91	88
T	87	91	102	124	128	109	89	87
	86	90	101	122	126	107	88	86
	85	88	99	121	124	105	87	85
	84	87	98	119	122	104	85	84
	83	86	96	117	120	102	84	83
	82	84	95	116	118	101	83	82
	81	83	93	114	116	99	82	81
	80	81	92	112	114	98	81	80
	79	80	91	111	112	96	80	79
	78	79	89	109	110	94	78	78
	77	77	88	107	108	93	77	77
	76	76	86	106	105	91	76	76
	75	74	85	104	103	90	75	75
	74	73	83	102	101	88	73	74
	73	71	82	101	99	86	72	73
G	72	70	81	99	97	85	71	72
O	71	69	79	97	95	83	70	71
O	70	67	78	96	93	82	68	70
D	69	66	76	94	91	80	67	69
	68	64	75	92	89	79	66	68
	67	63	73	91	87	77	65	67
	66	61	72	89	85	75	64	66
	65	60	71	87	83	74	62	65
	64	59	69	86	81	72	61	64
	63	57	68	84	79	71	60	63
	62	56	66	82	77	69	59	62
	61	54	65	81	75	68	57	61
	60	53	63	79	73	66	56	60
	59	52	62	77	71	64	55	59
	58	50	61	76	69	63	54	58
	57	49	59	74	67	61	53	57
	56	47	58	72	65	60	51	56
	55	46	56	71	63	58	50	55
	54	44	55	69	61	56	49	54
	53	43	53	67	59	55	48	53
F	52	42	52	66	57	53	46	52
A	51	40	51	64	55	52	45	51
I	50	39	49	63	53	50	44	50
R	49	37	48	61	51	49	43	49
	48	36	46	59	49	47	41	48
	47	35	45	58	47	45	40	47
	46	33	43	56	45	44	39	46
	45	32	42	54	43	42	38	45
	44	30	41	53	41	41	37	44
	43	29	39	51	38	39	35	43
	42	27	38	49	36	37	34	42
	41	26	36	48	34	36	33	41
	40	25	35	46	32	34	32	40
	39	23	33	44	30	33	30	39
	38	22	32	43	28	31	29	38
P	37	20	31	41	26	30	28	37
O	36	19	29	39	24	28	27	36
O	35	17	28	38	22	26	25	35
R	34	16	26	36	20	25	24	34
	33	15	25	34	18	23	23	33
	32	13	23	33	16	22	22	32
	31	12	22	31	14	20	21	31

administration of the test is the same for both boys and girls, the only difference being in the scoring. Table 19 for boys and Table 20 for girls have been constructed for this purpose. To score the test, it is first necessary to determine the classification index for each pupil, boys and girls

TABLE 20.   *(Continued)*

CLASSIFICATION INDEX GROUPINGS

Scale Score	Up to 609	610-644	645-679	680-714	715-749	750 and over	Scale Score
30	10	21	29	12	19	19	30
29	9	19	28	10	17	18	29
28	8	18	26	8	15	17	28
27	6	16	24	6	14	16	27 P
26	5	15	23	4	12	14	26 O
25	3	13	21	2	11	13	25 O
24	2	12	19	1	9	12	24 R
23		11	18		7	11	23
22		9	16		6	9	22
21		8	14		4	8	21
20		6	13		3	7	20
19		5	11		1	6	19
18		3	9			5	18
17		2	8			3	17
16		1	6			2	16
15			4			1	15
14			3				14 I
13			1				13 N
12							12 F
11							11 E
10							10 R
9							9 I
8							8 O
7							7 R
6							6
5							5
4							4
3							3
2							2
1							1

Courtesy of Franklin, C. C., and Lehsten, N. G.: Indiana Physical Fitness Tests for the Elementary Level (Grades 4–8). The Physical Educator 5:38–45, May, 1948.

alike; this may be obtained from Table 21. Then the scaled scores from either of the above tables, depending of course on whether the subject is a boy or girl, may be ascertained. For example, the following scores have been obtained from a high school boy:

Age	13 yrs.	Push-ups	12
Height	65 in.	Squat thrust (20 sec.)	14
Weight	100 lbs.	Straddle chins	10
		Vertical jump	16 in.

1. The sum of the straddle chins, squat thrusts, and push-ups is 36.

2. Multiplying this total (36) by the vertical jump (16 in.) gives 576. This is then divided by 10, giving 57.6.

3. Referring to Table 21, the classification index is found to be 750.

4. Entering Table 16 under the column 750 and over, in which the classification index of 750 falls, the obtained score of 57.6 is found to be in the FAIR category.

TABLE 21. *A Table for Computing Classification Index I for Boys and Girls**

Age in Years and Half Years

Height in inches	9	9.5	10	10.5	11	11.5	12	12.5	13	13.5	14	14.5	15	15.5	16	16.5	17
48	468	478	488	498	508	518	528	538	548	558	568	578	588	598	608	618	628
49	474	484	494	504	514	524	534	544	554	564	574	584	594	604	614	624	634
50	480	490	500	510	520	530	540	550	560	570	580	590	600	610	620	630	640
51	486	496	506	516	526	536	546	556	566	576	586	596	606	616	626	636	646
52	492	502	512	522	532	542	552	562	572	582	592	602	612	622	632	642	652
53	498	508	518	528	538	548	558	568	578	588	598	608	618	628	638	648	658
54	504	514	524	534	544	554	564	574	584	594	604	614	624	634	644	654	664
55	510	520	530	540	550	560	570	580	590	600	610	620	630	640	650	660	670
56	516	526	536	546	556	566	576	586	596	606	616	626	636	646	656	666	676
57	522	532	542	552	562	572	582	592	602	612	622	632	642	652	662	672	682
58	528	538	548	558	568	578	588	598	608	618	628	638	648	658	668	678	688
59	534	544	554	564	574	584	594	604	614	624	634	644	654	664	674	684	694
60	540	550	560	570	580	590	600	610	620	630	640	650	660	670	680	690	700
61	546	556	566	576	586	596	606	616	626	636	646	656	666	676	686	696	706
62	552	562	572	582	592	602	612	622	632	642	652	662	672	682	692	702	712
63	558	568	578	588	598	608	618	628	638	648	658	668	678	688	698	708	718
64	564	574	584	594	604	614	624	634	644	654	664	674	684	694	704	714	724
65	570	580	590	600	610	620	630	640	650	660	670	680	690	700	710	720	730
66	576	586	596	606	616	626	636	646	656	666	676	686	696	706	716	726	736
67	582	592	602	612	622	632	642	652	662	672	682	692	702	712	722	732	742
68	588	598	608	618	628	638	648	658	668	678	688	698	708	718	728	738	748
69	594	604	614	624	634	644	654	664	674	684	694	704	714	724	734	744	754
70	600	610	620	630	640	650	660	670	680	690	700	710	720	730	740	750	760
71	606	616	626	636	646	656	666	676	686	696	706	716	726	736	746	756	766
72	612	622	632	642	652	662	672	682	692	702	712	722	732	742	752	762	772
73	618	628	638	648	658	668	678	688	698	708	718	728	738	748	758	768	778
74	624	634	644	654	664	674	684	694	704	714	724	734	744	754	764	774	784
75	630	640	650	660	670	680	690	700	710	720	730	740	750	760	770	780	790
76	636	646	656	666	676	686	696	706	716	727	736	746	756	766	776	786	796
77	642	652	662	672	682	692	702	712	722	732	742	752	762	772	782	792	802
78	648	658	668	678	688	698	708	718	728	738	748	758	768	778	788	798	808

To use this table to compute Classification Index I, find the number *below* the age reckoned to the last half year, and to the *right* of the height taken at the last full inch, and add this to the weight, e.g., if the individual is 16 years and four months old, 66.7 inches tall and weighs 121 pounds, the result will be 716 + 121 = 837, which is his Classification Index I. All ages of 17 or more are calculated as for 17 years.

*Adapted from McCloy, C. H.: The Measurement of Athletic Power. A. S. Barnes & Co., New York, 1939, p. 119.

Youth Physical Fitness Test

"The strength of our democracy is no greater than the collective well-being of our people. The vigor of our country is no stronger than the vitality and will of all our countrymen. The level of physical, mental, moral and spiritual fitness of every American citizen must be our constant concern.

"It is of great importance, then, that we take immediate steps to ensure that every American child be given the opportunity to make and keep himself physically fit—fit to learn, fit to understand, to grow in grace and stature, to fully live."

These were the words of John F. Kennedy, President of the United States, in an address to schools on the physical fitness of American youth. He also strongly urged each school to adopt the three specific recommendations of his Council on Youth Fitness:

1. Identify the physically underdeveloped pupil and work with him to improve his physical capacity.

2. Provide a minimum of fifteen minutes of vigorous activity every day for all pupils.

3. Use valid fitness tests to determine pupils' physical abilities and evaluate their progress.

The following is the screening test suggested by the Council on Youth Fitness; it is designed to measure strength, flexibility, and agility.[20]

1. Pull-ups (arm and shoulder strength).

2. Sit-ups (flexibility and abdominal strength).

3. Squat thrusts (agility).

It is recommended that all pupils be screened at the beginning of the school year, and that those who fail any item be retested every six weeks until they can pass.

Instructions.   Divide the class into pairs. One pupil is scorer for his partner while the other performs the test. After each test, results are recorded by the teacher on the record form (Fig. 48). The equipment needed includes a chinning bar, a stopwatch, and record forms.

Pull-ups: boys (Fig. 34).   Subject grasps bar with palms facing forward, hangs with arms and legs fully extended, feet clear of floor. The partner stands slightly to one side of subject and counts each successful pull-up.

Action

1. Subject pulls body up with arms until chin is placed over bar.

2. Lowers body until elbows are fully extended.

3. Repeats as able up to required number of times.

Rules

1. Pull must not be a snap movement.

2. Knees must not be raised.

3. Kicking the legs is not permitted.

SAMPLE RECORD FORM FOR IDENTIFICATION OF PHYSICALLY UNDERDEVELOPED PUPILS

Teacher _Miss Jones_

Period or Section _4th Grade_

School _Cumberland_

School Year _Fall 1961_

Date of 1st Test _9/25/61_

GIRLS

Name of Pupil	Modified Pull Ups Ages 10-17; 8			Sit Ups Ages 10-17; 10			Squat Thrust Ages 10-17; 3			Remarks*
	1st Test		Retest	1st Test		Retest	1st Test		Retest	
	Pass	Fail	Date Passed	Pass	Fail	Date Passed	Pass	Fail	Date Passed	
Adams, Mary	✓			✓				✓	11/6/61	Overweight
Barry, Alice	✓			✓			✓			

* Enter here any conditions, e.g., obesity, posture, etc., that may affect physical performance.

Figure 48. Record form for Youth Physical Fitness Test. Boy's form is identical, except for norms.

4. The body must not swing. If pupils starts to swing, his partner stops the motion by holding an extended arm across the front of the pupil's thighs.

5. One complete pull-up is counted each time the subject places his chin over the bar.

To pass

Boys, ages 10 to 13: 1 pull-up.

Boys, ages 14 to 15: 2 pull-ups.

Boys, ages 16 to 17: 3 pull-ups.

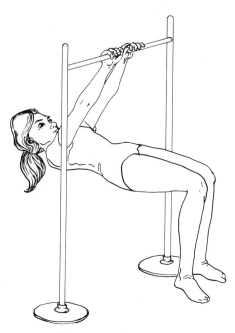

Figure 49. Pull-ups: girls.

Pull-ups: girls (Fig. 49).   Adjust height of bar to subject's chest level. Subject grasps bar with palms facing out, extends legs under the bar, keeping body and knees straight with heels on the floor. Subject fully extends arms so they form an angle of 90 degrees with the body line. The partner braces the subject's heels to prevent slipping.

Action

1. Subject pulls body up with the arms until chest touches the bar.
2. Lowers body until elbows are fully extended.
3. Repeats the exercise as able up to the required number of times.

Rules

1. The body must be kept straight.
2. The chest must touch the bar; the arms must be fully extended.
3. No resting is permitted.
4. One pull-up is counted each time the chest touches the bar.

To pass

Ages 10 to 17: eight modified pull-ups.

Sit-ups: boys and girls (Fig. 50).   Subject assumes a supine position, legs extended and feet about twelve inches apart. Subject's hands with fingers interlaced are grasped behind the neck. A partner holds the ankles of the subject to keep his heels in contact with the floor, and counts each successful sit-up.

Action

1. Subject sits up and turns trunk to left; touches right elbow to left knee.

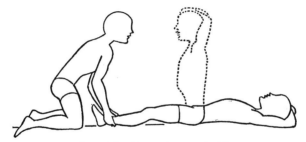

Figure 50. Sit-ups: boys and girls.

2. Returns to starting position.
3. Sits up and turns trunk to right; touches left elbow to right knee.
4. Returns to starting position.
5. Repeats as able up to required number of times.
6. One complete sit-up is counted each time the pupil returns to starting position.

To pass

Boys, ages 10 to 17: 14 sit-ups.

Girls, ages 10 to 17: 10 sit-ups.

Squat thrust: boys and girls (see Fig. 46, *D*).   Pupil stands at attention for the starting position of the squat thrust or Burpee test.

Action

1. Subject bends knees and places hands on the floor in front of feet. Arms may be between, outside, or in front of the bent knees.
2. Thrusts legs back far enough so that the body is perfectly straight from shoulders to feet (the push-up position).
3. Returns to squat position.
4. Returns to erect position.

Scoring.   The teacher instructs the subject on the correct procedure for squat thrusts, telling him to do as many correct squat thrusts as possible within a 10-second time limit. The teacher gives the starting signal, "Ready!—Go!" On "Go" the pupil begins; his partner counts each squat thrust. At the end of 10 seconds, the teacher says, "Stop."

Rules.   The pupil must return to the position of attention at the completion of each squat thrust.

To pass

Girls, ages 10 to 17: 3 squat thrusts in 10 seconds.

Boys, ages 10 to 17: 4 squat thrusts in 10 seconds.

The Youth Fitness Test is a minimal test of motor fitness; it is easy to administer, as it requires very little time or equipment. There is no evidence of reliability or validity presented for it. One might question the origin of the very minimal standards set for the test items, as, for example, the requirement that boys 10 to 13 years of age need complete only one pull-up to pass. The record forms, however, are good and can be adapted to most motor fitness tests. There also is an individual screening record, which includes the three test items and room for recording "pass" and "fail." A complete set of norms may be found in the reference cited.

JCR Test

The JCR is a three-item test using the vertical jump, chinning, and a 100-yard shuttle run in which the subject runs a 10-yard course ten times.[11] Bankboards, set at an angle of approximately 40 degrees with the floor, are used to assist the subject in making the 180-degree turn. The test was designed to measure total ability in the performance of fundamental motor skills, including jumping, running, and dodging, which in turn contain such basic elements of power as strength, speed, agility, and endurance.

The reliability of the test items, according to data collected on two groups of 135 men, is as follows:

	Jump	Chin	Run	JCR Score
Group A	.89	.92	.80	.91
Group B	.89	.95	.81	.94

Validity of the test was first determined by obtaining a multiple correlation of .81 with a 25-variable criterion; a second evidence of its validity was the multiple R of .90 obtained between it and a 19-variable criterion of physical fitness, consisting of vertical jump, chins, dodging run, sit-ups (speed), softball throw, 300-yard run, dips, standing broad jump, rope climb, vault, Burpee, total sit-ups, medicine ball put, push-ups, three broad jumps, flexion, extension, a 50-yard dash, and an endurance index. A third study of validity was completed between the JCR and the AAF motor fitness test which resulted in a corrected r of .78. Also an r of .66 was obtained between the JCR and a 17-obstacle, 670-yard obstacle course. On the basis of the validity studies and the high reliability of the items contained in the JCR, this test can contribute much in the way of motor fitness testing in the public school.

Administration of test items. *Vertical jump.* The same technique as described in the Indiana motor fitness test may be used. The best of three jumps is recorded as the score.

Chinning. The same technique employed in the Indiana Motor fitness test may be used. No partial scores are allowed.

Shuttle run (Fig. 51). The subject runs 100 yards over a 10-yard course; he runs 10 yards, makes a 180-degree turn, and returns to the starting line. He makes another 180-degree turn and continues for five complete round trips. Runners start and finish at the same line. They start "inside" the starting line with one foot on or touching the bankboard and are started by the conventional "On your mark, get set, go!" Runners may turn in either direction, but must touch the bankboard in making the turns.

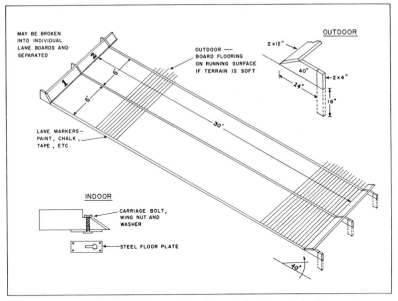

Figure 51. Running area and bankboards for 10-yard shuttle run.

Apparatus (Fig. 51).   Running lanes are approximately 6 feet wide and exactly 10 yards long. Bankboards, which are used to help the subject make the turns, are placed at both ends of the lanes so that their bottom inside edges are flush with the ends of the lanes. They are approximately 12 inches wide and are set at an angle of 40 degrees with the floor. Running is done on a hard and level surface that assures good footing. Practice lengths are permitted before the run for time. The examiner should watch to see that runners stay in their own lanes and are encouraged to go "all out" for the complete distance, that bankboards are used from which to "spring" and not to bounce, and that runners are given a few lengths in practice before running for time.

Scoring for the JCR Test.   Scoring tables for the JCR have been constructed from 3783 officer candidates and officer trainees between the ages of eighteen and forty-five years, and appear in reference 11. In constructing these tables, the raw scores were first changed into standard scores; the standard scores were then added in order to obtain a composite score, which was converted into a final standard score. This method for constructing norms is very practical and may be readily adapted by the physical educator for use in his own particular situation.

Division for Girls' and Women's Sports Tests (DGWS)

The Research Committee of the DGWS states that "one function of the physical education program for girls is to develop muscular control and coordination, speed, agility of movement, and strength to move the body and the implements used in work and play." The Committee further states that it is the responsibility of the teacher to provide the facilities and the necessary motivation, as well as to enable the youngster to measure her progress toward these objectives.

On the basis of past experience, the Research Committee empirically selected test items to measure these objectives.[9] To represent general motor ability, the standing broad jump, basketball throw, and potato race were selected. For purposes of measuring strength of specific muscle groups primarily used in moving the weight of the body, sit-ups for abdominal muscles, and pull-ups and push-ups for measuring arm and shoulder girdle strength were selected. As a measure of agility, the ability of the body to change directions rapidly, the ten-second squat thrust was included. The thirty-second squat thrust was added partially to measure endurance, the ability of the body to continue a strenuous activity for a specified period of time.

These eight test items were administered to 20,021 girls in a number of high schools. Using the data gathered from the twenty-five schools having the highest test results, a set of scales, employing three standard deviations above and below the mean, was constructed. Table 22 contains these scaled scores.

TABLE 22.   *Scoring Table for Physical Performance Levels (1945 Revision)*

Scale Score	Standing Broad Jump	Basketball Throw	Potato Race	Pull-ups	Push-ups	Sit-ups	10-Second Squat Thrust	30-Second Squat Thrust	Scale Score
100	7–9	78	8.4	47	61	65	9–1	24	100
95	7–7	75	8.6	45	58	61	9	23	95
90	7–4	72	8.8	42	54	57	8–3	22	90
85	7–2	68	9.0	39	51	54	8–1	21	85
80	6–11	65	9.4	37	47	50	8	20	80
75	6–9	62	9.6	34	43	46	7–3	19	75
70	6–7	59	10.0	32	39	43	7–1	18–2	70
65	6–4	56	10.2	29	36	39	7	18	65
60	6–2	53	10.4	26	32	36	6–2	17	60
55	6–0	50	10.6	24	28	33	6–1	16	55
50	5–9	46	11.0	21	25	29	6	15	50
45	5–7	43	11.2	18	21	25	5–2	14–2	45
40	5–5	40	11.6	16	17	22	5–1	14	40
35	5–2	37	11.8	13	13	18	4–3	13	35
30	5–0	34	12.0	10	10	15	4–2	12	30
25	4–9	31	12.4	8	6	11	4	11	25
20	4–7	27	12.6	5	2	7	3–3	10	20
15	4–4	24	13.0	3	1	3	3–2	9	15
10	4–2	21	13.2	1	0	1	3	8–2	10
5	4–0	18	13.4	0	0	0	2–3	7–2	5
0	3–9	15	13.6	0	0	0	2–2	7	0

Physical Performance Levels for High School Girls. J. Health & Phys. Educ., June, 1945, p. 309.

In situations where it is not possible to administer the eight-item test battery, the Committee recommends a short battery composed of the five following items:

1. Standing broad jump.
2. Basketball throw.
3. Potato race *or* ten-second squat thrust.
4. Sit-ups.
5. Push-ups or pull-ups.

Administration of test items. *Basketball throw.* Mark parallel lines on the floor at intervals of 5 feet. Number the lines 0, 5, 10, 15, and so on, up to about 80 feet.

The thrower stands one step behind the 0 line. She throws the ball (an official basketball, properly inflated) as far as possible, using any type one- or two-hand throw (preferably a one-hand over-arm, side-arm, or hook to get distance). She may take one step forward as she throws. Both feet must remain behind the starting line until the ball has left her hands.

Two observers are stationed at the approximate distance that the girl has thrown in practice. As the ball strikes the floor, the observers move quickly to the spot where the ball hits. They note in which zone the ball landed and whether it is 1, 2, 3, or 4 feet past the zone line. Two trials are given and the best is recorded.

The score is the length of the distance in feet that the ball traveled in the air.

Potato race. Draw two lines on the floor 30 feet apart. Place two small blocks of wood (approximately $2 \times 2 \times 4$ inches) just beyond the second line.

The runner stands behind the first line. On the signal "Are you ready?" (pause) "Go!" she runs to the second line, picks up one block of wood, runs back to the first line and places (not throws) the block behind the line; she then runs to the second line again, picks up the second block of wood and runs back to the first line, finishing as she crosses the line with the block in her hand. Two trials are given and the best one is recorded. Time will be saved by having girls start alternately from the first and second lines, as this makes it unnecessary to move the blocks between runners.

The score is the time in seconds and fifths of a second from the starting signal until the runner crosses the line on her second round trip.

Sit-ups. The subject begins supine with legs separated 2 to 2½ feet in a V-position and hands behind head, fingertips touching. The subject executes the sit-up by alternately touching her right knee with left elbow and her left knee with right elbow. A partner places her hands on the subject's ankles and holds the heels in contact with the floor. The knees are not permitted to come off the floor and fingertips of both hands must remain in contact. The back may be rounded and the head and elbows brought forward in sitting up and in touching the knee.

The score is the number of sit-ups executed.

Push-ups (Fig. 46, *C*).   The student lies face down on the floor with body straight and legs together. She bends her knees to a right angle and places her hands on the floor at shoulder level. She pushes up to a position in which the arms are straight and the weight is supported entirely on the hands and knees. Her body must be in a straight line from head to knees; she must not bend her hips, or round or hollow her back. Next she bends her arms until her chest touches the floor. Legs or waist should not be permitted to touch. The weight continues to be supported by the arms and knees. The entire exercise is repeated as many times as possible.

Pull-ups (Fig. 49).   Place 3½ feet from the floor a horizontal bar or one arm of parallel bars, or any securely supported rod. The student grasps the bar with both hands, palms upward, bends her arms and moves close to the bar and at the same time she extends her legs under the bar until the body is in a straight line from knees to shoulders. She extends her arms fully, bends her knees to a right angle, and keeps her feet on the floor. Her body should now be in a straight line from shoulders to knees and parallel to the floor. The weight is supported by the hands and feet. From this starting position, she pulls up with her arms until her chest touches the bar. Her body moves from the knees and she must not bend at the hips, or round or hollow the back. She returns to extended-arm position. She repeats as many times as possible.

Squat thrusts (Fig. 46, *D*).   From a standing position the student (1) takes a deep knee bend, placing her hands on the floor in front of her feet in a squat-rest position; (2) jumps and extends her legs backward to a front leaning-rest position, with the body resting on hands and toes; (3) returns to squat-rest position; (4) stands erect, head up. In the front leaning-rest position the back must not sway nor hollow, nor should the hips be raised above the line of the back. Repeat as many times as possible in the time allowed.

The score is the number of complete exercises plus extra quarter movements made in either ten or thirty seconds.

Instructions.   The following are instructions for giving the tests:

1. The tests should be administered only to girls who have been approved for strenuous exercise by the health-examining agency in the school. Girls restricted in activity for any reason (heart, postoperative, hernia, recent illness, structural defects) should not be permitted to take the tests.

2. No girl should be permitted to take the tests during her menstrual period.

3. The tests should be explained, demonstrated, and practiced during at least one class period prior to the testing. During the practice period, form rather than maximum performance should be stressed.

4. It is recommended that not more than two tests be given on any one day, and that, in general, not more than two official tests for record be given in any one week.

Scoring the DGWS test. To illustrate the use of the tables in scoring the DGWS test, let us assume that a girl received the following scores in the five-item test battery:

Test	Raw score	Scaled score
Standing broad jump	5-5	40
Basketball throw	46	50
Ten-second squat thrust	6-1	55
Sit-ups	25	45
Push-ups	32	60
Total		250

$$250 \text{ divided by the number of items or } \frac{250}{5} = 50$$

The index of this particular girl is 50, which is average. We know this to be true, for on our scaled scoring tables the mean is located at 50. To determine the amount of improvement we should expect this particular pupil to make, a specially prepared table that appears in reference 9 may be used.

It is the opinion of the Committee that the scoring tables may be used throughout the entire period of secondary school, for relatively few girls will reach the point at which no further improvement is possible. Furthermore, it was observed that eighth and ninth grade girls improve slightly more than do eleventh and twelfth grade girls. Because of these slight differences the preparation of separate tables for the two groups was avoided.

Interpretation of Scores. The average index score in the high school group should be 50 or more on the basis of the test data gathered. If the girls score exceedingly high in some of the items and low in others, the program should be studied in terms of emphasis. For example, the group may be exceptionally high in endurance items but extremely low in upper arm strength. If this is true, then activities should be introduced that will emphasize shoulder girdle development. Program redirection is much more prudent than having the girls practice the test items for which they received low scores.

At the end of the semester, retesting the group should result in an average over-all improvement of seven-scale points. This was found to be true for twenty-five high schools which were studied. Obviously, one cannot expect each individual to improve by seven-scale points or even score an average of 50 on the test. This is true because individuals differ markedly and fall heir to such limiting factors as obesity, poor coordination, certain structural deviations, and body type. However, an all-out effort on the part of the physical educator should be made to determine the cause or causes of low-scoring individuals. Careful case study procedures should be conducted, as well as personal interviews with the child, to help the girl understand her own limitations and potential. Thus, greater insight into the general physical fitness of the girl will be gained, enabling the physical educator to outline intelligently and scientifically an individualized program to help the pupil.

Army Air Force Physical Fitness Test (AAF Test)

In constructing this test the primary physical factors sampled included only the major organic constituents of fitness. The purpose of the test is to measure the type of fitness underlying aviation skills and wartime physical needs.[7] The following seven components of physical fitness were empirically selected and tested:

1. *Muscular endurance.** The capacity of the individual for long-continued contractions (submaximum) when a sufficient number of muscle groups are used with a sufficient duration and intensity to put a demand on the functions of circulation and respiration.

a. Endurance index: (time for 60-yard × 6)—time for 360-yard run.

2. *Muscular endurance.* The capacity of the individual to continue successive exertions under conditions where a load is placed on the muscle being tested.

a. Chinning.

b. Dipping.

c. Sit-ups.

d. Leg-lifts.

e. Floor push-ups.

3. *Muscular explosiveness or power.* The capacity of the individual to release maximum force in the shortest period of time.

a. Vertical jump.

b. Three standing broad jumps.

c. Shuttle race.

4. *Agility.* The capacity of the individual as measured by the rate of changing his position in space.

a. Agility test (Burpee).

5. *Speed.* The capacity of the individual in the rate of making successive movements of the same kind.

a. The 60-yard dash.

6. *Body coordination.* The capacity of the individual to integrate movements of different kinds (different requirements for each phase of the activity) into one pattern.

a. Cozens' dodge run.

b. Baseball throw for distance and accuracy.

c. Direction change.

---

* Although referred to as muscular endurance, this run is sufficiently demanding to be called cardiorespiratory, i.e., a test of cardiovascular endurance.

7. *Speed and endurance*. The capacity of the individual to sustain a maximum rate of speed over an extended distance.

a. The 360-yard run.

The selected tests were administered to a sample group of AAF personnel. The results were then intercorrelated with each other and with the criterion measure (sum of all test scores). The final statistical analysis resulted in the selection of chinning, sit-ups for two minutes, and a 300-yard shuttle run; the three items correlated .86 with the criterion measure. It was found that the 360-yard run correlated sufficiently high with the 300-yard shuttle run, so that it could be discarded in favor of the latter. In order to select a replacement for the 300-yard shuttle run, which would allow administration of the test indoors, shuttle runs of different lengths and distances were administered to AAF personnel selected at random. On the basis of this experiment, a 250-yard shutttle run of 25-yard shuttle distance was selected. The correlation between the outdoor (300-yard run, 60-yard shuttle) and the indoor tests was .90. Thus, either of the two runs may be permitted in combination with chinning and the two-minute sit-ups.

Administration of the Army Air Force Physical Fitness Test   *Chinning*. Same technique for chinning is employed as described under Indiana motor fitness test (p. 123).

Sit-ups. To start, the subject lies on his back on the floor, knees straight, feet approximately 12 inches apart. The hands are clasped behind the head. An assistant kneels on the floor and holds the soles of the subject's feet against his knees, preventing them from rising from the floor. At the command "go," the subject raises his back from the floor and touches his right elbow to his left knee (knees may bend slightly) and returns to the floor. The second time, the subject rises from the floor and touches his left elbow to his right knee and returns to a lying position. In this way, alternately touching left and right knees with the opposite elbow, the subject performs as many sit-ups as possible in a two-minute period. The examiner should announce the time at twenty-second intervals. The movement must be continuous, although rest periods are permitted within the two-minute period. One point is scored for each complete movement.

No score is permitted if the subject unclasps his hands from the head, keeps knees bent when lying on the back or when beginning the sit-up, or pushes off from the elbow.

The 300-yard shuttle. The lanes should be from 4 to 6 feet wide, marked out on level terrain. A stake 18 inches high is placed in the center of each lane on the beginning line and on the finish line that the subjects must round in performing the shuttle run.

The 250-yard shuttle. When testing in the gymnasium, a 25-yard course is laid out, with lanes 4 feet wide. Turning boards are placed at each end of the course, at an approximate angle of 45 degrees with the floor. A sprint start is used with the subject bracing one foot against the turning board. The runner traverses the 25-yard distance ten times, touching the turning board with one or both feet each time. The score in either of the running events is the number of seconds required to cover the distance. The Army scores the events by having the examiner call out the full seconds that have elapsed, while the performer catches his own time to the nearst second as he crosses the finishing line.

For public school use, it is recommended that the scoring be more precise and be recorded to the nearest tenth of a second. A large number of subjects may be tested in a relatively short period of time with minimum man power, by having subjects score themselves or by having partners score for each other. However, it is better, for more reliable results, to have experienced examiners do the testing and scoring. Competent student leaders may be trained to assist the physical educator in the administration of these tests, so that he need not rely upon the ability of the subjects to score themselves.

Tables containing the scaled scores for determining the PFR (Physical Fitness Rating) have been prepared and appear in the reference cited. The norms were constructed by use of the T-scale, five standard deviations above and below the mean.

The raw scores are converted to the scaled score, totaled, and then the total score is placed on a T-scale. In this way an index, or as it is called in the particular test, the PFR, may be obtained by dividing the total scaled score by three, the number of items.

To compute such classification for use in the school situation, a method similar to that employed in the Indiana motor fitness test may be used.

Navy Standard Physical Fitness Test

In order to determine the fitness status of Navy personnel, a five-item motor fitness test was developed.[12, 17] The validity of the test, as to its ability to reflect the type of fitness required of naval personnel, has not been reported. The items contained in the test battery are as follows: squat thrusts, sit-ups, push-ups, squat jumps, and pull-ups.

Test administration. As with most motor fitness tests, the subjects should have experienced taking the tests before data to be used are recorded. The Navy instructions indicate a five-minute rest period between the test events, as well as a warm-up calisthenic drill prior to the testing program.

Squat thrusts. The subject performs this exercise for one minute. Hips and knees are bent in a squatting position, with hands placed on the floor. It does not matter whether the arms are between, in front of, or outside the knees. The legs are then thrust in an extended position backward so that the body is in a push-up position. The subject returns his legs to a squat position and then stands to complete the event. In executing this four-part exercise the subject must come to a straight standing position with chest up. A slight, total body lean is permissible.

The score for the test is one point for each complete squat thrust. The exercise should be performed as rapidly as possible.

Sit-ups. This exercise is performed in the same manner as listed under the AAF test, with one exception. The sit-ups are performed continuously until exhaustion. One point is scored for each sit-up.

Push-ups. The exercise is begun by the subject in a prone position on the floor. The body is raised by straightening the arms. The body should be raised in a straight line, with no sagging or pumping action permitted. On the return, the subject's chest should touch the floor. The motion must be continuous and the exercise is performed until exhaustion. One point is scored for each complete push-up.

No scores are permitted if: (1) the subject's arms are bent at the top of the movement; (2) the hips sag; (3) a pumping motion in which the shoulders, then the hips, are raised, or vice versa, is noted.

Squat jumps. The subject stands in a comfortable position with heel of left foot even with toes of right foot. The hands are then interlocked with palms down and held on top of the head. From this position the subject drops to right heel and immediately springs with both feet to an upright position, interchanging feet and dropping to the left heel. This exercise is continued until exhaustion occurs.

The subject receives one point for each time he comes to the upright position. No credit is permitted if: (1) the subject fails to go all the way down to his heel; (2) the subject fails to extend his legs completely in the upright position; (3) the subject does not interchange his feet; or (4) the subject removes his hands from his head.

Pull-ups. These are the same as those described on page 85.

Scores. T-scores, constructed from data based upon a number of conditioned naval personnel, appear in references 12 and 17. In making application of this test to school groups, it would be advisable to construct the tables from data gathered upon youngsters to whom the norms are to be applied. Once the scales are computed, a common fitness index may be obtained by dividing the sum of the scores of the five events by five. This would be similar to the scoring system employed in the Indiana motor fitness test, in the AAF, and in the JCR.

Army Physical Efficiency Test

In an attempt to measure the basic elements of strength, endurance, agility, and coordination, the Army devised a ten-item test battery.[4, 19] Esslinger and McCloy validated the test by selecting from a number of tests those items that showed the greatest differences between conditioned and non-conditioned troops. To facilitate administrative economy, the test was finally reduced to the following five items: pull-ups, squat jumps, push-ups, sit-ups, and a 300-yard shuttle run.

In administering the test indoors, a 250-yard shuttle run or the 60-second squat thrust may be substituted for the 300-yard run. The method of administering the various test items has been reported on previous pages, as follows:

Pull-ups: as reported, page 85.

Squat jumps: as reported, page 147.

Push-ups: as reported, page 124.

Sit-ups (two-minute): as reported, page 147.

300-yard run: as reported, page 145; or 250-yard run: as reported, page 145; or squat thrusts: as reported, page 146.

Scoring tables for the Army Tests have been constructed, but as the data are not applicable to the public school situation, they have not been reproduced in this text.

Measurement of Power

Power is a prime requisite for success in athletics. It is defined as the rate of doing work. For example:

$$W = F \times D$$

in which

W = work
F = force
D = distance through which the force moves

If a 2-pound weight were raised a vertical distance of 4 feet, 8 foot-pounds of work would be done:

$$W = F \times D$$
$$F = 2 \text{ lbs.}$$
$$D = 4 \text{ feet}$$
$$W = 2 \times 4 \text{ or 8 foot-lbs. of work}$$

Provided the work were performed in one minute, power output would be 8 foot-lbs./min., as in:

$$P = \frac{W}{T}$$

in which

P = power
W = work
T = time

Time (T) may be expressed either in minutes or seconds and work in either foot-lbs. or kilogram-meters.

Physical Test of a Man.   The Physical Test of a Man was published by Sargent in 1921 as one of the first attempts at measuring this attribute. It was based upon the following equation:

$$\text{Efficiency Index} = \frac{\text{(Weight in pounds) (Height jumped in inches)}}{\text{Stature in inches}}$$

Sargent considered the test as a "a momentary try-out, combining one's strength, speed, energy and dexterity."[14] Weight and stature were later deleted from the equation, as it was felt that the height jumped was independent of both these measures. However, today it is recognized that the weight factor must be included to arrive at a more valid expression of the individual's power output. Presently known as the vertical jump or Sargent Jump, the test is usually administered as described on page 124.

Margaria-Kalamen Power Test.[8]   Margaria suggested an excellent test for power, which has been modified by J. Kalamen.[6] The test is designed for high school and college males, although there is no reason why it could not be adapted to women. The subject stands 6 meters in front of a staircase. When ready, he runs up the stairs as rapidly as possible, taking three at a time. Switchmats are placed on the third and ninth stairs. (An average stair is about 174 mm. high). A clock starts as the person steps on the first switchmat (on the third step) and stops as he steps on the second (ninth step). Time is recorded to a hundredth of a second. The test should be administered several times and the best score recorded. Power output is computed in the following manner:

$$P = \frac{W \times D}{T}$$

in which

P = Power
W = Weight of person
D = Vertical height between first and last test stairs
T = Time for first to last test stairs

A diagram of the test administration appears in Figure 52.

The test is scored as follows:

W = 75 kg.
D = 1.05 meters
T = 0.49 seconds
$$P = \frac{75 \times 1.05}{0.49} = 160.7 \text{ kg-meters per sec.}$$
P = P = 160.7 kg.-meters per sec.

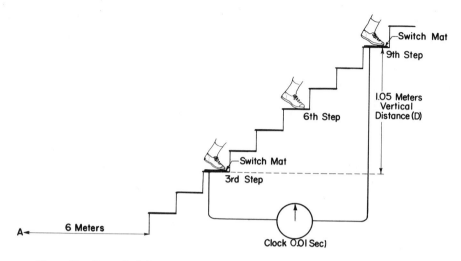

Figure 52. Margaria-Kalamen power test. (From Mathews, Donald K., and Fox, Edward L., The Physiological Basis of Physical Education and Athletics. Philadelphia, W. B. Saunders Company, 1971.)

Kalamen, using 23 non-athlete males in service classes at the Ohio State University, obtained a mean power output of 168.5 kg.-meters per second, with a standard deviation of 31. When evaluating seven sprinters from the Ohio State University track team he obtained a mean power output of 200 kg.-meters per second, with a standard deviation of 16. The greater power output of the trained athlete contributes evidence of the validity of this test.

Chaloupka's adaptation of Margaria Power Test (grades two through six). The youngster stands 6 meters in front of the steps and takes two, rather than three steps at a time. Switchmats are placed on the second and sixth steps. Chaloupka found that the average of the first five trials correlated .94 with the average of the second five. He also found that body weight correlated .797 with power output. Even though the correlation is statistically significant, it is not of sufficient magnitude to be used for predictive purposes ($r^2 = .63$). Consequently elementary children participating in contact sports would be better equated on the basis of power output in place of body weight; the latter method is presently used in the Pop Warner Football program. Table 23 contains data obtained from youngsters in grades two through six.

Oregon Motor Fitness Test.[10] This test was established for realization of the following functions: (1) to determine physical fitness status according to grade level; (2) to identify those below standard so that programs can be introduced to improve fitness; (3) to determine effectiveness of the physical education program in regard to fitness objective; and (4) to motivate youngsters to improve their fitness.

TABLE 23. *Means and Standard Deviations Obtained from the Performance of Elementary School Boys on Chaloupka's Adaptation of the Margaria-Kalamen Power Test**

Grade	Age (yrs.)	Height (cm.)	Weight (kg.)	Power (kg.-m./sec.)
Second		130.19	29.48	29.88
N = 27	7.8 ± .65	± 9.50	± 4.16	± 8.55
Third		134.63	30.75	34.13
N = 21	8.76 ± .55	± 7.07	± 5.81	± 6.59
Fourth		142.74	35.78	47.24
N = 25	9.76 ± .54	± 6.43	± 6.62	± 10.82
Fifth		144.85	38.17	63.25
N = 25	10.76 ± .60	± 5.18	± 7.20	± 10.38
Sixth		146.23	39.87	64.46
N = 38	11.76 ± .55	± 7.94	± 6.75	± 11.86

* O. S. U. Exercise Physiology Research Laboratory. The Ohio State University, Columbus, Ohio.

Test groups and respective batteries are as follows:

Test Group	Test Battery
Boys (grades 4–6)	Standing broad jump, push-ups, sit-ups
Boys (grades 7–12)	Jump and reach, pull-ups, potato race
Girls (grades 4–12)	Hanging in arm-flexed position, standing broad jump, crossed arm curl-ups.

Test items are administered in the following manner:

Standing broad jump.   Mat or floor is marked with parallel lines two inches apart. Student toes take-off line with both feet; crouching and swinging arms to aid in jump he takes off from both feet, jumping as far as possible. He must land on both feet and scoring is the nearest inch from take-off line to line nearest heel position.

Push-ups.   (See p. 124)

Sit-ups.   Student supine, knees straight, feet approximately 12 inches apart and hands clasped behind head; scorer kneels on floor and holds subject's soles against his knees. Subject sits up touching right elbow to left knee (knee may flex slightly) and returns to supine position; he repeats the exercise, alternating by touching left elbow to right knee. Scoring is one point for each complete movement of touching elbow to knee.

Hanging in arm-flexed position.   Pupil stands on support to grasp 1-inch horizontal bar; hands are a shoulder-width apart; elbows are flexed so that chin can be level with bar. Support is removed and the pupil maintains some flexion in arms; legs and thighs should remain extended throughout test. Score is the length of time (in seconds) that a degree of flexion at elbow is maintained.

Crossed arm curl-ups.   Pupil on back, knees bent at about 90° angle; feet flat on floor, arms folded across chest; partner holds feet on the ankles. Scoring is the number of times pupil comes to sitting position.

Jump and reach.   Pupil stands with right side (left if left-handed) against smooth wall. He reaches up and places a mark on the wall with chalk, as high as he can reach. Then, crouching, he jumps as high as possible, making a second mark. Distance measured to the nearest ½ inch between the first and second marks is the score. Three trials are allowed, with the best of three being recorded.

Potato race.   Figure 53 contains a diagram of this agility course. Three circles, one foot in diameter, are placed on the floor, with their centers forming a straight line. Circle 1 is behind and tangent to the

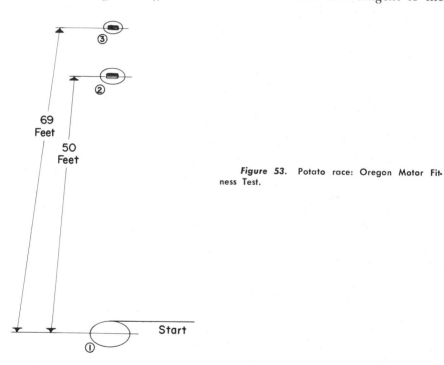

Figure 53.   Potato race: Oregon Motor Fitness Test.

starting line; the centers of circles 2 and 3 are 50 and 69½ feet respectively from starting line. Circles 2 and 3 each contain a wooden block 3 × 2 × 4 inches (two blackboard erasers may be substituted). Assuming a standing start position with one foot on starting line, at command "Go!" student runs to circle 2, picks up the block and brings it to circle 1. He then runs to circle 3 and brings that block to circle 1. He then picks up the first block from circle 1 and returns it to circle 2, picks up the second block from circle 1 and returns it to circle 3, returning to starting line as rapidly as possible. Pupil must place the blocks in the circles, not toss or drop them. Score is the elapsed time in seconds.

Norms for this test based upon the T-scale appear in Appendix F.

Boys Fitness Test (President's Council on Youth Fitness). Recent studies[19] have shown that the average high school pupil spends fifteen to thirty hours a week watching television and only two hours participating in physical activity. Consequently, one-third of 200,000 pupils tested on the President's Council on Physical Fitness failed a simple test of strength, stamina, and flexibility. Table 24 contains standards representing top level physical fitness for boys twelve through eighteen years of age.

Kirchner's Motor Fitness Test. This test was designed for use with boys and girls ages six to twelve. It contains the following five items: standing broad jump, bench push-ups, curl-ups, squat jumps and 30-yard dash.

Standing broad jump (p. 151). One practice jump is allowed. The jump is repeated if the pupil steps with one foot and then jumps, touches floor with hands before landing, or falls backward after landing.

Bench push-ups (Fig. 44). Seat of chair should be 14 to 17 inches above mat. Pupil grasps near corners using a front leaning rest position. Body in straight line, feet together, arms at right angles to body, youngster lowers himself so chest touches nearer edge of chair. Score is the number of push-ups performed up to 50, at which point the child is stopped.

Curl-ups (Fig. 54). Child in supine position with knees flexed and hands interlaced behind head. The examiner holds ankles and knees while child executes the curl-up. Each time the pupil touches examiner's arm with his forehead, score one point. Stop the pupil at 50.

Squat jump (Fig. 55). Child assumes a crouched position, hands placed in front, on floor and outside of knees. He jumps approximately 4 inches above mat with arms at sides to maintain balance, and returns to starting position. Count one point for each execution up to 50, at which point the pupil is stopped.

The 30-yard dash. Pupil commences in standing position at starting line. He runs as rapidly as possible upon command "Go!" through finish tape at 30-yard marker. Score is calculated to nearest tenth of a second.

Norms. Employing the T-scale, norms are available for boys and girls six to twelve years. Youngsters are classified as being superior, good,

TABLE 24. *For Boys Who Like a Challenge: Goals to Shoot For*

Age	12	13	14	15	16	17	18
Pull-ups	7	8	10	11	12	13	14
Sit-ups	50	55	60	65	70	75	80
Standing broad jump	6'2"	6'8"	7'2"	7'8"	8'0"	8'4"	8'6"
600-yard run-walk	2:05	2:01	1:50	1:43	1:40	1:36	1:30
Endurance swim	250 yards	440 yards			880 yards		

Vigor: A Complete Exercise Plan for Boys 12 to 18. Prepared by President's Council on Physical Fitness. Superintendent of Documents, U. S. Government Printing Office, Washington, D. C. 20402.

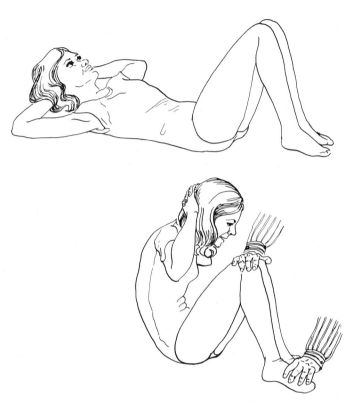

Figure 54. Curl-ups.

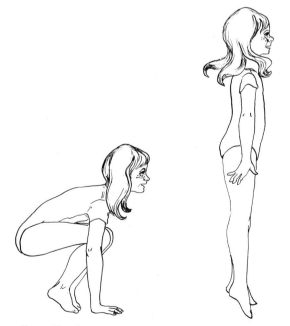

Figure 55. Squat jumps: Kirchner Motor Fitness Test.

average, below average, or poor on each item, as well as on the complete test battery. Data for construction of the norms were obtained from 30,000 children, representing rural and urban populations from six states. Appendix E contains a condensed form of the norms.

Summary and Conclusions

The motor fitness tests and the test items discussed in this chapter are an efficient means for evaluating one aspect of physical fitness in the elementary and junior and senior high schools. The utility of the test items makes their application within the reach of every physical education program.

Because the tests can be performed almost any place and because they are self-administered, the pupils can practice the test items on their own. A number of individual scoring cards can be made up for personal use by the youngster. In this way the pupil may keep track of his own performance record over a period of time.

Norms, scales, or decile tables may be posted on the bulletin board so that pupils may compare their records with the school standing as a whole. The norms may also serve as a means for marking in the area of fitness.

Those pupils with low scores should be studied individually, to determine the cause or causes of low fitness. Then a program based upon these pupils' needs may be constructed to aid in ameliorating their subfit condition.

It should be emphasized that norm tables constructed upon the scores of military personnel do not adequately serve as a basis for scoring school children. One should test a group of fairly well-conditioned pupils and use these data for constructing scales and norms. Although, in a number of the tests reported in this chapter, the authors have used T-scales or Sigma scales as the basis for constructing the norm, it is recommended that the Hull scale (3.5 standard deviations above and below the mean) be used for the public school situation, as discussed in Chapter 3.

Finally, one should remember that motor fitness testing is for purposes of evaluating the organic condition of the child. This is a part, a very important part, of measurement and evaluation. However, to round out the measurement schedule completely, evaluation should also be conducted in the areas of sport skills, body mechanics, knowledge, attitudes, and certain social objectives.

BIBLIOGRAPHY

1. AAHPER Youth Fitness Test Manual. AAHPER — NEA, Fitness Department, 1201 Sixteenth St., N.W., Washington 6, D.C., 1967.
2. Bookwalter, Karl W., and Bookwalter, Carolyn W.: A Measure of Motor Fitness for College. Bulletin of the School of Education, Indiana University, Vol. 19, No. 2, March, 1953.
3. Bookwalter, Karl W.: Test Manual for Indiana University Motor Fitness Indices for High School and College Men. Research Quart., Vol. 14, No. 4, December, 1943.
4. Esslinger, Arthur: Unpublished data. University of Oregon, Eugene, Oregon.
5. Franklin, C. C., and Lehsten, N. G.: Indiana Physical Fitness Tests for the Elementary Level (Grades 4–8). The Physical Educator, Vol. 5, No. 3, May, 1948.
6. Kalamen, J. L.: Measurement of Maximum Muscular Power in Man. Columbus, Ohio, The Ohio State University, Doctoral Dissertation, 1968.
7. Larson, Leonard A.: Some Findings Resulting from the Army Air Forces Physical Training Program. Research Quart., Vol. 17, No. 2, May, 1946.
8. Margaria, R., Aghemo, Piero, and Rovelli, E.: Appl. Physiol., 21:1662-1664, September, 1966.
9. Metheny, Eleanor (Chairman, Committee Report): Physical Performance Levels for High School Girls. J. Health & Phys. Educ., Vol. 16, No. 6, June, 1945.
10. Motor Fitness Tests for Oregon Schools. State Department of Education, Salem, Oregon, 1962.
11. Phillips, B. E.: The JCR Test. Research Quart., Vol. 18, No. 1, March, 1947.
12. Physical Fitness Manual for the U. S. Navy, Chapter IV. Bureau of Naval Personnel, Training Division, Physical Section, 1943.
13. Physical Performance Test for California (Revised). California State Department of Education, Sacramento, 1971.
14. Sargent, Dudley A.: The Physical Test of a Man. Am. Phys. Ed. Rev., 26:188–194, April, 1921.
15. State of Indiana: Physical Fitness Manual for High School Boys. Bulletin No. 136. Department of Public Instruction, Indiana, 1944.
16. State of Indiana: Physical Fitness Manual for High School Girls. Bulletin No. 137. (Revised). Department of Public Instruction, Indiana, 1944.
17. Tunney, J. J.: The Physical Fitness Program of the U. S. Navy. J. Health & Phys. Educ., Vol. 13, No. 10, December, 1942.
18. Vigor: A Complete Exercise Plan for Boys 12–18. Prepared by President's Council on Physical Fitness. Superintendent of Documents, U. S. Government Printing Office, Washington, D. C. 20402.
19. War Department Field Manual, FM 21–20.
20. Youth Physical Fitness Manual. President's Council on Youth Fitness. Superintendent of Documents, U. S. Government Printing Office, Washington, D. C. 20402, July, 1961.

chapter 6

general motor ability

Have you ever seen a deer effortlessly bounding across the fields? A dancer rhythmically executing intricate patterns of movement? Or a skier sailing down a mountain side through fresh, powdered snow, performing beautiful Christiana turns? These are examples of a highly trained body functioning at the epitome of movement. Think for a moment of the numerous and varied factors such as balance, flexibility, power, timing, and coordination, each contributing interdependently to the perfection of the total movement. Almost like the independent notes of a musical masterpiece, these specific factors combine to produce a symphony in movement.

The immediate capacity of an individual to perform in many varied stunts or athletic events is referred to as general motor ability; the term is used synonymously with general athletic ability. Although much work has been done in this area of measurement, it can be seen that a single test that adequately reflects all aspects of motor ability would be difficult to develop.

Motor ability factors.   We know there are many factors that contribute to successful performance in athletic skills. For example, in reviewing some twenty-eight factor analysis studies dealing with motor ability tests, the following factors appeared most frequently; strength, velocity, and muscular coordination. Other important factors identified were motor educability, body size, height, weight, force, endurance, balance, and agility.

Also, in a preliminary study related to the learning of motor skills, McCloy lists some of the most important factors as: muscular strength, dynamic energy, ability to change direction, flexibility, agility, peripheral vision, good vision, concentration, understanding of the mechanics of the techniques of the activities, absence of disturbing or inhibiting emotional complications, timing, rhythm, and coordination.[28]

Memory drum theory of neuromotor reaction.   Recent research has cast doubt on the widely accepted theory that motor ability is completely

157

general. We have let ourselves believe that if one excels in a certain sport, the ability shown there will carry over into other activities. In this connection, we often think, although perhaps erroneously, of the range of skills displayed by the multi-letter winner in high school athletics. Relying on the "obvious," we have permitted ourselves to conclude that motor ability is truly general or nonspecific, when the contrary is more likely true. The multi-letter winner may owe more to his motivation and to his numerous activity experiences than to any carry-over of acquired skills from one sport to another. Also, he may be endowed with numerous specific sports aptitudes, rather than any great amount of general motor ability.

Research by Franklin Henry and his colleagues[11, 14] at the University of California has shown that the simple ability to perform a given neuromotor skill well is no indication that the performer will be equally good in another; that is, motor ability is *specific* to a task rather than *general*. His reasoning led to the theory that neuromotor coordination patterns are stored in the mind on what we might call a memory drum. Whenever a specific movement pattern is needed, the stimulus causes the storage center or memory drum to "play back" the particular learned skill. Hence, the movement is performed automatically. Such learned skills as playing the piano, running, walking, throwing, and eating are all performed without conscious thought; the memory drum simply plays them back on demand.

The entire process might be likened to the functioning of an electronic computer. According to this theory, the program (or recorded movement pattern) has previously been learned and stored on the memory drum (motor memory) ready to be selected and released when needed. Such a program consists of a set of non-conscious instructions that direct the necessary nerve impulses to the appropriate muscles in a coordinated sequence, thus causing the desired movement. The "readout time," or performance time, varies somewhat, depending on the length and complexity of the movement. A program in process of being "read out" cannot be changed before it has been completed, in conformity with the all-or-none law of physiology. The following are among the findings that lend support to this theory:

1. Individual differences in ability to make a fast arm movement are about 70 per cent specific to the particular movement being made. That is to say, a person fast in one movement is not necessarily fast in other movements with the same arm.

2. Reaction time lengthens with increased movement complexity.

3. Very low relationships exist between static strength and speed of movement. This seems to indicate that speed of movement depends more upon the quality of the impression on the memory drum than on the muscular strength of the arm.

4. A fast limb movement, once under way, cannot be changed in its

direction. Nor can it be stopped part way through, unless it was originally programmed to be stopped rather than completed.

5. Motor-oriented programming results in slower movement and greater reaction latency than sensory-oriented programming. For instance, concentrating on the movement to be made (motor orientation) rather than on the starting signal (sensory orientation) tends to result in *slower* reaction time, as conscious control of motor movement interferes with the reading out of the programmed impulses.

6. The component parts of skill are first learned discretely and are gradually combined into a continuous pattern on the memory drum. When a skill deteriorates, as would be the case in aging or long disuse, one notices that the combined pattern breaks up and reverts to the separate movements.

7. Research over a period of many years has shown that the interaction between motor skills is usually quite low.

Application of this knowledge may be made in interpreting motor ability scores. For example, those children scoring high on a motor ability test do so because they have learned certain skills and stored them on their memory drums. Initiation and control of the desired movements is therefore automatic, and results in a good score. One might say that a pupil's abilities, as determined by the motor ability test, are reflections of the extent of the child's previous experience in the elements of the item being tested, rather than of an improvement in his general coordination.

Constructing motor ability tests. To help us to understand motor ability measurement more fully, Larson[23] has made an excellent classification of the general methods employed in constructing tests for this broad area. His first classification consists of studies pertaining to cause, that is, to the fundamental elements underlying the performance of the skill, such as accuracy, speed, endurance, control of voluntary movements, agility, balance, body condition, sensory motor coordination, rhythm, body structure, dodging ability, and strength.

The second group of studies deals with the fundamental skills themselves—one might say the effect, as contrasted with the cause. The primary skills contained in such tests include abilities in running, jumping, vaulting, throwing, kicking, climbing, and catching.

The third area of test construction in general motor ability is associated with specific sport skills, as in gymnastics, basketball, and football.

Use of motor ability tests. It becomes obvious that there are many components involved when one attempts to measure the ability of a pupil to participate in skills. Rather than employ all factors in motor ability evaluation, the instructor must select the single test or test battery that is most valid in representing the type of general motor ability that he is interested in measuring. Such testing is worthwhile, for, knowing the motor ability of the pupils, he may classify groups according to proficiency for participation in physical education classes. It stands to reason that, if the physical education program is made up mostly of skill activities, it is most practical to place pupils of nearly the same general athletic ability together. As we know, this type of classification is referred to as homogeneous grouping, and is important for two major reasons: it permits a more desirable teaching situation from the standpoint of presenting the materials efficiently; and it creates a social atmosphere more conducive to instruction.

Let us consider for a moment the value of placing pupils of like ability in the same group in terms of teaching efficiency. Were you to conduct a single tennis class made up of beginners, intermediates, and advanced players, one lesson plan could not possibly satisfy the situation. For example, you would not spend a great deal of time on the fundamentals with the advanced players, nor would you begin discussing theory and strategy of play with the novice group. Instead, the lesson would be planned with reference to the strengths and weaknesses of the individual pupils in the group. Thus, if you were teaching all advanced pupils, or all beginners, your instructional program would be greatly facilitated by homogeneous grouping.

Unconsciously the physical educator may create an undesirable social atmosphere in the classroom, causing a number of the pupils to dislike the program. For instance, if you were exceptionally good in a sport you would not enjoy playing with a dub, and by the same token the novice would not enjoy participating with you. To be sure, most of us enjoy playing with someone just a little better than ourselves, for then the competition is keen. Actually it is possible for the instructor to create a feeling of distaste for physical education among certain pupils of low motor ability who have inadvertently been placed in a gym class with highly skilled individuals. No one can deny that everyone likes success on occasion, and this can be made possible through equating the competition. As a matter of fact, pupils sometimes effect homogeneous grouping themselves by "choosing sides" before the start of a game.

Youngsters appreciate fairness and enjoy competing with other pupils of similar athletic ability. As proof of this statement, Lockhart and Mott,[25] in surveying physical education classes that had been equated on motor ability, found that 98 per cent of the girls placed in the highly skilled group favored such classification, and that 89 per cent of the girls placed in the less skilled groups were also in favor of such grouping.

Classification types. Classification or grouping may take place in two forms, general and specific. General classification refers to the technique of placing pupils of like athletic ability into groups for purposes of instruction throughout the entire school year. As an illustration, pupils might be measured on a test of general motor ability in the spring of the year and, on the basis of the test results, they could be scheduled in classes of like ability for the coming fall term. This, of course, would be an ideal situation, and to realize it would require considerable salesmanship and planning on the part of the physical education instructor, working with the principal or his class scheduling committee. A physical education director in a large city system obtained such a schedule by convincing the high school faculty of the advantages of double class periods. He first discussed the values of such a plan with the music director, the physics teacher, the chemistry teacher, the home economics instructor, and the manual arts teacher. Each of these instructors saw immediately the advantage of a double class period for his or her course. Since this group constituted a major portion of the faculty, the double class period was voted into effect. The instructor's next move was to have himself placed on the scheduling committee, in which position he succeeded in scheduling his physical education classes into homogeneous groups.

Specific classification is the grouping of pupils of like ability within particular sports areas, such as volleyball, tennis, or badminton. The instructor administers the skill test to the class at the beginning of the instructional unit. Then, using the test results, the youngsters are grouped within the class according to their ability in the specific activity.

In addition to grouping pupils in a general as well as a specific classification for instructions, homogeneous grouping works well in the intramural program. By equating the teams, the greater interest stimulated by keener competition adds much to the program. If a youngster feels that there is a fifty-fifty chance of his team's winning, he will be much more interested in being dressed and in the gym on time. For small schools in which only one league of about four or five teams is involved, the youngsters should be paired according to their test scores. If the sport is basketball, then the total of the basketball test scores should be about equal among the teams that are participating. In a large school it is advisable to have more than one league, if at all possible. The teams within each of the leagues should be equated as described above.

Classification methods.   There are two general methods of classifying youngsters for participation in physical education. One method is to group the children according to age, height, and weight. The second method is to group them on the basis of test scores as mentioned above. The former method is quite a rough measure when compared with the latter. This is true for several reasons, the most obvious being that chronological age does not always correlate directly with maturation age. That is to say, one boy may be old physiologically at twelve years of age as another boy is at sixteen. Although weight usually correlates quite high with strength, this relationship is not valid in all cases, particularly with girls. Obviously then, these factors place serious limitations on the use of age, height, and weight levels when grouping youngsters for participation in physical education activities. The most important use of such a classification scheme seems to be in conjunction with the construction of scales or norms. As indicated in Chapter 5, it is most advisable for the instructor to construct his own norms based upon data obtained at hand. When he is making use of such a test as motor fitness, greater reliability of the scaled scores may be gained by taking into consideration the age, height, and weight of the child in constructing norms or scaling the scores. The Indiana physical fitness test (p. 122) is an excellent example of the application of this technique.

For direct classification on the basis of general motor ability, it is recommended that one of the motor ability tests be used rather than a scheme based upon age, height, and weight. The tests that follow have been carefully selected, taking into consideration their utility to the teaching program as well as the scientic manner in which they were constructed. Some of the tests are more complex than others, some require less equipment than others; it is the responsibility of the physical educator to decide what the test will be used for and to select the test that he feels best serves his purposes.

Classification Indexes

McCloy's Classification Index. McCloy[31, 32] has devised a classification index based upon age, height, and weight. This index correlates .81 with track and field events and .57 with a selected group of sports skills. For the purpose of grouping youngsters to form homogeneous physical education classes it is a rather rough measure. However, in preparing norms for tests measuring motor fitness and general motor ability, the scheme has excellent application. Certainly, by taking into consideration the body size of the child, a much fairer test score can be obtained.

McCloy proposes the following three classification indexes:

High school
Classification Index I = (20 × age) + (6 × height) + weight.

College men
Classification Index II = (6 × height) + weight.

Elementary school
Classification Index III = (10 × age) + weight.

In the elementary school (Index III), height is omitted, as it was found to be a negligible factor. For high school (Index I), height is an important factor. In college (Index II) it was found that, after seventeen, age failed to make a difference. Table 21 for computing Classification Index I may be found on page 133. The remaining Indexes will be found in references 31 and 32.

Neilson and Cozens Classification Index. Working with age, height, and weight, Neilson and Cozens[34] have proposed a classification formula. It is computed as follows:

Classication Index = (20 × age) + (5.55 × height) + weight.

TABLE 25. *The Neilson and Cozens Classification Chart for Boys and Girls (Elementary and Junior High School)*

Exponent	Height in Inches	Age in Months	Weight in Pounds
1	50 to 51	120–125	60 to 65
2	52 to 53	126–131	66 to 70
3		132–137	71 to 75
4	54 to 55	138–143	76 to 80
5		144–149	81 to 85
6	56 to 57	150–155	86 to 90
7		156–161	91 to 95
8	58 to 59	162–167	96 to 100
9		168–173	101 to 105
10	60 to 61	174–179	106 to 110
11		180–185	111 to 115
12	62 to 63	186–191	116 to 120
13		192–197	121 to 125
14	64 to 65	198–203	126 to 130
15	66 to 67	204–209	131 to 133
16	68	210–215	134 to 136
17	69 & over	216 & over	137 & over

Sum of exponents	Class	Sum of exponents	Class
9 and below	A	25 to 29	E
10 to 14	B	30 to 34	F
15 to 19	C	35 to 38	G
20 to 24	D	39 and above	H

Neilson, N. P., and Cozens, F. W.: Achievement Scales in Physical Education Activities. California Department of Education, Sacramento, 1934.

This index, designed to be used with high school groups, correlates .983 with McCloy's Index I, indicating that either formula may be used. Tables 25 and 26 contain the classification charts for the Neilson and Cozens classification index.

Tests of Motor Ability

The motor ability test developed by Humiston[15, 16] measures the present status of college women in terms of motor ability. After a detailed analysis by experts, relative to the basic factors of motor ability, fifteen items were selected to represent the criterion measure. As a result of the statistical analysis it was found that seven items, when used as an index, correlated .81 with the criterion. If the same seven items are administered separately, the validity coefficient with the criterion becomes .92. The

TABLE 26. *Classification Index for Boys*
Grades 10, 11, 12

Exponent	Age (Months)	Height (Inches)	Weight (Pounds)	Sum of Exponents	Class
9			53-59	88 and over	A
10			60-65	83-87	B
11			66-71	82 and below	C
12			72-78		
13			79-84		
14			85-90		
15			91-96		
16			97-103		
17			104-109		
18			110-115		
19			116-121		
20			122-128		
21			129-134		
22		0-47	135-140		
23		47.5-49	141-146		
24		49.5-51.5	147-153		
25		52-53.5	154-159		
26		54-55.5	160-165		
27	159-164	56-57.5	166-171		
28	165-170	58-59.5	172-178		
29	171-176	60-62	179-184		
30	177-182	62.5-64	185-190		
31	183-188	64.5-66	191-		
32	189-194	66.5-68			
33	195-200	68.5-70.5			
34	201-206	71-72.5			
35	207-212	73-74.5			
36	213-218	75-			
37	219-224				
38	225-230				

AAHPER Youth Fitness Test Manual. Revised ed. Washington, D. C. 20036, 1965, p. 42.

seven items contained in this test are as follows: a dodging run, sideward roll on a mat, climb over a box, turn in a circle and continue on between barriers, ladder climb, basketball throw over a rope, and a short straight-away run.

It is recommended that the test be used for classifying students for instruction, for equating in intramural games, for determining progress, and as a partial means for selecting physical education majors.

NEWTON MOTOR ABILITY TEST

The Newton motor ability test, constructed to be used with high school girls, establishes three motor ability criteria: (1) a score based upon six sports skill tests; (2) a score based upon a series of tests devised to measure various fundamental skills and various aspects of motor ability; and (3) a subjective rating by a jury of competent judges who observe the students in action, one at a time, as they run an obstacle race.[35]

The second criterion, consisting of eighteen objective tests, is classified into three areas: power and strength, speed, and coordination. After the raw scores were converted into T-scores, the items were averaged for each of the three motor ability elements and used as the objective criterion of general motor ability.

For the third criterion, judges, using a ten-point rating scale, rate the subjects as they perform: (1) a 30-inch running high jump; (2) a basketball toss and catch over a 7-foot net; (3) rolling the base of a jumping standard around a stool 15 feet away; and (4) climbing a high obstacle constructed from gymnasium apparatus and mats. The composite rating by the whole jury is used as the subjective criterion score.

As a result of statistical analysis it was found that the scramble test, the wall pass, the broad jump, and the velocity throw and hurdles correlated highest with the sports criterion, while the hurdles and broad jump correlated highest with the subjective ratings.

On the basis of this analysis the following items are suggested for testing general motor ability: broad jump, hurdles, and scramble.

To compare the effectiveness of the best four Newton motor ability tests in terms of predictive ability, the Rogers PFI was administered. The predictive efficiency of the Newton test batteries was found to be about three and a half times as good as the Rogers indexes. This study apparently indicates the inadequacies of strength as a measure of motor ability for high school girls. In fact, the broad jump alone (PI .36) was more than twice as effective in predicting motor ability as the SI (PI .16). Anderson,[1] in a similar study, found the Sargent jump a superior measure of athletic ability for high school girls to either the PFI or SI, which corroborates the results of Powell and Howe.

Test administration *Broad Jump*. This is performed as described on page 124.

Hurdles. The equipment consists of ten gymnasium benches and five split bamboo sticks for setting up the hurdles, an Indian club, and a stop watch. The first hurdle is placed 5 yards from the starting line, the others at 3-yard intervals beyond it, with the Indian club 3 yards beyond the last hurdle. The height of the hurdles is 15 inches.

The subject is instructed to run at top speed over the hurdles, around the Indian club, and back over the hurdles to the starting line. No penalty is made for displacing a hurdle. The score is recorded to the nearest fifth of a second.

Scramble. The equipment consists of a jumping standard with a small shelf 4 feet above the floor, a tap bell, and a stop watch. The tap bell is fastened securely to the shelf on the jumping standard and placed 10 feet away from the wall.

The subject starts from a supine position on the floor with both feet against the wall and arms stretched sideways at shoulder level, palms down. The subject must scramble to her feet and run to tap the bell twice and then return to the starting position, clap her hands on the floor twice, and repeat the entire performance as rapidly as possible until she has made the fourth double tap of the bell. The time is recorded to the nearest fifth of a second.

The authors recommend that the tests be administered twice in order to increase the reliability of the resulting score, the second series being given on a subsequent day, allowing the students an opportunity to improve their initial scores.

Scoring. Achievement scales for the broad jump, hurdles, scramble, and the battery composed of these three tests were worked out upon data obtained from 812 Newton High School pupils. Decile scores as well as standard deviation point scores appear in the achievement scales in reference 35.

The authors suggest that pupils scoring in the ninth and tenth deciles might well receive special attention and instruction. It appears that the Newton motor ability test is of value chiefly because it permits the instructor to identify the inferior as well as the superior pupils early in the fall. In this way, instruction may be adapted to individual needs, as well as to the needs of the majority.

SCOTT MOTOR ABILITY TEST

Scott,[38] in a rather extensive study of motor ability items, used the following four items in constructing a test for high school and college women:

1. Subjective ratings of sports ability.
2. Skill items associated with most common sports.
3. McCloy general motor ability items for girls.
4. A composite score composed of the above three criteria.

As a result of statistical analysis the following items are proposed as a measure of motor ability: (1) obstacle race; (2) basketball throw; (3) standing broad jump; (4) wall pass;* (5) 4-second dash.*

Test administration *Dash.* The running lane (85 to 90 feet long and 4 feet wide) is marked by either a white line or cards placed every yard. The subject assumes any starting position she desires; the starter, with

---

* Items 4 and 5 may be added if time permits. The obstacle race may be omitted if this is done.

stop watch and whistle, stands at the starting line. The starter commands "ready," then blows the whistle, at which time the runner starts; at the end of four seconds, the starter again blows the whistle. An assistant records the distance in yards from the starting line to the place the girl had reached at the sound of the second whistle.

Basketball throw. The subject throws a basketball from behind a line, for distance; a running approach is allowed if desired. Three trials are given and the best recorded to the nearest foot.

Standing broad jump. This is executed as described on page 115. The best of three trials is recorded to the nearest inch.

Wall Pass. A flat wall at least 8 feet square is used. A line is drawn 9 feet from the wall and parallel to it. The subject stands facing the wall (behind the line) and rebounds the ball off the wall as rapidly as possible. The throw may be of any type and the score is recorded as the number of hits in a fifteen-second period. If the ball goes out of control, or if the subject must step over the line to retrieve the ball, the subject must immediately return to behind the line before the next throw. Three or four practice throws are allowed.

Obstacle Race (Fig. 56). The space required for the obstacle course is 55 feet along and 12 feet wide. The equipment consists of three jumping standards and a crossbar at least 6 feet long.

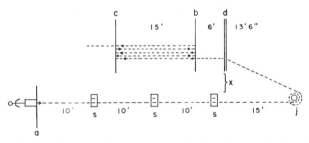

Figure 56. Diagram for Scott obstacle race. *a*, Starting line; *b*, line for shuttle; *c*, finish line; *d*, crossbar (18″ high); *j*, jump standard; *s*, spot on floor (12″ × 18″); *dotted line*, path of runner in direction of arrows; *x*, distance from end of crossbar to line of inner sides of spots (4′ 4″). (Courtesy of Gladys Scott.)

Figure 56 depicts the layout of the obstacle course. The subject, in supine position, heels touching line *a*, gets up and runs toward *j* at the command "go." As the subject reaches each square she must step on it with both feet. She runs twice around *j* and then crawls under the crossbar at *d*. Rising on the other side, she runs to line *c* and continues to shuttle between *c* and *b* until she comes to *c* the third time. The score is the time to the nearest tenth of a second required to run the course.

In marking the ability of the performer to step with both feet on the square, do not discredit the runner if the toe or heel extends outside the square. Some feet may be too large to fit inside the square when the feet are lowered. The examiner should be concerned as to whether the stride is adjusted to contact the square and whether a transfer of weight takes place in the square.

Scoring. Norms for high school and college women, based upon T-scores, have been constructed for the Scott motor ability test. Table 27 for high school girls has been reproduced; the tables for college women appear in reference 38. The simplest method of computing a girl's score is to take the average of the T-scores earned on the three or four tests given. Figure 57 contains a score card and hypothetical data to illustrate the scoring procedures.

Name_____Age_____Grade_____		
Test	*Raw Score*	*T-Score*
Basketball Throw	52.0	68
Obstacle Race	19.7	67
Standing Broad Jump	76.0	57
	Total	192

Average Score $= \dfrac{192}{3} = 64$

Figure 57. Scoring card for Scott motor ability test.

TABLE 27.   *T-Scales for Motor Ability Tests for High School Girls*

T-Score	Wall Pass (410)*	Basketball Throw (Ft.) (310)*	Broad Jump (In.) (287)*	4-Sec. Dash (Yd.) (398)*	Obstacle Race (Sec.) (374)*
80	16	71			
79			96		
78					
77	15	68	94	27	
76		66			18.5–18.9
75		65			
74		64	92		
73	14	63			
72		61			
71		59	90	26	
70		55	88		19.0–19.4
69	13	54			
68		52	86	25	
67		51			19.5–19.9
66		50			
65		49			
64		48	84	24	20.0–20.4
63	12	47			
62		46	82		20.5–20.9

TABLE 27. *(Continued)*

T-Score	Wall Pass (410)*	Basketball Throw (Ft.) (310)*	Broad Jump (In.) (287)*	4-Sec. Dash (Yd.) (398)*	Obstacle Race (Sec.) (374)*
61			80		
60		45		23	
59		44	78		21.0–21.4
58	11	43			
57		42	76		21.5–21.9
56		41			
55		40	74	22	
54					22.0–22.4
53		39			
52	10		72		
51		37			22.5–22.9
50		36		21	
49		35	70		
48			68		23.0–23.4
47		34	66		
46	9	33			23.5–23.9
45		32	64	20	
44		31			24.0–24.4
43			62		
42		30			24.5–24.9
41	8	29	60	19	
40		28			
39			58		25.0–25.4
38		27	56		
37	7		54		25.5–25.9
36		26			26.0–26.4
35			52	18	26.5–26.9
34		25	50		27.0–27.4
33					
32		24	47		27.5–27.9
31	6	23			
30			44		
29		22		17	28.5–28.9
28					29.0–29.4
27		21			29.5–29.9
26			40		30.0–30.4
25	5	20			
24				16	30.5–30.4
23		19	36		31.5–32.4
22				15	32.5–34.9
21		16			
20	4			14	35.0–36.0

Scott, M. Gladys, and French, Esther: Evaluation in Physical Education. St. Louis, C. V. Mosby Co., 1950, pp. 200-202.

* Indicates the number of subjects on which the scale is based.

The average motor ability score may be used to section classes, to make up teams, or to obtain an approximation of the level of achievement that might be expected in future work. Also the bottom 15 to 25 per cent may be sorted out for special help in developing skills proficiency. Then too, the members of the top scoring group may be given additional work requiring greater tests of their ability. These highly skilled pupils, in most cases, will serve as excellent student leaders. They may well be asked to work with pupils of low motor ability or to lend a hand in the developmental and remedial phase of the physical education program.

BARROW MOTOR ABILITY TEST

Barrow has constructed a test of motor ability for college men in which expert opinion is used in the validation process.[2,3] First, an analysis of a number of recognized tests of motor performance was made to determine what test items had been found to be the most valid measures of motor ability. These were submitted to a jury and, as a result of the jury's analysis, eight factors of motor ability and twenty-nine items measuring these factors were selected for study. The items were administered to 222 college men; the resulting data were subjected to statistical analysis, including item reliability, objectivity, and correlations with the criterion. Upon conclusion of the statistical treatment of the data, two test batteries, including one short indoor test, were devised.

Test number one. The first test is a six-item battery that may be considered as most valid in that it yielded a multiple R of .950, with a standard error of estimate of 3.16 in terms of the twenty-nine item criterion. The items included are: standing broad jump, softball throw, zigzag run, wall pass, medicine ball put, and 60-yard dash.

Test number two. This test is a three-item indoor battery, consisting of standing broad jump, medicine ball put, and zigzag run. The three-item battery has a validity coefficient of .920 with the criterion, and a standard error of estimate of 3.968.

Norms for the two general motor ability tests have been constructed for both college students and physical education majors. They appear in reference 2.

Test administration. *Standing broad jump.* A 5- by 20-foot tumbling mat is used for administration of this test in the gymnasium. A warm-up jump is permitted; then three successive trials are given. Scoring is the distance of the best jump measured to the nearest inch.

The 60-yard dash. One trial is permitted and scoring is to the nearest tenth of a second.

Wall pass. A restraining line is marked on the floor 9 feet from a smooth wall. The subject stands behind the restraining line with a regulation basketball. On the signal to start, the ball is passed against the wall in any manner desired. It is caught on the rebound and returned to the wall as rapidly as possible for fifteen seconds. Both feet of the subject must remain behind the restraining line, and, if the ball is missed, the subject must retrieve it and return to the starting line before continuing the test. Scoring is the number of times the ball hits the wall in the fifteen-second time allotment.

Softball throw.   The field is marked in 5-yard intervals, with football sideline markers placed at each interval to designate distance. A regulation softball (12-inch inseam) is used for the test. Each subject is allowed three throws, with a short run to the starting line permitted. Scoring is to the nearest foot for the best of three throws.

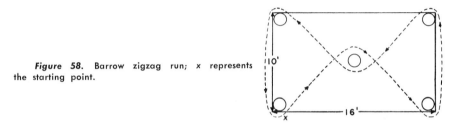

Figure 58. Barrow zigzag run; x represents the starting point.

Zigzag run.   A course is laid out as depicted in Figure 58. The subject starts at point *x* in a semi-crouched position. He traverses the course three times and must not grasp the standards or chairs that have been placed in the circles as obstacles. If a foul is committed, as, for example, knocking over an obstacle, a second trial is permitted. Scoring is to the nearest tenth of a second. (Standards commonly used for high jumping or volleyball supports, or chairs, or even Indian clubs may be employed as obstacles.)

Medicine ball putt.   The subject stands behind a restraining line and is permitted three successive trials in putting a 6-pound medicine ball. A distance of 15 feet behind the restraining line is designated as the area in which a run may be made up to the restraining line in performing the medicine ball put. Scoring is to the nearest one-half foot, the best of the three trials being recorded.

COZENS' TEST OF GENERAL ATHLETIC ABILITY

Cozens,[4] securing judgments from fifty-two physical educators as to the elements comprising general athletic ability, arrived at the following seven basic components: (1) arm and shoulder girdle strength; (2) arm and shoulder girdle coordination; (3) hand-eye, foot-eye, arm-eye coordination; (4) jumping strength, leg strength, and leg flexibility; (5) endurance; (6) body coordination, agility, and control; and (7) speed of legs. Some forty tests were then collected and categorized under these seven headings, and, after experimentation, one test for each element was retained.

TABLE 28.   *Test Items and Weights for Cozens' Test of General Athletic Ability*

Test Item	Weight or Multiplier
1. Dips	0.8
2. Baseball throw for distance	1.5
3. Football punt for distance	1.0
4. Standing broad jump	0.9
5. Bar snap	0.5
6. Dodging	1.0
7. Quarter-mile run	1.3

Bovard, John F., Cozens, Frederick, W., and Hagman, E. Patricia: Tests and Measurements in Physical Education. 3rd ed. Philadelphia, W. B. Saunders Co., 1949.

Table 28 contains the test items and scoring weights for each of the seven tests. The validity and reliability of the test are high, indicating that the test may be satisfactorily used for classification as well as for diagnostic purposes on the college level.

Rouhlac, in analyzing the Cozens test by means of factor analysis, found the following four factors: speed, coordination, power, and endurance.[37] As these factors are recognized to be basic elements of general athletic ability, the results lend further validity to the Cozens test.

Test administration.   *Baseball throw.*   Three throws for distance are allowed, with one minute for warm-up. The ball used is a 12-inch outseam softball. Markers are placed every 5 feet and the first bounce of the ball is estimated to the nearest foot. The best score of the three throws is recorded.

Football punt.   No warming-up punts are permitted, and only three punts for distance are allowed. The field is divided by 5-yard markers, and the best of the three punts is estimated to the nearest yard.

Bar snap.   The bar height is 4½ feet from the ground or floor. The stunt is performed by standing on the floor or ground facing the bar; the bar is grasped and the body swung underneath, with the feet close to the bar; the feet are shot upward at an angle approximating 45 degrees; the back is arched and the student lets go of the bar at the right moment to give distance, landing on his feet. Three trials are allowed and the best of three is recorded in feet and inches. Measurements are taken on the floor or ground from the plane of the bar to the point nearest the bar where any part of the student's body touched the ground or mat.

Standing broad jump.   This is performed as described on page 124.

Dip (on Parallels).   The description of this item appears on page 81.

Dodging.   Five 3-foot track lanes are laid out, 11 yards in length. Hurdles are placed as indicated.

Starting from point A the runner goes straight ahead, turns right at hurdle 2, left at hurdle 3, right at 4, and runs around 5, coming to the far point of B, then following the same path back to A as was originally taken.

Two complete round trips are made, starting at A and ending at A. Time is taken from the word "go" until the finish line is crossed. Only one trial is allowed unless a runner becomes confused and runs incorrectly. The subject should jog over the course twice before running it for time.

Quarter mile. Time is recorded to the nearest second.

Scoring. To score the test, raw scores are transposed into Sigma scale scores; the Sigma values are then multiplied by the weights appearing in Table 28, which results in the relative value that each test item contributes to the total general athletic ability score.

Figure 59 is a sample classification test record card containing hypothetical data to illustrate the proper procedures in scoring the test.

COZENS' CLASSIFICATION TEST RECORD CARD

Name   Robert Brown   Height   5'10"   Weight   155   Date_____

Class Division   MH

	Raw Score	Sigma Score	Weight	Final	Classification	
Baseball throw	196 ft.	66	1.5	99	Superior	496–up
Football punt	50 yds.	86	1.0	86	Ab. Av.	399–495
Bar snap	6 ft.	57	.5	28.5	Average	302–398
Standing broad jump	8' 4"	69	.9	62.1	Blw. Av.	205–301
Dip	12	63	.8	50.4	Inferior	204–down
Dodging	22.2	84	1.0	84	Assignment: Track, Games, Gymnastics, Handball, Tennis, Swimming, Wrestling, Boxing, Elective	
Quarter-mile	59.8	81	1.3	105.3		
			Total	515.3		

Figure 59. Classification test record. (Adapted from Bovard, John F., Cozens, Frederick W., and Hagman, E. Patricia: Tests and Measurements in Physical Education. 3rd ed.)

Obviously, the student whose record appears on the score card has excellent general athletic ability. On this basis he would be permitted an elective course in physical education. Students scoring low on the test might be placed in sections where greater individual attention can be given them. In such cases, all possible information relative to the cause or causes of low scores should be gathered. This information may then be effectively used in constructing the proper program for the student. Tables of norms for scoring the various activities and directions for computing the scores may be found in Cozens' Achievement Scales in Physical Education for College Men, published by Lea & Febiger in 1936.

LARSON MOTOR ABILITY TEST

After experimenting with twenty-five motor ability items, Larson[22] constructed an indoor and outdoor test of motor ability for secondary school and college men. The test items are as follows:

Indoor test	Outdoor test
Dodging run	Baseball throw
Chinning	Bar snap
Dipping	Chinning
Vertical jump	Vertical jump
Bar snap	

Using the total score for the twenty-five motor ability items, a multiple R of .97 was obtained for the indoor test and a multiple R of .98 for the outdoor test.

Larson indicates that the tests do not reflect specific skills ability, but rather correlate with the basic elements underlying sports skills. The application of the test results may be used for classification purposes in physical education.

Test administration. *Dodging run.* This is executed as described under Cozens' test, page 172. Five parallel lanes are constructed 3 feet wide and 11 yards long. Five low hurdles are placed in the first, second, third, fourth, and fifth lanes (see Fig. 72). The runner starts at the starting point and runs as indicated by the broken line. The time necessary for *two complete* runs is the score. The subject should not touch the hurdles when circling them.

Bar snap. This test is administered in the same manner as described on page 172. Measurement is made in inches from the plane of the horizontal bar to the back of the heels at the point where the subject lands. Three trials are given and the maximum score is recorded. Care should be taken to see that the subjects have first mastered the skill before test data are gathered.

Chinning. This is administered in the same manner as described on page 85. However, no partial score is permitted; the count is one for each full chin completed.

Dips. There should be a ten-minute rest period between dips and chinning. The dips are administered, in the same manner as described on page 88, from parallel bars. However, no partial dips are permitted. The count is one for the jump into the first position, then one for each complete dip.

Vertical jump. This item is executed as described on page 124.

Baseball throw for distance. A 12-inch inseam ball is used. The subject is allowed to run to the throwing line, but must not overstep the line. The field is marked at 5-foot intervals to facilitate measurement. The examiner estimates the distance between the markers when the ball hits the ground. A warm-up period should be allowed, and the best throw of three trials is scored in feet.

Scoring.   The indoor and the outdoor tests are scored in the same manner. If, for example, the indoor test is used, the first step is to change the raw scores into "weighted standard scores"; next, these "weighted standard scores" are totaled; the result is referred to as the "index score."

Tables for making the computations appear in the reference cited.

STRENGTH TESTS OF MOTOR ABILITY

Larson's Muscular Strength Test.   Larson's[23] strength test for secondary school and college men is composed of three items: chins (description p. 85); dips (description p. 88); and vertical jump (description p. 124).

Through a factor analysis study of strength items as related to motor ability, Larson found two components of muscular strength: (1) dynamic strength, defined as the ability to raise body weight and propel it upward; and (2) static dynamometrical strength, that strength registered by use of a dynamometer. This study revealed that dynamic strength has almost three times the predictive value of static dynamometrical strength when related to motor ability. This was also verified in another study by Dunder, who found that back and leg strength in a combination with other strength factors contributes little to the relationship between a gross strength test and general motor ability.

Scoring the Larson strength test.   Larson's proposed strength test is computed as an index score by converting the raw scores into weighted standard scores. The scoring tables for men seventeen to twenty-four years of age appear in reference 23.

The Physical Fitness Index and the Strength Index.   The PFI and the SI, discussed in Chapter 5, have been used rather extensively as measures of motor ability to classify pupils into homogeneous groups.[36]

Wellman[41] set up quite an interesting study to discover, among a group of tests of speed, agility, balance, strength, and native motor ability, a test or battery of tests that might be used in restricting admissions of women to professional physical education programs in teacher-training schools. The criterion selected as a measure of skills necessary for success in physical education was a high level of grades received in physical activity classes.

The following tests were used: (1) Brace test; (2) Burpee test (ten-second squat thrusts); (3) Physical Fitness Index; (4) other activity tests of speed, agility, and balance.

The following coefficients of correlation between grades and the selected tests were obtained (predictive indices shown as PI):

Test	Correlation with criterion	PI
Physical fitness index	.53	.15
Speed test	.39	.08
Agility test	.38	.07
Burpee test	.37	.07
Brace test	.35	.06
Balance test	.23	.003

From the tests studied, the PFI appears to be the best indication of success in motor skills for boys. It is interesting to note that the PFI correlates with the criterion more closely than does the Brace test; in fact, according to the Predictive Indices, the PFI is more than twice as good as the Brace test in predictive value.

Wellman suggests that the PFI, which is actually gross strength related to body size, should correlate high with motor ability, because the relationships obtained between strength and speed of running and skating and team abilities for boys are high.

In support of this rationale, Shay[39] using as a criterion speed in learning the kip or upstart on the horizontal bar, and fitness scores, found the following relationships (predictive indices shown as PI):

Test	Correlation with criterion	PI
Physical fitness index	.83	.45
Strength index	.78	.37
Brace test	.52	.16

It seems quite apparent from Shay's data that the PFI is almost three times as good as the Brace test in predicting ability to learn the kip.

Use of the SI in equating opponents in sports. Clarke and Bonesteel,[6] using six intramural teams of eleven players each, equated them by use of the SI. The six teams were then arranged in three groups of two teams each, and a series of intramural contests was conducted within each group. The sports played were touch football, speedball, field hockey, and indoor soccer. It was found that of sixty-four games played by all teams in the four sports, twenty-nine, or 45 per cent, were tie games.

The authors observed that it was evident that all the boys were enthusiastic and active participants. Apparently as a result of the intense interest in the competition, no disciplinary problems arose and no boy was absent from any of the games in which his team was scheduled to play. This, the authors concluded, was a very desirable teaching situation, from which educational objectives as well as recreational pleasures should be realized.

To validate the SI as a measure of general athletic ability, Rogers obtained a correlation of .76 between the SI and the weighted score for the 100-yard dash, running high jump, and the bar vault. He also obtained an r of .81 between the SI and ability in a two-lap run, standing broad jump, running high jump, 8-pound shot-put, basketball free throw, and baseball and football target throws.[36]

In another validation study, Rogers compared the SI's of varsity lettermen with those scored by all other boys in the school. The assumption underlying this investigation was that "making the school team" should be a satisfactory criterion of athletic ability. Rogers found that half of the football players scored above 95 per cent of the boys in the upper three grades of high school. For the 390 boys studied, nineteen scored above the ninety-fifth percentile, of which only nine were not among the best football players.

From a study of many investigations, it appears that researchers are in agreement that strength is the most important single element contributing to success in performing motor activities. On this basis, tests of strength can be used with satisfactory precision in the equating of teams, and placing youngsters into homogeneous groups for participation in athletic sports skills.

How to equate teams using the SI. On the basis of the SI, physical education classes may be divided into teams of equal ability for competition in team games, as well as for classroom instruction. Once the scores are obtained, Rogers suggests that in order to group them, simply arrange the pupils' names in the order of their respective strength indices, with the largest at the top. The next step is to deal out the names into as many piles as there are to be teams, dealing first to the right, then to the left, then to the right until all cards are dealt out. It is suggested that, in order to protect the weaker boys, there should be at least two or preferably three levels of ability for each class. Assuming a class of forty-eight pupils and two levels of ability, the mean Strength Indices for each group might be as follows:

Team A	Team B	Team X	Team Y
1,860	1,825	1,398	1,380

The final step is to total the SI's for each team and make any necessary adjustments to provide nearly equal totals (within fifty to one hundred points if possible).

OBERLIN COLLEGE TEST

The department of Physical Education for Men at Oberlin College has developed a general motor ability test to be used as a means of qualifying students for the elective program in physical education.[8] The ten-item test is scored on the basis of one hundred points—ten points are credited for the successful performance of each of the following items:

Element	Test Item	Standard
1. Running	176 yards (2 laps, indoor track)	24 sec.
2. Jumping	Running high jump	4 feet, 10 in.
3. Vaulting	On low horizontal bar from standing position	Height 47 in.
4. Climbing	20 foot rope, kneeling start	12 sec.
5. Pulling and lifting	Two backward circles on high horizontal; hanging start, arms extended, body motionless	Continuous movement for each
6. Pushing	Dips on parallel bar	10 times
7. Throwing	Baseball target throw for accuracy, 18-inch circle	3 hits out of 5 throws at 60 feet
8. Swimming	100 yards, free style	1 min., 45 sec.
9. Tumbling	Hand spring	
10. Balancing	Hand stand; movement confined to 4-foot diameter circle	10 sec.

SIGMA DELTA PSI TEST

The Sigma Delta Psi is a national athletic fraternity organized in 1912 at the University of Indiana to stimulate interest in all-round athletics.[4] The requirements for membership to this fraternity are as follows:

1.	100-yard dash	11⅗ sec.
2.	120-yard low hurdles	16 sec.
3.	Running high jump	5 feet
4.	Running broad jump	17 feet
5.	16-pound shot-put	Distance according to man's weight; 30 ft. for 160 lbs. or over
6.	Rope climb	20 ft. in 12 sec.
7.	Baseball throw	250 ft. on fly
8.	Football punt	120 ft. on fly
9.	Swimming	100 yards in 1 min., 45 sec.
10.	One-mile run	6 min.
11.	Tumbling:	
	a. Front handspring	
	b. Frence vault, bar at chin height	
	c. Hand stand	10 sec.
12.	Posture	Erect carriage
13.	Scholarship	C

NOTE: A varsity sport in which a letter has been earned may be substituted for any one of the above, with the exception of swimming.

McCLOY'S GENERAL MOTOR ABILITY TESTS

General Motor Ability Score (GMAS).   In this instance, McCloy[31, 32] refers to general motor ability as developed capacity, the present ability of an individual to perform in a variety of sports activities. In the development of this particular test battery, studies were made in which test elements were correlated against the total score of a large battery of achievement tests. As a result the studies indicated two types of tests that could be expected to measure motor ability. These were: (1) a combination of three or four track and field events; and (2) strength. The items contained in McCloy's general motor ability test are as follows:

Boys:

1. Arm strength computed by McCloy's formula as follows:

Chinning or Dipping strength $= 1.77$ (Weight) $+ 3.42$ (Chins or dips) $- 46$.

2. Track and field events, depending upon age and experience of the group. Including at least:
   a. A sprint, varying from 50 to 100 yards.
   b. Broad jump, standing or running.
   c. Running high jump.
   d. One weight-throwing event, shot-put, basketball or baseball throw for distance.

The four events should be scored on McCloy's scoring tables, which appear in reference 32, and the sum of these scores taken as total track and field points. The elements are then combined in the following formula:

General Motor Ability Score (GMAS) $= .1022$ (Total track and field points) $+ .3928$ (Chinning strength).

Girls: In the girls' GMAS, the actual number of pull-ups is used, rather than pull-up strength. The following test items are used:

1. Sprint.
2. Broad jump.
3. Throw for distance.

These items are scored on McCloy's scoring tables for *boys,* which appear in reference 32. The formula for combining the elements is as follows:

GMAS $= .42$ (Total track and field points) $+ 9.6$ (Number of chins).

McCloy's Universal Scoring Tables.   McCloy[31, 32] has constructed scoring tables for a number of track and field events. These tables were developed on the theory that the closer a boy approaches peak performance, the more difficult it becomes to increase his score. As an illustration, according to the Universal Scoring Tables, which appear in reference 31, a person increasing his time in the 100-yard dash from fifteen to fourteen seconds receives a score of 52 points, whereas a pupil increasing his time from eleven seconds to ten seconds would receive 191 points. There are contained in the Universal Scoring Tables twenty-seven track and field events as well as floor push-ups and chins. The tables permit comparison of the various events, and hence scores may be added to one another as well as averaged to obtain a single score for several of the events.

McCloy's Athletics Quotient. Using the Universal Scoring Tables and the Classification Index, McCloy[31, 32] in order to equalize the effects of age and size in performing tests of track and field ability, devised the Athletics Quotient for secondary school boys. This quotient is the percentage relation the actual performance bears to the average performance of a well-selected sampling of performers of the same sex, age, height, and weight.

It is for this reason that the Athletics Quotient has application to the physical education program. In the first place, pupils may be classified into homogeneous groups according to the quotient score. Second, this score may serve as an excellent means of marking in the area of motor ability, for the pupil can be graded according to his body size and capacity. Third, the obtained score serves as tangible evidence of the boy's athletic ability, a mark which the pupil, individually, can attempt to improve upon.

McCloy's General Motor Capacity Test. McCloy[31, 32] refers to general motor capacity as inborn, hereditary potentialities for general motor performance. The author indicates that the test is not a measure of specific skill, such as basketball ability. This is demonstrated by the fact that events requiring specialized ability have a lower correlation with the general motor capacity score than do events requiring motor ability of general nature. Hence track and field ability are highly correlated with the general capacity score, whereas specific skills such as basketball and football are not. The test correlates about .70 with football and basketball. It must be recognized that this test may be used only as a prediction of motor capacity, the potential levels to which the individual may attain.

The test was validated against a battery of motor tests and against teachers' judgments for both boys and girls. On the basis of the results, a battery was devised containing the following items:

1. The Classification Index (measure of size and maturity).
2. The Sargent jump (measure of power).
3. Ten-second squat thrusts (measure of agility and large muscle coordination).

The items were weighted and resulted in the following regression equations for computing the general motor capacity (GMC) of pupils at the different age levels:

Elementary school boys

$$\text{GMC} = 0.181 \text{ (Classification Index)} + 0.769 \text{ (Sargent jump in cm.)}$$
$$+ 0.510 \text{ (Brace test T-score)} + 2.187 \text{ (Burpee test)} - 62$$

Junior and senior high school boys

GMC = 0.329 (Classification Index) + 1.446 (Sargent jump in cm.)
+ 0.926 (Brace test T-score) + 3.973 (Burpee test) − 202

Elementary school girls

GMC = 3.576 (Sargent jump in cm.) + 2.20 (Brace test T-score)
+ 19.12 (Burpee test) + 29

Junior and senior high school girls

GMC = 3.576 (Sargent jump in cm.) + 2.20 (Brace test T-score)
+ 19.12 (Burpee test) + 119

The correlations with the teachers' ratings were .512 for boys and .734 for girls, and, with the criterion score, .969 for boys and .921 for girls. Remembering that the test is restricted to the measurement of the subject's potential motor ability, the results may be used in the following manner:

1. *General Motor Capacity Score (GMCS).* This is the total score of the test and may be used as a measure of motor capacity. McCloy defines it as the motor analogue of the raw score of an intelligence test, which is usually expressed as mental age.

2. *The Motor Quotient (MQ).* The GMCS, when divided by the norm for the subject, expresses his capacity as a percentage of the norm or Motor Quotient. This quotient is the motor analogue of the IQ score used in the measurement of intelligence. The score, based upon the Classification Index for boys, and on age for girls, represents the individual's motor capacity relative to size and general maturity. A boy achieving an MQ of 100 would be average for boys his age and size, whereas an MQ of 120 would indicate a very superior ability to acquire new motor skills. A boy scoring an MQ of 80 would find great difficulty in learning new motor skills. The MQ indicates how the individual ranks when compared with others of equal size and maturity. To facilitate computation of the scores, tables have been prepared and appear in reference 32.

General Motor Achievement Quotient (GMAQ). The GMAQ may be obtained by dividing the GMAS by the GMCS, and multiplying the result by 100. This quotient will be in terms of the percentage relationship of the actual ability to the predicted or standard ability. A GMAQ of 90 indicates an achievement that is 90 per cent of what it should be if the individual were developed as well as he could be, with reference to his capacity, age, size, and general maturity. Hence it should be recognized that the GMAQ represents achievement, the relationship existing between the individual's developed ability and his potential capacity. Thus, the GMAQ is subject to change with the individual's increased ability in motor skills.

The computation of these four tests requires a number of tables, which appear in references 31 and 32.

TEST OF RUNNING ENDURANCE

Distance running is frequently used as a measure of cardiorespiratory endurance.[28] A shortcoming of this type of test lies in the difference between the innate running abilities of the pupils taking the test. For example, in the 200-yard run, one boy may be exceptionally fast in terms of running speed, whereas another boy may be slow but actually may possess greater endurance. The score of the latter boy would suffer as a result of his innate slowness.

To circumvent this problem, McCloy has devised a system whereby the time for a distance run is divided by the time for a sprint. This results in a quotient that can be interpreted in terms of endurance points.

Administration of running endurance tests. *Six-second run.* Markers of heavy cardboard about 9 inches square, with proper yardages painted on them, are first prepared. One marker should be made for each distance, at units of 2 yards, from 34 to 56 yards. These are then fastened to the ground at their proper distances. The test may be greatly facilitated if chalk lines are drawn on the ground at 2-yard intervals. Also a number of pupils should be trained to act as inspectors, one for each running lane. The inspectors, holding recording cards, are placed approximately 45 yards from the starting line. Using a hand signal the "starter" starts the group with the conventional "get set" and "go" signals. At "go" the timer starts his watch and continues to observe the watch, not the runners. He counts aloud by seconds—"three," "four," "five"—and when the second hand has reached exactly six seconds, he blows his whistle. Each inspector notes the place that his boy has reached, using the chest of the boy as the point of measurement. The inspector then marks the spot and observes where it is relative to the cards or chalk lines marking the distance. The score to the nearest foot is recorded. It is recommended to give two trials, which may be administered five minutes apart.

The 200-yard run. This event is executed on a 100-yard straightaway. It is started in the same manner as the six-second run. The timer observes his watch, and, as the first runner approaches the finish line, he counts the seconds in a loud voice, with the accented syllable corresponding to the full second in the count and a "hup" for the half-second; thus twenty-*six*, hup, twenty-*seven*, hup, twenty-*eight*, hup, where six, seven, and eight, respectively, mark the seconds and "hup" marks the half-seconds. Tables containing the data for scoring the running endurance test appear in reference 28.

The 300-yard run. McCloy computed a factor analysis on twelve athletic events administered to 400 well-conditioned soldiers.[26] Four of the events could be considered as tests of circulorespiratory endurance; four, muscular endurance; and the remainder, tests of speed. In addition, four combinations of tests were included. The most important finding of this research was the high factor weighting of the endurance index (300-yard run divided by the six-second run) with circulorespiratory endurance

(.8835). This was found to be almost as high as that for the entire endurance combination (.8964).

The 300-yard run may be performed on a 60-yard course. The administration of the test is the same as for the 200-yard run. Tables containing the scoring standards similar to the 200-yard run, for computing the running endurance quotient, may be found in reference 26.

Henry and Kleeberger have questioned the use of such endurance indexes.[13] Their research shows that the time scores of subjects on the long distance runs correlated quite well with those recorded for the shorter distances. This apparently demonstrates that the index is not achieving its purpose to a satisfactory degree, which would be the elimination of a bias in favor of running skill. To obtain a more refined measurement of endurance, it has been proposed that the subject be scored on a 70-yard run, and that the result be used to calculate a predicted score for his 300-yard run.[12] The subject would then have two scores for the 300-yard run, one actual and one predicted. Henry suggests that a *residual* score, based on the difference between the actual and the predicted scores, would be more purely a measure of endurance, as the factor of the subject's running ability has been largely eliminated from it.

Individual skill in running and the desire to go "all out" are variables in an endurance event, and detract from the validity of these endurance measures.

Motor Educability

The ease with which a person learns new skills is referred to as motor educability. The principle or theory involved in the application of such a test to the physical education program may be compared to intelligence measurement in the field of psychology or education.

Tests of motor educability may be used as a method to place pupils in homogeneous groups for physical education classes. Also, because of the wide variety of skills taught in a professional school of physical education, such tests may prove helpful in selecting prospective candidates.

Brace, in 1927, was the first researcher to publish a description of a test attempting to measure motor educability.[5] Twenty self-testing stunts, some easy and some difficult, scored on pass-or-fail basis, comprised the battery. The number of items passed was interpreted from scaled scores. However, no consideration was given to differences in age or body size, which doubtlessly contributed to the low reliability of the test.

IOWA-BRACE TEST

McCloy,[29] in an attempt to secure a test of motor educability, studied forty stunts and eliminated them one by one until twenty-one remained, all of which met the following criteria:

1. The percentage of individuals passing the stunt increased proportionately as age increased.

2. The items had low correlation with measures of strength, size, maturity, and power.

3. The test correlated relatively high with track and field athletic ability in the form of "total points" when the Classification Index, the Sargent jump, and strength were held constant to the athletic events, but not to the stunt. The theory involved here was that if age, size, speed, and strength were held constant in the correlations with athletic events, individuals more adept in track and field skills would be so because of their greater degree of motor educability.

From the twenty-one stunts, six groups of ten stunts each were included in a battery for the upper three grades of elementary school, for junior high school, and for senior high school. Batteries of tests are constructed for both sexes.

Stunts. The stunts used in the Iowa-Brace test are as follows (the asterisk [*] indicates those ten stunts that were originally included in the Brace test):

Test 1. One foot-touch head. Stand on left foot. Bend forward and place both hands on the floor. Raise the right leg and stretch it back. Touch the head to the floor and regain the standing position without losing balance. It is a failure:

    1. Not to touch head to the floor.

    2. Losing the balance and having to touch the right foot down or step about.

Test 2. Side leaning rest. Sit down on the floor, legs straight out and feet together. Put the right hand on the floor behind you. Turn to the right and take a side leaning-rest position, resting on the right hand and the right foot. Raise the left arm and keep this position for five counts. It is a failure:

    1. Not to take the proper position.

    2. Not to hold the position for five counts.

Test 3. Grapevine. Stand with both heels tight together. Bend down, extend both arms down between the knees, around behind the ankles, and hold the fingers together in front of the ankles without losing the balance. Hold this position for five seconds. It is a failure:

    1. To fall over.

    2. Not to touch and hold the fingers of both hands together.

    3. Not to hold the position for five seconds.

Test 4. One-knee balance. Face to the right. Kneel down on one knee with the other leg raised from the floor and arms stretched out at the side. Hold your balance for five counts. It is a failure:

    1. To touch the floor with any other part of the body than the one leg and knee.

    2. To fall over.

Test 5. Stork stand. Stand on the left foot. Hold the bottom of the right foot against the inside of the left knee. Place the hands on the hips. Shut both eyes and hold the position for ten seconds without shifting the left foot about on the floor. It is a failure:

1. To lose the balance.
2. To take the right foot down.
3. To open the eyes or remove the hands from the hips.

Test 6. Double heel click. Jump into the air and clap the feet together twice and land with the feet apart (any distance). It is a failure:

1. Not to clap the feet together twice.
2. To land with the feet touching each other.

Test 7. Cross-leg squat. Fold the arms across the chest. Cross the feet and sit down cross-legged. Get up without unfolding the arms or having to move the feet about to regain the balance. It is a failure:

1. To unfold the arms.
2. To lose the balance.
3. To be unable to get up.

Test 8. Full left turn. Stand with feet together. Jump into the air and make a full turn to the left, landing on the same spot. Do not lose the balance or move the feet after they strike the floor. It is a failure:

1. Not to turn all the way around.
2. To move the feet after they strike the floor.

Test 9. One knee-head to floor. Kneel on one knee with the other leg stretched out behind, not touching the floor, the arms out at side parallel to the floor; bend forward and touch the head to the floor and raise the head from the floor without losing the balance. It is a failure:

1. To touch the floor with the raised leg or with any other part of the body before completing the stunt.
2. Not to touch the head to the floor.
3. To drop the hands.

Test 10. Hop backward. Stand on either foot. Close the eyes and take five hops backward. It is a failure:

1. To open the eyes.
2. To drop the other foot.

Test 11. Forward hand kick. Jump upward, swinging the legs forward, bend forward and touch the toes with both hands before landing. Keep the knees as straight as possible. It is a failure:

1. Not to touch both feet while in the air.
2. To bend the knees more than 45 degrees.

Test 12. Full squat-arm circles. Take a full squat position with arms out sidewise. Wave the arms so that the hands make a circle about 12 inches across, and jiggle up and down at the same time for ten counts. It is a failure:

1. To move the feet about on the floor.
2. To lose the balance and fall.

Test 13. Half-turn jump—left foot. Stand on the left foot and jump one-half turn to the left, keeping the balance. It is a failure:

1. To lose the balance.
2. To fail to complete the half turn.
3. To touch the floor with the other foot.

Test 14. Three dips. Take a front leaning-rest position, i.e., place the hands on the floor, with arms straight, extend the feet back along the floor until the body is straight (in an inclined position to the floor). Bend the arms, touching the chest to the floor, and push up again until the arms are straight. Do this three times in succession. Do not touch the floor with the legs or waist. It is a failure:

1. Not to push up three times.
2. Not to touch the chest to the floor each time.
3. To rest the knees, thighs, or waist on the floor at any time.

Test 15. Side kick. Throw the left foot sideways to the left, jumping upward from the right foot; strike the feet together in the air and land with the feet apart. The feet should strike outside the left shoulder line. It is a failure:

1. Not to swing the feet enough to the side.
2. Not to strike the feet together in the air.
3. Not to land with the feet apart.

Test 16. Kneel, jump to feet. Kneel on both knees. Extend the toes of both feet out flat behind. Swing the arms and jump to the feet without rocking back on the toes or losing the balance. It is a failure:

1. To have the toes curled under and rock back on them.
2. Not to execute the jump, and not to stand still on both feet.

Test 17. Russian dance. Squat as far down as possible; stretch one leg forward; do a Russian dance step by hopping to this position with first one leg extended, then the other; do this twice with each leg. The heel of the forward foot may touch the floor. It is a failure:

1. To lose the balance.
2. Not to do the stunt twice with each leg.

Test 18. Full right turn. Stand with both feet together. Swing the arms and jump up in the air, making a full turn to the right. Land on the same spot and do not lose the balance, that is, do not move the feet after they first strike the floor. It is a failure:

1. Not to make a full turn and to land facing in the same direction as at the start.
2. To lose the balance and have to step about to keep from falling.

Test 19. The top. Sit down; put the arms between the legs and under and behind the knees; grasp the ankles; roll rapidly around to the right with the weight first over the right knee, then the right shoulder, then on the back, then left shoulder, then left knee; then sit up facing in the opposite direction from that in which you started. Repeat from this position and finish facing in the same direction from which you started. It is a failure:

1. To let go of the ankles.

2. Not to complete the circle.

Test 20. Single squat balance.   Squat as far down as possible on either foot. Stretch the other leg forward off the floor, hands on hips. Hold this position for five counts. It is a failure:

1. To remove the hands from the hips.

2. To touch the floor with the extended foot.

3. To lose the balance.

*Test 21. Jump foot.   Hold the toes of either foot in the opposite hand. Jump up and jump the free foot over the foot that is held, without letting go. It is a failure:

1. To let go of the foot that is held.

2. Not to jump through the loop made by holding the foot.

Administration of the Iowa-Brace Test.   The pupils should be divided in two rows facing each other, about 10 feet apart. There should be at least 3 feet between pupils. One group is seated while the other remains standing. Direction cards should be prepared in advance for the particular age group to be tested. The stunt should be read from the card exactly as it appears in the text by the examiner. While the directions are being read, it is advisable to have an assistant (who has previously shown competence in the tests) demonstrate the proper way in which the stunt is to be performed. Also, the common faults that result in a failure should be executed by the assistant as the examiner reads from the direction card. Once the demonstration is completed the examiner should ask if there are any questions. If not, the group of pupils standing performs the stunt. In this manner each of the first five stunts is performed by the first group. At the completion of the fifth stunt, this group sits down and the second group stands. The second group starts with the first stunt and continues until the entire ten stunts are completed. The first group then stands and completes the remaining five stunts. In this manner both groups have the opportunity to witness five of the stunts before being asked to perform them.

The following are the stunts used for the various grades:

	Boys				
Elementary Grades 4–6		Junior high school Grades 7–9		Senior high school Grades 10–12	
1st half	2nd half	1st half	2nd half	1st half	2nd half
10	2	1	2	1	3
4	3	14	3	11	14
13	7	13	12	16	15
11	16	19	16	5	17
8	17	6	17	20	21
		Girls			
10	1	2	1	3	2
18	3	12	13	11	18
8	16	15	11	7	16
19	15	19	16	17	9
11	6	17	20	19	20

Scoring Iowa-Brace Test.   The pupil is given two points for successful completion of each stunt on the first trial, one point for success on the second trial, and zero points if he fails to pass the test in two attempts.

Obviously, the scores on stunt tests of this nature can be greatly affected through practice. McCloy recommends that the test be used once every three years for the same group.

JOHNSON TEST OF MOTOR EDUCABILITY

Johnson, in 1932, published a description of a test of motor educability to be used for homogeneous grouping of pupils in physical education classes.[17] The validity of the test is .69; however, the criterion measure is not mentioned. In another study, Koob, using the number of trials necessary for junior high school boys to learn ten tumbling stunts, obtained an *r* of .95 between the Johnson test and motor educability. Koob[21] also obtained a correlation of .81 between this test and three track and field events.

Using the Johnson test with girls, Gire and Espenschade[9] report a reliability coefficient of .61. Hatlestad,[10] studying motor educability of college women, indicates a need for greater objectivity in the Johnson test.

Administration of Johnson Test.   A target is drawn on a canvas 4½ feet wide and 15 feet long, the length of which is divided into three squares, 18 inches wide (Fig. 60). The outline of the target and the lines marking the 18-inch squares are painted black and are ¾ of an inch wide. The two outside lanes are divided into ten 18-inch squares. The second,

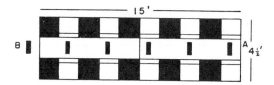

Figure 60. Canvas markings for Johnson test. A, Start. B, Finish.

fourth, and alternate squares in the two outside lanes are painted black. The center lane is not marked off in squares, but the first, third, and other alternate spaces in this lane each contain a "target" 12 inches by 3 inches in the center of the square. There is an additional "target" placed outside the canvas on the finish side. There is another lane 2 feet wide, marked in red down the center of the canvas, divided half way by a cross line of red; this is used only for the rolling exercises.

The target should be placed over two joined mats and the ends of the canvas tucked under the mats. Preferably, the canvas, after it is folded under the mats, should be laced to insure a smooth and taut surface.

The test consists of the following ten stunts:

1. *Straddle jump.*   Hands on hips. Start with feet together in first center target (*A*). Jump astraddle to first two black squares. Return to

feet-together position on second target. Proceed thus across mat in regular jumps, finishing on the finish target.

2. *Stagger skip.*   Hands on hips. Start with feet together in front of right lane (*B*). Step with left foot on first center target and hop, still on left foot, to first black square on left. Step with right foot to second center target and hop, still on right foot, to second black square on right. Continue in regular skips across mat.

3. *Stagger jump.*   Hands on hips. Feet together throughout exercise. Start with feet together in front of right lane (*B*). Jump obliquely with both feet to first black square on right, then to second white square on left, finishing on finish target.

4. *Forward skip, holding opposite foot from behind.*   Start with feet together before either right or left lane (optional), hop with right foot into first white space, raising left foot behind and taking it with right hand behind right thigh at the same time. Hop in this position on right foot to first black space. Release left foot and leap with left foot to second white space, lifting right foot behind and taking it with left hand behind left thigh. Hop in this position on left foot to second black space. Continue thus across mat.

5. *Front roll.*   Disregard all black markings and perform in red lane. Start outside of chart in front of center lane. Perform two front rolls, the first within the limits of the first half of the lane, the second within the limits of the second half, never touching or overreaching the red lanes.

6. *Jumping half turns, right or left.*   Start with feet together on first target, hands free. Jump, feet together, to second target while executing a half turn to the right or left, ending on second target facing starting end. Jump to third target, executing another half turn, rotating in the same direction (as a barrel would be rolled along upright), ending on third target facing the finish. Continue across mat, ending on finish target facing starting end.

7. *Back roll.*   Perform in red lane. Start in front of red lane with back to pattern. Execute two back rolls, one on each half of the lane.

8. *Jumping half turns, right and left alternately.*   Start as in 6, on first target. Jump with both feet, as in 6, to third target, executing half turn in the opposite direction. Continue across mat, alternating the direction of rotation, finishing as in 6.

9. *Front and back roll combination.*   Perform in red lane. Start as in 5, facing red lane. Perform a front roll in the first half of the lane, finishing with legs crossed at ankles and executing a pivot with both feet, turning either right or left. Perform a back roll in second half of the lane.

10. *Jumping full turns.*   Start outside of chart in front of first white space in either outside lane. Jump with feet together into first black space in same lane, executing a full right or left turn with the body. Continue across mat, executing full turns, rotating in the same direction, being sure to land on both feet in back spaces.

Scoring the Johnson Test. A maximum of 100 points may be scored, with a range of 0 to 10 for each stunt.

In executing a step, skip, or jump into white or black squares one or both feet must land entirely within the particular square; however, no part of the foot may touch the outside square. Furthermore, in executing the step, skip, or jump, the feet or foot, whichever the case may be, must land on the target without touching the side lines or outside lanes. In performing the rolls, the subject must not touch or overreach the red lines, and must complete the roll within the prescribed half limits. All the exercises must be performed with reasonably erect and dignified posture. The jumps must be performed with regular rhythm, approximately two short jumps per second, or five seconds for each exercise.

Penalty points are deducted for the following reasons:

Exercise 1. Deduct 1 from the score for each jump in which the feet overstep the squares or miss the target; 1 for each jump in which the feet do not land at the same time; 1 if the hands are removed from the hips at some point during the exercise; and 1 if rhythm is not maintained. Even if rhythm is broken more than once, a person is penalized only for the first time.

Exercise 2. Score as for Exercise 1, except that the feet need not come down together.

Exercise 3. Score as in Exercise 1.

Exercise 4. Deduct 1 for each step or jump in which the subject oversteps a square or in which he does not have the proper position of hand and opposite foot or both. (Only one penalty is given for each square.) Deduct 1 for lack of rhythm.

Exercise 5. Count 5 for each roll. Deduct 2 for overreaching the red line at the right or left in each roll. (If the subject overreaches both sides, deduct 4.) Deduct 1 for overreaching the limit on each roll. For failure to perform a true roll, deduct 5. If the subject fails on first roll, he should be permitted to take his position and try the second roll.

Exercise 6. Deduct 2 for each jump in which the subject does not land with both feet on the target, or turns the wrong way, or both. Since the half-turn jumps are in the same direction, the scorer should not be too critical of the subject if he does not turn exactly 180 degrees.

Exercise 7. Score as in Exercise 5.

Exercise 8. Score as in Exercise 6, except that, since the subject turns alternately to right and left, the turn must be made approximately 180 degrees. If the subject lands on the target and makes no other error except that the turn is not quite 180 degrees, subtract 1 point. (This is a variant from Johnson's scoring technique, recommended by McCloy.)

Exercise 9. Score as in Exercise 5, deducting 1 if the subject oversteps the border or executes the turn incorrectly.

Exercise 10. Score as in Exercise 6. Deduct 2 if the subject fails to land on both feet simultaneously, if he oversteps the black square, or turns too far or not far enough, or loses his balance before starting the next jump. If the only error is in not making a complete 360-degree turn, but if the subject makes a turn of more than three-fourths of a circle, deduct 1 point. (This is a variant from Johnson's scoring technique, recommended by McCloy.)

Organization of subjects. It is recommended that about twenty pupils be tested in a forty-minute period. Ten pupils can be conveniently tested at a time. The subjects should be lined up facing the mats; the examiner reads the test while an assistant demonstrates the first event. The errors are indicated by the examiner and demonstrated by the assistant, in the manner similar to that employed for the administration of the Iowa-Brace test. The test is demonstrated once, and all pupils perform each stunt before the next one is read and demonstrated.

Some authors suggest the use of student scorers. However, unless they have exhibited their abilities in practice sessions under the supervision of the physical educator, it is best not to rely upon students for scoring this particular test.

To weight the effect of the same subjects always performing the test first or last, the pupils should be rotated. The rotation for ten pupils would be as follows:

TEST NUMBER	ORDER OF SUBJECTS
1	1, 2, 3, 4, 5
2	2, 3, 4, 5, 1
3	3, 4, 5, 1, 2
4	4, 5, 1, 2, 3
5	5, 1, 2, 3, 4

JOHNSON-METHENY TEST

Metheny,[33] in a study of the Johnson test, found that tests 5, 7, 8, and 10 (p. 185) for boys correlated .977 with the total Johnson score. In addition, she found that these four items correlated .934 against the criterion of learning tumbling stunts. For girls, the Metheny revision, using tests 5, 7, and 8 (p. 185), correlated .868 with the entire Johnson test. By eliminating six of the original items, Metheny was able to simplify considerably the target used in performing the tests. Figure 61 illustrates the canvas markings for the Johnson-Metheny test. The canvas is 15 feet long with a lane 24 inches wide, marked down the middle. This lane is divided

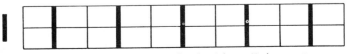

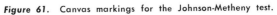

Figure 61. Canvas markings for the Johnson-Metheny test.

in two by a center line running the entire length of the mat. The lane is then divided into ten equal parts by lines running parallel, every 18 inches, the width of the target. These lines are alternately ¾ of an inch wide and 3 inches wide, with the centers 18 inches apart.

LATCHAW MOTOR SKILLS TEST

After examining the physical education curriculum at the fourth, fifth, and sixth grade levels for boys and girls, Latchaw[24] concluded that running, jumping, throwing, catching, striking, and kicking were fundamental to the activities taught.

The following test items were selected to measure these fundamental skills:

1. Shuttle run to measure agility and speed in running.
2. Vertical jump for height.
3. Standing broad jump for distance.
4. Basketball wall pass ⎫ to demonstrate the ability of the child
5. Softball repeated throws ⎭ to manipulate two different sized balls.
6. Volleyball wall volley for striking ability.
7. Soccer wall volley for kicking.

Reliability of the test items was determined by administering them to approximately 50 boys and 50 girls at each grade level. What is referred to as *face validity* was claimed for each of the seven items. For example, the standing broad jump is a test that measures one's ability to stand and jump; so too with the vertical jump for height. As a result, no statistical study using a criterion measure was employed to establish validity for each item.

The reliability coefficients ranged from .77 for the soccer wall volley and softball repeated throws to .97 for the standing broad jump. That the major portion of the correlations were in the upper 80's and middle 90's indicates quite satisfactory results regarding reliability.

Latchaw, after careful analysis of her data, concluded:

1. The relationship between age, height, and weight and performance as measured by these tests was relatively low.

2. Generally, the scores were higher from grade to grade with the following exceptions:

a. For the fifth and sixth grade boys there was no significant difference in the vertical jump, standing broad jump, and shuttle run.

b. There was no significant difference between the mean scores of fourth and fifth grade girls, and fifth and sixth grade girls, in the standing broad jump and the shuttle run.

3. Apparently, experience or maturation was a more significant factor in determining performance in these test items than was age for the group studied.

Test administration. *Basketball wall pass.* This test measures the ability of the subject to throw a basketball successively into a given target area from a specified distance.

The equipment consists of a regulation basketball and a stop watch. On a flat wall space, a target area is marked 8 feet wide and 4 feet high, at a distance of 3 feet from the floor. A restraining line 8 feet long is drawn on the floor 4 feet from the wall and parallel to the wall target.

The subject stands at any position he chooses in back of the restraining line. On the signal "go," he throws the ball against the wall into the target area in any manner that he chooses, and continues successive throws until the signal "stop" is given. If the ball gets out of control at any time, he must recover it without assistance. A throw is considered successful when the ball, thrown from behind the restraining line, hits the target area. Balls hitting the target line are not fair hits. The ball may be caught on a bounce if the subject so chooses. However, the ball need not be caught to constitute a successful throw.

One point is given for each successful throw. The subject is given a ten-second practice trial, for which the score is not recorded. The test administrator scores verbally during this trial, and encourages the subject to retrieve lost balls rapidly and to throw the ball as fast as he can successfully manipulate it. Two 15-second trials are given after the practice trial. The total number of points is recorded for *each* trial. The better of the two trials is the final score for the test.

Volleyball wall volley. This test measures the ability of the subject to strike a volleyball with his hands successively against the wall within a given target area and from a specified distance on the floor.

The equipment consists of a regulation volleyball and a stop watch. On a flat wall space, a target area is marked 8 feet wide and at least 4 feet high, at a distance of 3 feet from the floor. A restraining line 8 feet long is drawn on the floor 4 feet from the wall and parallel to the wall target.

The subject stands at any position he chooses in back of the restraining line. On the signal "go," he tosses or throws the ball against the wall into the target area, and as it rebounds he continues to bat it repeatedly against the wall. The ball may be tossed against the wall when it is necessary to start again. If the ball gets out of control, the subject retrieves it, brings it back to the restraining line, and starts again. In a successful hit, the ball, upon rebounding from the wall, is clearly batted into the target area from behind the restraining line on the floor. The hit is not considered successful if the ball is thrown or pushed against the wall. Balls hitting the target line are not fair hits.

One point is given for each successful hit. The subject is given a ten-second practice trial. The test administrator scores verbally during this trial, calling the attention of the subject to balls that are not legal hits if he pushes the ball at any time. This score is not recorded. Four 15-second trials are given after the practice trial. The total number of points is recorded for *each* trial. The best of the four trials is the final score for the test.

Vertical jump.   This test measures the ability of the subject to jump vertically from a stationary position on the floor.

One-inch cloth strips are suspended from a horizontal bar, and spaced at 1-inch intervals from each other. The longest strip is 5 feet from the floor and the shortest strip is 8 feet 11 inches from the floor. Each strip is weighted with a penny at the end nearest the floor to insure even hanging.

The subject stands with both heels on the floor under the suspended strips, and, reaching with one hand, touches the highest strip that he can. This is recorded under "reaching height." The subject then jumps from a stationary position under the bar, and reaches the highest strip that he can. He may start from a crouch if he wishes, but he may not take any steps or preliminary bounces. Any number of trials is allowed, but it is advisable to estimate where the subject's best jump will be, in order to avoid fatigue from too many trials.

The score is the difference in inches between the height of the reach and the height of the best jump.

Standing broad jump.   This test measures the ability of the subject to jump horizontally from a standing position.

The equipment consists of a tumbling mat, 9 feet long, and a measuring tape, unless the mat is permanently ruled.

The subject stands with the toes of both feet touching the restraining line that marks the take-off area, and from this standing position jumps as far forward as he can. Any preliminary movement must be executed with some part of both feet in contact with take-off area. The subject is given three successive trials and measurement is taken to the last inch. For example, if the subject jumps 5 feet 2½ inches, the jump is recorded as 5 feet 2 inches. This distance is measured from the restraining line of the take-off area to the nearest contact made on landing. (This measurement is usually to the first heel mark made on landing; but if the subject loses balance, falls backward, and catches himself with his hand or body, the mark nearest the restraining line is used in measuring the distance of the jump.)

The best of three trials, in feet and inches, is the score for the test.

Shuttle run.   This test, which necessitates quick stops and changes of direction, measures the ability of the subject to run rapidly between two given marks.

A stop watch, calibrated in 1/10-second intervals, is the equipment used. Two 12-inch lines are marked on the floor, parallel to each other and 20 feet apart. One of these lines is the starting line, which should have an unobstructed area behind it at least 20 feet long to give the runner an opportunity to check his speed *after* passing this line upon completing his run.

The subject stands with the toes of his forward foot on the starting line. On the signal "go," he runs to the opposite line, touches it (or the area beyond it) with one or both feet, and returns to touch the starting line. This constitutes one complete trip. The subject does not stop, but continues running to the opposite line until he has completed three trips. or a total of 120 feet. If the subject fails to touch or step over a line at any time during the run, he is stopped at once and no score is recorded for the trial. After a brief resting period he is given one opportunity to repeat this performance, and if he fails again to execute the test correctly, the test score is rejected.

The time in tenths of a second is recorded from the signal "go" to the crossing of the starting line upon completing the three trips.

Two trials are given in this test. Subjects are tested in pairs, with two children running alternately, one resting while the other is performing.

The score for this test is the better of the two trials, recorded in seconds to the nearest tenth.

Soccer wall volley.   This test measures the ability of the subject to kick a soccer ball successively against the wall within a given target area and from a specified distance on the floor.

The equipment consists of a regulation soccer ball and a stop watch. On a flat wall space, a target area 4 feet wide is marked at $2\frac{1}{2}$ feet from the floor. On the floor, extending from and parallel to the wall target, a similar area (4 feet wide and $2\frac{1}{2}$ feet long) is marked. The 4-foot line on the floor at the greatest distance from the wall target is extended 1 foot on either side, and constitutes the restraining line.

The ball is placed behind the restraining line at any position the subject chooses (usually toward the center of the line). On the signal "go," the subject kicks the ball against the wall into the target area, and as it rebounds he continues to kick it repeatedly against the wall. If the ball gets out of control, the subject retrieves it, brings it back to the restraining line, and starts again. The subject may not touch the ball with his hands while it is in the rectangular floor area between the re-straining line and the target. If the ball stops within this area, he must remove it with his foot. Whenever the ball goes outside of this rectangular floor area, the subject may use his hands in retrieving or moving it.

A successful hit is one in which the ball is kicked into the target area on the wall from *behind* the restraining line on the floor. Balls hitting the target line are not fair hits. To score a fair hit, the subject must kick the ball from in back of the restraining line (not *on* it), and the ball must land between the lines that bound the wall target.

One point is given for each successful hit. Each time that the ball is touched with the hands when it is inside the rectangular floor area, one point is subtracted from the score. The subject is given a 15-second practice trial, for which the score is not recorded. The test administrator scores verbally during this trial, calling attention to illegal hits. Four

15-second trials are given after the practice trial. The total number of points is recorded for *each* trial. The best of the four trials is the final score for the test.

Softball repeated throws. This test measures the ability of the subject to throw a softball, using an overhand throw, into a given target area from a specified distance.

A regulation 12-inch inseam softball and a stop watch are used for this test.

On a flat wall space, a target area is marked 5½ feet wide and at least 10 feet high, at a distance of 6 inches from the floor. A throwing area, 5½ feet square, is marked on the floor at a distance of 9 feet from the target and parallel to it. A backstop, 12 feet long and at least 2½ feet high, is placed 15 feet in back of the throwing area.

The subject stands at any position he chooses inside the throwing area. On the signal "go," he throws the ball against wall into the target area, using an overhand throw, and continues successive throws until the signal "stop" is given. The balls may be received from the target on either the bounce or the fly. If the ball gets out of control at any time, the subject must recover it without assistance. Most of these balls will be stopped by the backstop; if not, the subject must chase the balls himself. A successful throw is made from inside the throwing area, and is an overhand throw by which the ball goes into the target area. Balls hitting the target line are not fair hits.

One point is given for each successful throw. The subject is given a ten-second practice trial. The test administrator scores verbally during this trial. This score is not recorded. Two 15-second trials are given after the practice trial. The total number of points is recorded for *each* trial. The better of the two trials is the final score for the test.

Perceptual Motor Evaluation

There is evidence that the efficiency of the higher thought processes can be no better than the basic motor abilities upon which they are based; that is, for his higher thought processes to function at their best, a child's neuromuscular development must be adequate. Both Kephart[18] and Delacato[7] emphasize the close relationship between difficulty in learning and the inability of slow learners to perform neuromuscularly. Neuromuscular development can be attained only through the physical activity experiences provided in a good physical education program. Neuromuscular activities are definitely associated with learning in the classroom; thus there is a vital reason for elementary school physical education.

Steinhaus[40] reports that in a small French town roughly half of the time that elementary school children had spent in the classroom was freed in their final year for all forms of sports and gymnastic activities;

88.8 per cent of these children passed the final government examination, whereas only 60 per cent of the other children passed these examinations.

The child's entire physical and physiological orientation to his immediate environment must progress within normal limits or difficulties in learning to read are liable to present themselves. For example, the child obviously must know left from right, or as Kephart suggests, how will he know the difference between the letters "b" or "d" while learning to read?

Kephart[19] states that many of the children who show difficulty in school learning in grades one through three will also show difficulties in perceptual motor development, and that these perceptual motor difficulties are fundamentally related to school achievement. He further points out the need to identify these children and the point of breakdown as early as possible. A perceptual motor screening test is used for this purpose.

The perceptual motor survey includes physical activities ranging from such simple movements as walking, to complex activities such as performance on a balance beam or trampoline. The objective for the physical education teacher is to find those children whose motor development is retarded. The teacher must watch the child carefully, observing not only the youngster's success in executing the skill, but also the particular way in which he accomplishes or attempts to accomplish the task. With experience in the use of the perceptual motor survey, the examiner will become proficient in detecting motor retardation. There is no statistical norm for this test; one must evaluate a single child's performance as it is related to the class as a whole. To be sure, a child can be marked "pass" or "fail" if he does not successfully walk a balance beam, for example. However, you as the teacher should watch not only for the "pass" or "fail," but also for the way in which the task is accomplished. Does the child perform in easy, relaxed, coordinated movements? Or is he stiff, fearful, and unrelaxed? Such observations are necessary to determine the level of his success as compared with the success of his peers. Furthermore, it again must be emphasized that practice in such observations results in a more skillful examiner. It has been estimated that as many as 20 per cent of school children in the first three grades are to some degree retarded in motor development.

Selection of the skills which should be included in the perceptual survey is limited only by the imagination of the teacher. However, the survey should at least include activities which will permit appraisal of: laterality, directionality, balance, hand-eye coordination, and conceptualization.

Laterality.   The child should know his left side from his right side. For example, he must learn to move laterally both his right arm and his left arm. He must learn to move simultaneously both arms, an arm and a leg, and the opposite arms and legs. In other words, he must learn to control the two sides of his body both separately and simultaneously.

Directionality.   The child must learn to orient himself with reference to the space and objects in his immediate environment. For example, the dimensions of height, breadth, and depth are learned in relation to objects in his immediate environment, such as chairs, tables, and boxes. The child will understand his environment more completely when his neuromuscular system interprets the images that his eyes receive.

Hand-eye coordination.   The ability of the child to throw, to catch, and to strike requires a close working relationship between the eyes and the neuromuscular system.

Balance.   Balance is maintained by the neuromuscular system, which receives information regarding one's position in space by a so-called transistorized relay system. The semicircular canals in the ears and the proprioceptors in muscles keep one constantly informed with regard to both position and the relationship of one appendage to another. Experts in gymnastics, diving, and trampoline performance possess well-developed neuromuscular balance systems.

Conceptualization (solution of movement pattern problems).   This skill is observed through the use of an obstacle course, which may be as elaborately arranged as time, money, and imagination permit. To get the job done, one needs merely wands and chairs. The examiner's objective is to watch how the child manipulates his entire body and its individual parts as he walks forward and sideways, stepping over and crawling under obstacles, to negotiate the course. Here the youngster is observed as he solves movement pattern problems. As he turns sideways, for example, to pass through a narrow corridor (chairs lined up—see Figure 64) does he repeatedly bang into the chairs? Does he touch one chair and then continue on without hitting any more? His ability to solve the pattern problem successfully is dependent on how well he can conceptualize (understand the problem) and his neuromuscular execution.

Following are examples of activities that the survey might include.

Balance beam (Fig. 62).   With the beam in the widest position, the child performs the following maneuvers:

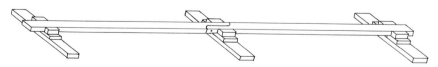

Figure 62. Wellnitz Portable Balance Beam. Manufactured by The Wellnitz Company, Columbus, Ohio.

1. Walks length of beam.
2. Walks backward on beam.
3. Slides sideways to the left.
4. Slides sideways to the right.

5. Walks sideways to the left, crossing right foot over left.
6. Walks sideways to the right, crossing left foot over right.
7. Hops length of beam on right foot.
8. Hops length of beam on left foot.
9. Repeats exercises one through six with the beam in the narrow position.
10. Repeats exercises one through six carrying a 1- to 2-pound weight, first in his right hand, then in his left.

Observe the child in terms of how relaxed he is, whether he skillfully uses both arms for balancing or only one arm, whether he moves rapidly to avoid balancing, and how perfectly he controls his body. Those children who fail the items must be forced to perform even if the instructor has to hold them while they practice. Such cases suggest that it is perhaps much easier to work with the truly motor retarded singularly or in very small groups (of less than five children).

Evaluation: Mark each maneuver on the following scale, recording also the grade, name, and age of the child and the date of the examination.

> 0—Failure
> 1—Fair
> 2—Average
> 3—Superior

Motor coordination and balance. On the floor, two parallel lines 3 inches wide and 10 feet long are marked at a distance of 15 feet from each other. Several 3-inch wooden cubes are used for this exercise.

1. The child stands on one line, from which he walks to the second line, picks up a 3-inch cube, walks back, and places the cube on the starting line. Instructions should require that the cube be placed precisely on the line.

2. The child repeats exercise 1 using his other hand.

Observe handedness, any hesitancy in retrieving the cubes, ability to place the cubes perfectly on the line, and ease or difficulty in retrieving the cubes (e.g., balance).

3. The child jumps the length of the line with his feet together.
4. The child hops the length of the line on his left foot.
5. The child hops the length of the line on his right foot.
6. The child hops the length of the line twice on each foot, alternately.
7. The child skips down the line and back.

Observe the child's balance and his ability to execute the stunts smoothly and without extraneous movements. Observe also his ability to distinguish right and left and to hop equally well on his right and left feet.

Obstacle course (Fig. 63). Chairs are placed 16 inches apart for forward and backward walking, and 12 inches apart for walking sideways. Some wands may be placed on the chairs at a height that requires the children to duck in order to negotiate the course; other wands may be

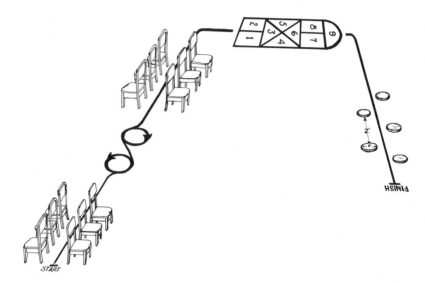

Figure 63.   Obstacle course for perceptual motor evaluation.

placed at a height requiring the children to step over the obstacles. The objective here is to evaluate the child's knowledge of his relationship to the objects about him. Does he move through the corridor without touching the chairs? Can he step over a wand and duck under it without knocking the object from the chair?

Exercises using a hopscotch target and stepping stone diagram require considerable neuromuscular skill, involving total body coordination. These are entertaining activities and can help in motivating the children. A motor perceptual obstacle course can be varied in order to maintain the children's interest and encourage them to practice.

Angels in the snow.   This activity is used to evaluate the child's ability to use both sides of his body.

The youngster, in a supine position, is asked to raise both hands over his head, sliding his arms across the floor. The exercise is repeated with the legs, an arm and a leg on the same side, and arm and a leg on the opposite side, and finally with both arms and legs.

Oseretsky Test—K.D.K. Revision.[20]   A Russian, N. Oseretsky, published one of the first scales of motor development organized by age levels from four to sixteen years. The test was designed to measure general static coordination, dynamic manual coordination, general dynamic coordination, motor speed, simultaneous voluntary movements, and asynkinesia (lack of precision in movement). The items contained in the test were selected primarily through clinical observation; the tasks chosen were ones which would aid in diagnosis of motor and neurological deficiencies. Since Oseretsky published his test there have been several revisions, the most recent one by Kershner and Dusewicz. Their version reduces the time required for administration through the use of group techniques. Forty-six items constitute the complete test battery, among them the following:

Task. Hop on one foot completely around a chair in a counter-clockwise direction. Then repeat using other foot.

Criterion. Score positive if subject is able to hop around chair as directed without suspended foot touching floor and without any part of body touching chair. (One success in four trials = ½ point per leg)

Task. Walk backwards, heel to toe with hands on hips, along a straight line 2 yards long and 2 inches wide.

Criterion. Score positive if subject is able to walk the length of the line backwards as directed, touching toe of moving foot to heel of stationary foot on each step taken and keeping both feet continually on the line. (One success in four trials = 1 point)

Task. Balance a yardstick on end, vertically, on the palm side of the tip of one forefinger.

Criterion. Score positive if subject is able to initiate balancing of yardstick and then maintain balance for ten seconds. (One success in four trials = 1 point)

Task. Extending arms out to sides and holding arm and wrist joints rigid, describe circles with forefingers.

Criterion. Score positive if subject can continue circular movement of forefingers for ten seconds without moving hands, wrists, or arms. (One success in four trials = 1 point)

Task. Rub abdomen with one hand, with circular motion of arm. Pat top of head with the other hand, using up and down motion of arm.

Criterion. Score positive if both actions can be performed simultaneously without interruption for ten seconds. (One success in four trials = 1 point).

Kraus-Weber tests (Page 97). Good muscular tonus is essential for learning motor movements. The Kraus-Weber tests provide an easy way of evaluating minimum muscular fitness.

The stunts and exercises contained in the perceptual survey may also be used as activities for the development of neuromuscular coordination.

The stunts and exercises which have been mentioned here are only a few of the infinite combinations of activities which may be employed. You as a teacher should evaluate the neuromuscular status of your pupils.

BIBLIOGRAPHY

1. Anderson, Theresa W.: Weighted Strength Tests for the Prediction of Athletic Ability in High School Girls. Research Quart., Vol. 7, No. 1, March, 1936.

2. Barrow, Harold: A Test of Motor Ability for College Men. Doctoral Dissertation, University of Indiana, 1953.

3. Barrow, Harold M.: Test of Motor Ability for College Men. Research Quart., 25: 253–260, 1954.

4. Bovard, John F., Cozens, Frederick W., and Hagman, E. Patricia: Tests and Measurements in Physical Education. 3rd ed. Philadelphia, W. B. Saunders Company, 1949.

5. Brace, David K.: Measuring Motor Ability. New York, A. S. Barnes & Co., 1927.

6. Clarke, H. Harrison, and Bonesteel, Harold A.: Equalizing the Abilities of Intramural Teams in a Small High School. Supplement to Research Quart., March, 1935.

7. Delacato, Carl H.: The Diagnosis and Treatment of Speech and Reading Problems. Springfield, Illinois, Charles C Thomas, 1963.

8. Department of Physical Education for Men, Oberlin College: Qualifying Test for Elective Program in Physical Education. J. Health & Phys. Educ., Vol. 7, No. 8, October, 1936.

9. Gire, Eugenia, and Espenschade, Anna: The Relationship between Measures of Motor Educability and the Learning of Specific Skills. Research Quart., Vol. 13, No. 1, March, 1942.

10. Hatlestad, Lucile: Motor Educability Tests for Women College Students. Research Quart., Vol. 13, No. 1, March, 1942.

11. Henry, Franklin M.: Influence of Motor and Sensory Sets on Reaction Latency and Speed of Discrete Movements. Research Quart., October, 1960.

12. Henry, Franklin M., and Farmer, S. Daniel: Condition Ratings and Endurance Measures. Research Quart., 20:2, 126–133, May, 1949.

13. Henry, Franklin M., and Kleeberger, F. L.: The Validity of the Pulse-Ratio Test of Cardiac Efficiency. Research Quart., 9:1, 32–46, 1938.

14. Henry, Franklin M., and Rogers, Donald E.: Increased Response Latency for Complicated Movements and a "Memory Drum" Theory of Neuromotor Reaction. Research Quart., October, 1960.

15. Humiston, Dorothy: A Measurement of Motor Ability in College Women. Research Quart., 8:181–185, 1937.

16. Humiston, Dorothy: A Measurement of Motor Ability in Women. Unpublished Doctor's Dissertation, New York University, 1936.

17. Johnson, Granville B.: Physical Skill Tests for Sectioning Classes into Homogeneous Units. Research Quart., Vol. 3, No. 1, March, 1932.

18. Kephart, Newell C.: The Slow Learner in the Classroom. Columbus, Ohio, Charles E. Merrill Books, Inc., 1960, p. 37.

19. Kephart, Newell C.: Ibid., p. 121.

20. Kershner, K. M., and Dusewicz, R.: "K. D. K.—Oseretsky Tests of Motor Development." Perceptual and Motor Skills, 1970.

21. Koob, Clarence G.: A Study of the Johnson Skills Test as a Measure of Motor Educability. Unpublished Master's Thesis, State University of Iowa, Iowa City, Iowa, 1937.

22. Larson, Leonard A.: A Factor Analysis of Motor Ability Variables and Test, with Tests for College Men. Research Quart., Vol. 12, No. 3, October, 1941.

23. Larson, Leonard A.: A Factor and Validity Analysis of Strength Variables and Tests with a Test Combination of Chinning, Dipping, and Vertical Jump. Research Quart., Vol. 11, No. 4, December, 1940.

24. Latchaw, Marjorie: Measuring Selected Motor Skills in Fourth, Fifth, and Sixth Grades. Research Quart., 24:4, 439, December, 1954.

25. Lockhart, Aileen, and Mott, Jane A.: An Experiment in Homogeneous Grouping and Its Effect on Achievement in Sports Fundamentals. Research Quart., Vol. 22, No. 1, March, 1951.

26. McCloy, C. H.: A Factor Analysis of Tests of Endurance. Research Quart., Vol. 27, No. 2, May, 1956.

27. McCloy, C. H.: A New Method of Scoring Chinning and Dipping. Research Quart., Vol. 2, No. 4, December, 1931.

28. McCloy, C. H.: A Preliminary Study of Factors in Motor Educability. Research Quart., Vol. 11, No. 2, May, 1940.
29. McCloy, C. H.: An Analytical Study of the Stunt Type Tests as a Measure of Motor Educability. Research Quart., Vol. 8, No. 3, October, 1937.
30. McCloy, C. H.: The Measurement of Athletic Power. New York, A. S. Barnes & Co., 1932.
31. McCloy, C. H.: The Measurement of General Motor Capacity and General Motor Ability. Supplement to Research Quart., March, 1934.
32. McCloy, C. H., and Young, Norma Dorothy: Tests and Measurements in Health and Physical Education. 3rd ed. New York, Appleton-Century-Crofts, Inc., 1954.
33. Metheny, Eleanor: Studies of the Johnson Test as a Test of Motor Educability. Research Quart., Vol. 9, No. 4, December, 1938.
34. Neilson, N. P., and Cozens, F. W.: Achievement Scales in Physical Education Activities for Boys and Girls in Elementary and Junior High Schools. New York, A. S. Barnes & Co., 1934.
35. Powell, Elizabeth, and Howe, E. C.: Motor Ability Tests for High School Girls. Research Quart., Vol. 10, No. 4, December, 1939.
36. Rogers, Frederick Rand: Physical Capacity Tests in the Administration of Physical Education. New York, Bureau of Publications, Teachers College, Columbia University, 1925.
37. Rouhlac, C. M.: A Factor Analysis of Cozens' General Athletic Ability Test. Springfield, Mass., Springfield College, Unpublished Master's Thesis, 1940.
38. Scott, Gladys M.: The Assessment of Motor Ability of College Women. Research Quart., Vol. 10, No. 3, October, 1939.
39. Shay, Clayton T.: The Progressive Part versus the Whole Method of Learning Motor Skills. Research Quart., Vol. 5, No. 4, December, 1934.
40. Steinhaus, Arthur: Your Muscles See More Than Your Eyes. Journal AAHPER, p. 38, September, 1966.
41. Welman, Elizabeth B.: The Validity of Various Tests as Measures of Motor Ability. Supplement to Research Quart., March, 1935.

chapter 7

sports skill testing

Application of skill tests. Skill tests reflect the ability of the pupil to perform in a specified sport such as badminton, handball, or basketball. By knowing the level of ability of a youngster in a particular sport, it becomes possible to use his ability score for purposes of classification, determining progress, and marking.

For example, the first time a teacher meets a class in tennis it would be advisable for him to place the pupils in groups of like ability in order to facilitate teaching. Administering the tennis skill test during the first meeting of the class permits the teacher to group the youngsters immediately. With a large number of pupils, it would probably take the instructor three or four days or even a week to become sufficiently familiar with the ability of the pupils to place them subjectively in homogeneous groups.

In team selection the skill test can prove of considerable worth. When a large number of players turn out for a first practice, the coach may administer the skill test, place the players into homogeneous groups, and then, through his subjective evaluation, more efficiently select a final squad.

When it becomes necessary to equate teams, as in intramural and interclass groups, the skill test for the particular activity is again a very effective tool. Simply placing participants with similar scores on opposite teams is an effective way of equating the teams.

Administering the skill test at the beginning and end of the course permits the instructor to observe the progression of the class, and provides a means for marking the pupils.

Validity of skill tests. A word of caution should be injected here as to the amount of confidence that can be placed in the results of the skill test, particularly in respect to marking. In Chapter 2 the criteria used in determining the statistical value of a test—objectivity, reliability, and validity—were given. With these three criteria in mind it might be well to discuss briefly how skill tests are constructed, in order to gain a greater understanding of their application.

Skill tests are constructed in most cases by careful studies of the various components or specific skills of the sport, that is, those deemed vital for successful performance. As an illustration, a test for basketball might proceed in accordance with the following general outline:

1. Critically examine the sport to determine the skills most essential for successful performance in the activity. In basketball, skills such as shooting, passing, dribbling, and pivoting would be highly important to playing ability. Therefore, you might select these skills as variables to be measured in making up a basketball skill test.

2. The variables selected for measurement are administered as a test to a large sample of the group of subjects to whom the results are to be applied, say, for example, junior varsity and varsity high school basketball players.

3. The final step is to ascertain whether those who scored high on the test were also the better basketball players. This may be done by having the coaches (board of experts) rank each of the players in regard to his basketball playing ability. If there is a close relationship—that is, a high correlation between the experts' ratings and the test scores—you may then conclude that the test is valid, as it measures what it purports to measure.

If you were constructing a test for an individual rather than a team sport, say a test for tennis, you would most likely proceed in a manner similar to the first two steps mentioned above. However, in determining validity of the test it would be better to have the selected subjects play a round-robin tournament. If the pupils' scores on the test prove to be closely related to the number of games won in the round-robin tournament, the test may be considered valid.

In selecting skill tests for use in the physical education program you must be careful to make certain that they are reliable, objective, and valid before using them. Furthermore, they should not be overly time-consuming. In some instances it might be better to rely upon rating sheets and the subjective opinion of the examiner rather than upon a long, tedious skill test. Still, it might be recognized that, when possible, the skill test should be employed, as it is more objective and meaningful to the pupil as well as to the instructor, provided it has been scientifically constructed. Although there are skill tests for almost every sport, only those tests that meet the statistical criteria for test selection, and are practical in terms of administration, have been included in this chapter.

Hyde Archery Test

The purpose of this test was to establish standards of achievement for college women in the Columbia Round. The norms or standards were constructed using approximately 1400 scores collected from twenty-seven colleges in sixteen different states.[9, 10] As the scales are sufficiently wide in range, it provides a means for evaluating the success of both beginning and advanced archers.

The norms are made in such a way that a scale score of 50 represents the average performance. A scale score of 100 is three standard deviations above the mean, while a scale score of zero is three standard deviations below the mean. This type of scaling of test scores enables one to add or average separate scale scores to obtain a total achievement score, if such is desired.

The archery scale[9] consists of three parts:

1. A scale for evaluating the total achievement in the *first* Columbia Round. This scale is the total score made in the first round ever shot by a student.

2. A scale used to evaluate the total score made in the *final* Columbia Round after an unlimited amount of practice in the event. It may be best used toward the end of the archery season in evaluating the highest or best score that the student has made during the semester.

3. A scale consisting of three separate sections for evaluating the achievement made at each of the distances (50, 40, and 30 yards) included in the round. This scale may also be used to evaluate success in shooting during a practice session in which 24 arrows constitute the practice unit. This part of the scale was constructed from the final or highest Columbia Round scores. Hence, if used to measure beginners, the achievement levels should naturally be expected to fall relatively low on the scale.

Test administration.   The author suggests that the test be given for the first time after a minimum of practice, which might include 120 arrows shot at each distance—30, 40, and 50 yards. The final round should be shot at the conclusion of the archery course as a final test of achievement. By following this procedure the beginning as well as the advanced students may be evaluated in terms of achievement.

The Columbia Round used in competition for women is as follows:

> First range: 24 arrows at 50 yards.
> Second range: 24 arrows at 40 yards.
> Third range: 24 arrows at 30 yards.

The directions for administering the test are as follows:

1. All scores shall be made on standard 48-inch target face, placed so that the center of the gold is 4 feet from the ground.

2. Not more than one practice end may be shot before beginning to record the score at each distance. The practice end may not be used in scoring.

3. At least one distance must be completed in each session.

Lockhart and McPherson Badminton Test

This volley test of badminton playing ability was established for sophomore college women.[16] Mathews, however, in using the test with freshman and sophomore men, has found it to work equally well for men as for women.[18]

The validity of the test was determined as follows:

1. Three experienced judges graded the badminton playing ability of sixty-eight girls on a 1- to 10-point scale. The total of the judges' opinions was correlated with the total scores that these players made on the badminton volleying test. The resultant coefficient of correlation was .71 ± .06.

2. Next a round-robin tournament was conducted with twenty-seven girls. The percentage of the total games won was correlated with each score the girl made on the badminton volleying test. The resultant r was .60 ± .12.

3. A third confirmation of validity was computed by correlating the total judges' opinions with the percentage of total games won by each girl in the round-robin tournament. The resulting r equalled .90 ± .03.

By the test-retest method of determining reliability, the authors obtained a correlation of .90 in administering the test twice to fifty players, within an interim of three days.

Administration of the test. The equipment consists of a badminton racket, a shuttlecock (bird), a wall space 10 feet high and 10 feet in length, a stop watch, score sheets, a 1-inch net line marked on the wall 5 feet above and parallel to the floor, a starting line drawn on the floor 6½ feet from the base of the wall, and a restraining line marked on the floor 3 feet from the base wall and parallel to the starting line (Fig. 64).

The player taking the test stands behind the starting line, holding the badminton racket in one hand and the shuttlecock in the other. On

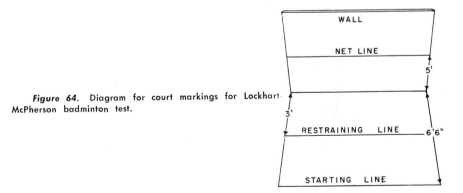

Figure 64. Diagram for court markings for Lockhart-McPherson badminton test.

the signal "ready, go" the shuttlecock is served in a legal manner against the wall on or above the net line. The shuttlecock is played as many times as possible against the wall in thirty seconds. Three trials are given to each player. Rest is allowed between trials and a practice period of fifteen seconds is given before the first trial.

Only hits that place the shuttlecock on or above the net line are considered good; one point is counted for each good hit. After the shuttlecock has been served the player may move up to the restraining line if he wishes. If the restraining line is crossed the hit is not counted, but the shuttlecock is still in play. If the bird is missed or goes out of control, the player must retrieve it and continue by putting it back in play with a serve from behind the starting line.

Scoring.   The score is the number of legal hits made on or above the backboard net line in the three trials. Tables containing T-scales based upon scores made by 178 University of Nebraska women appear in the article cited.[16]

Miller Wall Volley Test

At an amateur badminton championship tournament, a careful study was made of the number of times services, drop shots, clears, smashes, drives, and half-court drives were used during a badminton game.[19] It was found that the finalists in both men's and women's singles used clears more often than any other stroke. On this basis a cinematographical analysis of the clear shot was made to ascertain the proper distance from the wall for the wall volley test.

As a result of this analysis the following court dimensions for the test were arrived at:

1. Wall: a 1-inch line is extended across the wall 7½ feet from the floor and parallel to the floor. The width of the wall space should be at least 10 feet and the height preferably 15 feet or more.

2. Floor: a straight line 10 feet from the wall is extended the length of the wall distance and parallel to the wall.

Test administration.   The subject is permitted a one-minute practice period before the first trial. On the signal "ready, go" the subject serves the shuttlecock in a legal manner against the wall from behind the 10-foot floor line. The serve puts the shuttlecock in a position to be rallied with a clear on each rebound. If the serve hits on or above the 7½-foot wall line, that hit counts as one point and each following rebound hit made on or above the 7½-foot wall line, when the subject is behind the 10-foot floor line, counts as one point. The hit is not counted if any part of his foot goes over the 10-foot restraining line. The scorer should say "back" whenever the subject consistently goes over the line. The hit is not counted if the shuttlecock goes below the 7½-foot wall line. However, if either the foot goes over the 10-foot line or the shuttlecock hits below the 7½-foot line, the subject is permitted to keep the shuttlecock in play. The bird may be stopped at any time and restarted with a legal service from behind the 10-foot line. If the shuttlecock is missed and falls to the floor, the subject must pick it up as quickly as possible, get behind the 10-foot line, and put it into play with a legal service.

Scoring.   An accumulative number of hits made within thirty seconds is given to the recorder by the scorer for each individual. When the timer gives the signal "stop" a total number of hits is given to the recorder. Three (thirty-second) trials are given. Any stroke may be used to keep the shuttlecock in play. A "carried bird" or a double hit is counted as good if the shuttlecock eventually goes on or goes above the 7½-foot wall line. The subject may step in front of the 10-foot line in order to keep the shuttlecock in play, but hits failing to follow the stated specifications do not count. The sponge-end shuttlecock will bounce if the shuttlecock falls to the floor. The subject does not have to pick up the bird if he can keep it in play in any other manner. The score consists of the sum of the three trials.

The reliability of the test was determined by the test-retest method. One hundred college girls of all ranges of ability were given the test one day, and within a period of one week the same players were tested again. The reliability coefficient obtained was .94 ± .008.

To determine validity, the scores on the wall volley test were correlated with the results of the round-robin tournament. The resulting coefficient was .83 ± .047.

Boys' Baseball Classification Plan

Using sixty-four subjects, ages eight to twelve years, Kelson has established a practical and seemingly worth-while measure in classifying boys for baseball participation.[12] Five qualities were selected as essential to performance in baseball: batting ability; ability to throw for distance; ability to throw for accuracy; ability to catch fly balls; and ability to catch ground balls.

The boys' seasonal batting averages were used for determining batting ability. Ability to throw for distance was recorded in feet, the best of three trials being used as the score. A run was permitted in executing the throw, but the subjects were not allowed to cross a restraining line.

Ability to run bases was determined by measuring the time in tenths of a second, starting from home plate to first base, second, third, and home—a distance of 60 yards.

The remaining abilities were subjectively rated on a scale of 1 to 5 by twelve judges who took into consideration the boys' coordination and ability to handle themselves with ease in performing the skills.

Multiple correlations were computed to find the best classification index from the measures used in the study. For practical purposes it was found the baseball throw for distance could be used alone for classification, as the correlation for this event was .850. Time in running the bases raised the correlation to .853, which is a negligible increase.

Achievement Level in Basketball Skills for Women

The purpose of this study was to determine achievement levels in basketball skills based on the accomplishments of women students majoring in physical education in colleges and universities located throughout the country.[20] The three tests used for the construction of the scales were chosen on the basis of results obtained by Leilich[15] in a factor analysis study covering all the basketball skill tests that have appeared in the literature.

The scales, which appear in reference 20, have been constructed in the form of T-scores and percentile ranks based upon data gathered from fifty-nine colleges. These standards are designed particularly for use in the professional physical education curriculum.

The three basketball tests selected were the bounce and shoot, the half-minute shooting, and the push pass. Leilich, in a factor analysis study, found four factors to be basic to these tests: basketball motor ability; speed; ball handling involving passing accuracy and speed; and ball handling involving accuracy in goal throwing.

Administration of test items. *Bounce and shoot.* The equipment consists of two chairs, two basketballs, a stop watch, a regulation backboard and rim, and a floor diagram as shown in Figure 65.

On either side of the basket, at an angle of 45 degrees, an 18-foot

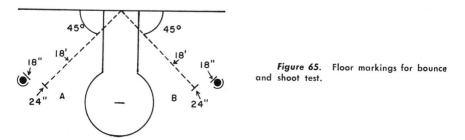

Figure 65. Floor markings for bounce and shoot test.

dotted line is drawn from the center of the end line. Perpendicular to the 18-foot line, a 24-inch line is added. Starting from a point 1 foot behind and 30 inches to the outside of the 18-foot line, additional lines of 18 inches are drawn. On each of the 18-inch lines, a chair with a ball is placed.

A ball catcher stands behind each chair and replaces the ball on the chair after each pass from the subject.

The subject starts on the 24-inch line at the B side of the basket. On the signal "go" from the timer, the subject picks up the ball from the chair, bounces, shoots, recovers the rebound, and passes the ball back to the catcher at B. She runs immediately to A, picks up the ball from the chair and repeats the sequence, passing the recovered shot back to the catcher at A. (This procedure is repeated, alternating five times on each side, making a total of ten shots.) Each bounce must start from behind the 24-inch line on the proper side. The timer keeps the time from the signal "go" and notes and records all fouls. The scorer records the points made on the basket shots, keeps a record of the number of shots and notifies the timer on the ninth shot.

Fouls. The fouls are: running with the ball; double bounce; failure to start from behind the 24-inch line.

Scoring. The score combines time and accuracy.

1. The time to the nearest tenth of a second from the signal "go" until the subject has caught the ball after the tenth shot at the basket.

2. The accuracy score for shooting on the following basis: two points for baskets made, one point for hitting the rim but missing the basket, nothing for missing the basket and the rim.

3. The addition of one second to the time score for any foul.

Final score. The time and accuracy scores are combined for each trial as described previously. The subject's final score is the sum of the best two out of three complete trials, given at least two minutes apart.

Half-minute shooting. The player stands at any position she selects near the basket, with a ball in her hands. On the signal "ready, go" she starts shooting and continues to shoot until the signal to stop is given, attempting to make as many baskets as possible within the thirty seconds. If the ball has left her hands when the signal to stop sounds, the basket counts, if made. Two trials are given to each player.

Scoring. The number of baskets made in thirty seconds is the score for each trial. The better of the two trials is given each player.

Push-pass. The target is shown in Figure 66. The contestant, with basketball in hand, stands behind a line drawn 10 feet from the target. On the signal "go" she makes a push-pass (two-hand chest pass) to the

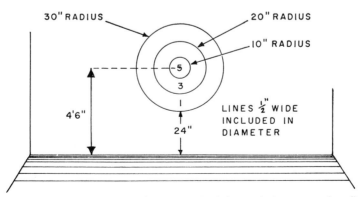

Figure 66. Push-pass target: three concentric circles marked on a smooth wall.

target, recovering the ball on the rebound (either fly or bounce) and continues to pass until time is called. Her score at the end of one-half minute represents the total of her target "hits." Inner circle counts 5, middle circle 3, and outer circle 1. A "liner" counts for the inside circle. Any throw hitting outside the large circle is recorded as zero.

Rules

1. Time is counted from the word "go," when the watch is started, until the word "stop," at the end of the thirty seconds. No score counts after the word "stop" is given. The score recorded is the total number of points made in thirty seconds.

2. The contestant must at all times have both feet back of the passing line, though she may reach over it to get the ball. No points are counted on a pass in which this rule is violated.

3. Two trials are allowed, and the best score is recorded.

The primary use of this particular test, as indicated by the author, is to aid teachers in the professional physical education curriculum to judge the adequacy of achievements of their students in basketball skills. Also it should be of assistance to students in diagnosing their own strength and weaknesses in basketball.

Johnson Basketball Ability Test

This basketball test, for high school boys, is composed of three items: field-goal speed test, basketball throw for accuracy, and dribble.[11] Johnson determined the validity by first dividing his test sample into two groups. Those who made the squad were the "good" group, while those who did not were referred to as the "poor" group. The biserial method of correlation permitted Johnson to determine the relationship between test scores and making the squad. The resulting validity coefficient of the test battery, with 50 boys in the "good" group and 130 boys in the "poor" group, was .880. The reliability of the test battery was computed to be .890.

Test administration. *Field-goal speed test.* The subject assumes any position that he desires under the basket. At the signal "go" he begins to make "lay-up" shots as rapidly as possible for a period of thirty seconds. Score one for each basket.

Throw for accuracy. A target (Fig. 67) is either hung or marked on a wall. Three rectangles, one inside the other, appear on the target; their sizes are 60 × 40 feet; 40 × 25 feet; and 20 × 10 feet. The target is placed on the wall, with the length of the rectangles parallel to the floor and the bottom of the largest rectangle 14 inches from the floor. The subject is permitted ten trials at a distance of 40 feet from the target, using either a hook or a baseball-type pass. The score is the total points made in the ten trials as follows: three points for the inner rectangle; two points for the middle; and one point for the outer rectangle and line.

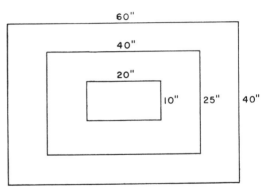

Figure 67. Target used in basket-ball throw for accuracy test.

Dribble test. Place chairs or hurdles as illustrated in Figure 68. The starting line is placed 12 feet from the first hurdle. Three more hurdles are placed in line, with 6 feet between them. The subject begins at the starting line, which is 6 feet long. He dribbles through the prescribed route as rapidly as possible for thirty seconds. The player's score is the number of hurdles or chairs that he passes in thirty seconds.

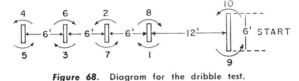

Figure 68. Diagram for the dribble test.

The three tests may be scored as a battery by totaling the three test scores after they have been scaled.

Knox Basketball Test

The Knox test[13] consists of four items: dribble shoot, speed dribble, penny-cup, and speed pass. The reliability of the test items was determined by the test-retest method, using fifty high school boys. The coefficients of correlation were found to be as follows:

Test item	Correlation
Dribble shoot	.579
Speed dribble	.71
Penny-cup	.904
Speed pass	.784
Total score	.88

In determining validity, the test was administered to 260 boys in eight "B" league high schools. The criterion established was success in becoming a member of the ten-man squad brought to the district tournament by each school. The test was administered during the second week of basketball practice.

The results of the study are as follows: (1) varsity players, with but two exceptions, made total scores of forty-six seconds or better. (2) Of 138 boys who made scores of forty-six seconds or better, 66 were players and 72 were non-players. (3) Twenty-four players and only one non-player made scores of thirty-eight seconds or better. (4) Of twenty-four players who made thirty-eight seconds or better, twenty were first-team members and four were substitutes. (5) The ten best total scores in each school were made by the ten boys who were players, and the five best total scores were made by members of the first team. (6) Knox, by using the total scores of the four test items, predicted sixty-one out of sixty-eight squad members, and twenty-nine out of thirty-six first-team members.

Test administration.   The equipment needed includes seven obstacles (chairs may be used), a basketball inflated to 13 pounds, a stop watch, and three tin cups, one painted blue, one red, and one white (coffee cans may be used).

Speed dribble (Fig. 69)   The subject places the ball on the start-finish line and then stands back of it, with hands on knees. With the signal

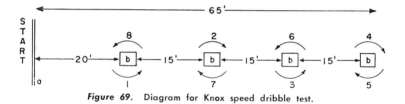

Figure 69.   Diagram for Knox speed dribble test.

"go" the subject picks up the ball and dribbles down and back through the line of chairs (obstacles) as indicated in Figure 69. The watch is started with the signal "go" and is stopped as the subject returns to the start-finish line. The score is the total number of seconds from the command "go" until the subject returns to the start-finish line.

Speed pass.   A line is marked on the floor 5 feet from the wall and parallel to it. The subject stands behind the line and rebounds the basketball from the wall as rapidly as possible fifteen times, using the chest pass. The score is the number of seconds from the signal "go" until the ball hits the wall the fifteenth time. If any rebound requires the subject to take more than one step for recovery, the test is repeated.

Dribble shoot (Fig. 70).   The same testing procedure is followed as required in the speed dribble test, with the exceptions that three obstacles instead of four are used and that the subject must make a basket before he returns. If he fails to make a basket on his first attempt he must continue shooting until he is successful. Any type of shot may be used; however, the one-handed lay-up seems most appropriate. The score is the number of seconds required to complete the test.

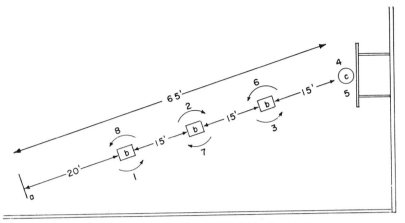

Figure 70. Diagram for Knox dribble shoot test.

Penny-cup test (Fig. 71). The subject stands on the starting line with his back to the cups and a penny in one hand. At the starting signal he turns and runs toward the cups. As he crosses the signal line he is given a direction signal by the examiner. He continues to the cup indicated by the direction signal and places the penny in that cup. The direction signal is one of three commands: "red," "white," or "blue." The time elapsing between the starting signal and the sound of the penny striking in the cup is measured with a stop watch. The test is repeated four times and the total time for each of the four tests constitutes the score. In testing a group of subjects it would perhaps be better to test one at a time privately, so that the same sequence of direction signals may be called; for example, red, blue, red, and white. In this way, each subject would be tested under the identical conditions.

The final score is the total number of seconds required to perform each of the four tests.

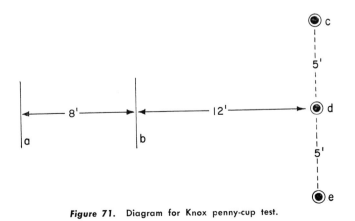

Figure 71. Diagram for Knox penny-cup test.

Lehsten Basketball Test

In establishing this test, various motor skills as well as activities fundamental to the game of basketball were included in the initial investigation. As a result, eight items were finally selected to comprise the original test battery. The test items were administered to eighty-six pupils in physical education classes.[14]

To determine the validity of the eight items, ratings made by five judges were correlated with the test scores, resulting in a correlation of .80. In order to ascertain whether or not the battery of eight tests could be cut down to facilitate testing, a composite score of the five items that had the highest individual validity coefficients was correlated against the total of the eight tests. A correlation of .968 was obtained, indicating that the five selected tests together were measuring to a high degree the same thing which the battery of eight tests was measuring.

On this basis the following five items are recommended for use as a measurement of basketball playing ability in high school boys: dodging run; 40-foot dash; baskets per minute; wall bounce; and vertical jump.

Test administration. *Dodging run* (Fig. 72). The runner begins at A and follows the course as indicated by the broken lines until he returns again to point A. The subject must traverse the outlined course twice, without stopping. The score is recorded to the nearest tenth of a second. Only one attempt is allowed.

The 40-foot dash. The subject takes a position behind the out-of-bounds line at the end of the floor. He begins from an upright position on the signal "go" and runs the 40-foot course across the finish line as fast as possible. The score is recorded to the nearest tenth of a second.

Wall bounce. A rectangular target is painted on a smooth-surfaced wall, 2 feet wide by 4 feet high with the lower limit of the rectangle 3 feet above the floor. At a point 6 feet from the wall target the subject on the command "go" bounces the basketball against the wall target and

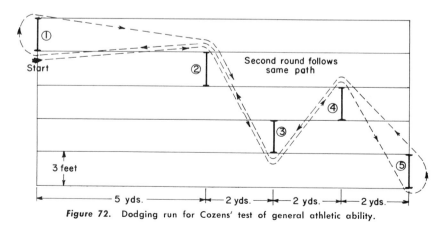

Figure 72. Dodging run for Cozens' test of general athletic ability.

catches the rebound (without the ball touching the floor following the rebound) as many times as possible in ten seconds. The ball must hit the wall inside the borders of the rectangular target. The score is the number of times that the ball is caught in rebound from the wall within the ten seconds allotted.

Vertical jump. This is performed as described on page 124.

Scaled scores for the five items and the composite score appear in reference 14.

Bowling Norms

Phillips and Summers have developed bowling norms and analyzed learning curves in bowling for college women.[21] Twenty-two colleges with a total of 3634 students who had completed ten to twenty-five lines of bowling constitute the data from which the norms were constructed.

The average of the first five lines bowled was eventually selected as the criterion for classifying students according to ability. On the basis of an earlier study, the authors established their norms at ten-point intervals. Thus, all students whose first five game average was between 50 and 59.9 were considered as one ability level, those whose average was between 60 and 69.9 constituted the second level of ability, and so on, for every ten points difference. In all, the authors constructed norms for eight different ability groups from 50 to 129.9 inclusive.

Norms were established at each of the eight levels of ability, at the end of ten lines of bowling, and for five-line intervals up to twenty-five lines of bowling. Norms for the first ten lines are based upon a cumulative average; for succeeding five-line intervals, the average score of each five lines was used.

To establish the qualitative ratings of inferior, poor, average, good, and superior, the distribution of six standard deviations was divided into fifths. Thus, each rating is separated by 1.2 standard deviations. For example, an individual rated as inferior would have obtained a score at least 1.8 standard deviations below the mean score at her level of ability. By the same token, a student considered as "average" would have a score between ± .6 standard deviations either side of the mean.

The authors found significant differences between the means of the adjacent skill levels, indicating that the selected levels of ability are significantly different as regards bowling skill at the end of twenty-five lines of bowling.

Phillips and Summers volunteer that the greatest weakness of the norms lies in the insufficient number of cases at the extreme levels of ability, and, in many cases, beyond the ten lines of bowling. Table 29 (p. 218) contains the norms for the eight levels of ability.

TABLE 29.   *Bowling Norms for College Women**

LEVEL OF ABILITY, 50–59.9

Rating	Lines 1–10	Lines 11–15	Lines 16–20	Lines 21–25
Superior	75 and up	102 and up	109 and up	113 and up
Good	69–74	89–101	96–108	99–112
Average	61–68	75–88	81–95	84–98
Poor	55–60	62–74	67–80	70–83
Inferior	54 and below	61 and below	66 and below	69 and below
N	99	64	59	40
M	64.5	81.4	87.8	90.1
S.D.	5.1	10.7	11.5	11.7

LEVEL OF ABILITY, 60–69.9

Rating	Lines 1–10	Lines 11–15	Lines 16–20	Lines 21–25
Superior	85 and up	109 and up	114 and up	115 and up
Good	78–84	96–108	100–113	102–114
Average	70–77	81–95	85–99	88–101
Poor	63–69	68–80	71–84	76–87
Inferior	62 and below	67 and below	70 and below	75 and below
N	322	206	151	114
M	73.5	88.0	92.2	94.8
S.D.	6.0	11.3	11.6	10.7

LEVEL OF ABILITY, 70–79.9

Rating	Lines 1–10	Lines 11–15	Lines 16–20	Lines 21–25
Superior	93 and up	117 and up	118 and up	124 and up
Good	86–92	101–116	103–117	109–123
Average	78–85	85–100	88–102	92–108
Poor	71–77	70–84	74–87	76–91
Inferior	70 and below	69 and below	73 and below	75 and below
N	611	378	280	213
M	81.3	92.7	95.2	99.7
S.D.	5.7	12.7	12.0	13.1

LEVEL OF ABILITY, 80–89.9

Rating	Lines 1–10	Lines 11–15	Lines 16–20	Lines 20–25
Superior	101 and up	119 and up	120 and up	125 and up
Good	94–100	106–118	106–119	111–124
Average	86–93	91–105	91–105	96–110
Poor	79–85	78–90	77–90	82–95
Inferior	78 and below	77 and below	76 and below	81 and below
N	818	492	337	249
M	89.3	97.8	98.2	102.8
S.D.	5.8	11.1	11.6	11.7

* Based on scores for 3634 students from twenty-two colleges and universities.

Borleske Touch Football Test

In establishing this test, a judgment was obtained from a group of forty-six physical education instructors as to the elements contained in the game. The composite judgment of the forty-six men gave a final classification with objective tests as follows: passing, catching, kicking, running, and pass defense. In determining the validity of the test items the battery of tests was administered to eighty-seven college men. Each subject was then evaluated subjectively by a trained group of examiners in terms of

TABLE 29. *(Continued)*

LEVEL OF ABILITY, 90–99.9

Rating	Lines 1–10	Lines 11–15	Lines 16–20	Lines 20–25
Superior	110 and up	126 and up	127 and up	131 and up
Good	102–109	111–125	112–126	116–130
Average	93–101	96–110	97–111	100–115
Poor	86–92	82–95	82–96	86–99
Inferior	85 and below	81 and below	81 and below	85 and below
N	797	502	342	255
M	97.2	103.4	104.2	107.8
S.D.	6.5	11.8	12.1	12.2

LEVEL OF ABILITY, 100–109.9

Rating	Lines 1–10	Lines 11–15	Lines 16–20	Lines 21–25
Superior	117 and up	130 and up	134 and up	134 and up
Good	110–116	117–129	119–133	120–133
Average	102–109	103–116	104–118	105–119
Poor	95–101	89–102	90–103	91–104
Inferior	94 and below	88 and below	89 and below	90 and below
N	552	369	247	200
M	105.6	109.1	111.1	112.1
S.D.	6.0	11.0	11.9	11.6

LEVEL OF ABILITY, 110–119.9

Rating	Lines 1–10	Lines 11–15	Lines 16–20	Lines 21–25
Superior	125 and up	135 and up	139 and up	139 and up
Good	118–124	122–134	125–138	124–138
Average	110–117	107–121	110–124	109–123
Poor	103–109	94–106	96–109	95–108
Inferior	102 and below	93 and below	95 and below	94 and below
N	310	209	153	119
M	113.6	114.1	116.8	116.3
S.D.	5.8	11.2	11.8	11.8

LEVEL OF ABILITY, 120–129.9

Rating	Lines 1–10	Lines 11–15	Lines 16–20	Lines 21–25
Superior	135 and up	145 and up	146 and up	150 and up
Good	127–134	132–144	133–145	135–149
Average	118–126	117–131	120–132	118–134
Poor	110–117	104–116	107–119	103–117
Inferior	109 and below	103 and below	106 and below	102 and below
N	125	93	60	50
M	122.4	124.0	126.0	126.0
S.D.	6.6	11.0	10.4	12.8

Phillips, Marjorie, and Summers, Dean: Bowling Norms and Learning Curves for College Women. Research Quart., 21:382–384, 1950.

performance in each of the objective tests. The coefficient of correlation was .851, indicating that the objective score was measuring to a reasonable degree the quality indicated by the judgment criterion.[5]

In the final analysis the five test items that produced the highest correlation with the objective criterion ($r = .925$) were:

1. Forward pass for distance.
2. Catching forward pass.
3. Punting for distance.

4. Running 50 yards carrying a ball.

5. Pass defense.

A battery of three tests produced a correlation of .880 with the criterion and may be regarded as a fairly valid measure. It includes:

1. Forward pass for distance.

2. Punt for distance.

3. Running 50 yards carrying a ball.

The catching forward pass test and the pass defense test have been excluded in discussing the administration of the Borleske test as they are quite time-consuming.

Test administration. *Forward pass for distance.* Lines are marked every 5 yards, with markers every 10 yards, so that men may throw from both ends of the field. Each contestant is allowed three throws after one minute has been allowed for warming up. The best distance of three throws is scored in yards. Each throw must be preceded by a catch of a pass from the center.

Punt for distance. Each kick is to be preceded by a catch of a pass from center, and the ball is to be kicked within two seconds after the snap. Each man is allowed three punts for distance, the best punt to be the final score in yards.

Running 50 yards. The contestant starts on snap of ball by center from point 5 yards back of center and from a backfield stance, i.e., three-point stance, catches the ball and carries it a total distance of 50 yards, running as fast as possible. Any form of carrying the ball used in football is permissible. T-scores for these three events appear in reference 5.

Cornish Handball Test

After a review of the literature dealing with handball tests, Cornish selected five handball test items for further investigation. His objective was twofold: to determine validity of certain skills in measuring ability in handball; and to select tests that would duplicate game situations for purpose of measurement. Five tests were selected for study: thirty-second volley, front wall placement, back wall placement, service placement, and power test.[4]

In determining the validity of the test items the scores obtained on the five tests by 134 college students were correlated against the total number of points scored by each student, minus those scored by his opponents in twenty-three games. A multiple correlation of the five tests with the total number of plus points on games won yielded an r of .694. To facilitate testing procedures, Cornish recommends using either the power test alone, as it had a correlation of .58 with the criterion; or the power test in combination with the thirty-second volley, as together they have a correlation of .667 with the criterion measure (total number of points scored).

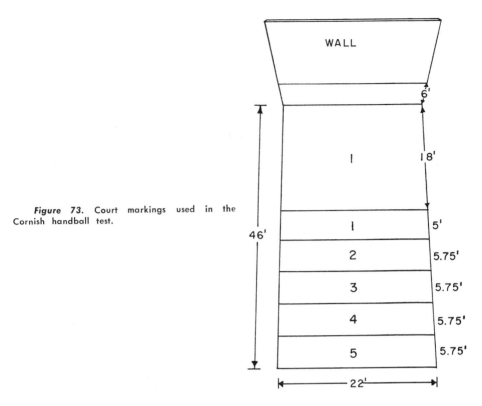

Figure 73. Court markings used in the Cornish handball test.

Administration of the test. *Power test.* The floor of the court is divided into five areas as shown in Figure 73. One point is scored if the ball strikes in front of the service line. Standing in the service zone the subject tosses the ball to the front wall, allowing it to bounce before playing it. The ball, after being stroked, must strike the front wall below the 6-foot line above the floor. If it strikes the front wall above the line or the subject steps into the front court, another trial is allowed. Five strokes with each hand are made, and the total number of points is recorded as the score.

Thirty-second volley. The subject commences by standing behind the service line. He drops the ball to the floor and strokes it continuously for thirty seconds. The ball must rebound far enough from the wall so that the subject remains behind the service line during the volley. In the event the ball fails to return, the subject is permitted to step into the front court to stroke the ball; however, he must return for the succeeding stroke. If the subject misses the ball, another is handed to him by the judge and the play is continued. A point is recorded each time the ball strikes the front wall, and the total points at the end of thirty seconds constitute the score.

McDonald Soccer Test

This test was constructed, using college freshmen, junior varsity, and varsity soccer players as subjects, for the purpose of predicting game proficiency. The test consists of kicking a soccer ball at a kickboard 11½ feet in height by 30 feet long from a distance of 9 feet in front of the kickboard. The score is the number of volleys performed in a thirty-second period.[17]

In computing validity of the test, the subjective ratings of three coaches were correlated against the test scores. The following are the obtained coefficients of correlation:

NUMBER OF SUBJECTS	GROUP	CORRELATIONS WITH SUBJECTIVE RATINGS
17	Varsity players	.94
18	Junior varsity players	.63
18	Freshman varsity players	.76
53	Combined groups	.85

Test administration. A restraining line is drawn 9 feet from and parallel to the kickboard. Three balls inflated to 13 pounds are used; one ball is placed on the restraining line for the subject to begin kicking, while the other two balls are placed 9 feet behind the restraining line and in the center of the testing area. This arrangement permits the subject to make a recovery in event of losing control of the original ball, the penalty being a reduction in scored kicks that would be occasioned by the loss of time in recovery.

When starting the test, the subject at the command "go" begins to kick the ball from behind the restraining line, and continues to rebound the ball from the kickboard as rapidly as possible for thirty seconds. Any type kick and any control methods are permissible; however, the kicking, to be scored, has to be done with the supporting leg on or behind the restraining line. The subject may retrieve a lost ball with either hands or feet, but must place it behind the restraining line before continuing the test; an alternative is to play one of the spare balls, using hands or feet to get the ball into the desired kicking position behind the restraining line.

The score is the number of "fair" kicks accomplished in thirty seconds. Four trials are permitted, and the highest total of any three trials constitutes the score.

Broer-Miller Tennis Test

The purpose of this test is to classify and grade women students; it also may be used for pointing up relative weakness and strength in both forehand and backhand drives. The test consists of hitting a given number of balls so that they pass between the top of the net and a restraining

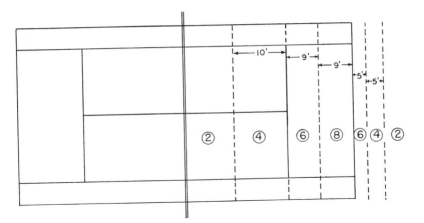

Figure 74. Special court markings for the Broer-Miller forehand-backhand drive test.

rope placed above the net, and of attempting to place these balls into the back 9 feet of the court. The ball is put into play by the student bouncing her own ball.[3]

The equipment required for this test includes a regulation net with a rope stretched 4 feet above the top of the net and fifteen to twenty balls in good condition. In addition, the tennis court must have special markings as seen in Figure 74. Two chalk lines are drawn across the court 10 feet inside the service line and 9 feet outside the service line and parallel to it. Two chalk lines are drawn across the court 5 feet and 10 feet respectively outside the base line and parallel to it. The chalked numbers in the center of each area indicate the scoring value.

The player taking the test stands behind the base line, bounces the balls to herself, hits the balls, and attempts to place them in the back 9 feet of the opposite court. Each player is allowed fourteen trials on the forehand and fourteen trials on the backhand.

In order to score the values as illustrated in Figure 74, balls must go between the top of the net and the rope and land in the designated area or on lines bounding the area. Balls that land on a line receive the highest score for that area. Balls that go over the rope score one-half the value of that area in which they land. If the player misses the ball in attempting to strike it, this is considered a trial. All "let" balls are taken over.

In scoring the test, cards wtih the diagram of the court markings facilitate the procedure. For example, the number of each trial is marked on the score card diagram in the same relative position as the ball landing on the court. Each ball hit is scored 2-4-6-8-6-4-2, depending upon the area in which it lands. The total score equals the sum of fourteen balls on the forehand and fourteen balls on the backhand.

The reliability of the test for twenty-seven intermediate players and thirty-two beginners was .80 ± .043 and .80 ± .047 respectively. The validity of the test was determined by correlating the test scores with the ratings of experienced tennis instructors. For the intermediate group the combined ratings of two judges with the tennis test results was .85. In the beginning group the correlation with the combined judges' rating and the skill test was .61.

The authors conclude that the test appears to be more valid with the intermediate group than with the beginners. However, they found that the ratings of the judges, who were the tennis instructors for the two groups employed in the study, correlated higher with the test results than did the combined judges' rating. A correlation of .87 was obtained by the judge for the intermediate group and an r of .66 for the judge of the beginning group when the respective individual ratings were correlated against the test scores.

Dyer Tennis Test

This test has been designed to measure ability in tennis for classification purposes. It consists of rallying a tennis ball against a backboard, attempting to score as many hits as possible within a thirty-second time limit.[6,7]

The initial study contains 736 cases, from representative women's tennis groups in nineteen colleges. Validity of the test was determined by two methods: correlating the test scores with judgments of three experts; and correlating the test scores with standings of the subjects in a number of round-robin tournaments. A coefficient of .85 was obtained in the first study and coefficients ranging from .85 to .92 were obtained in the second validity study.

Reliability of the test was determined first by correlating chance halves of the test that resulted in an r of .85; secondly, reliability was computed by the test-retest method, which resulted in a range of coefficients from .86 to .92.

Test administration. To administer the test it is necessary to have a backboard or wall, approximately 10 feet in height and about 15 feet in width, for each person taking the test at one time. A clearly visible line, 3 inches in width and 3 feet from the floor, should be drawn on the wall to represent the net. A restraining line, 5 feet from the base of the wall, should be drawn on the floor (masking or adhesive tape works very well for the lines). The subject should have two tennis balls at least in fair condition and a tennis racket without flaws.

A box for extra balls, about 12 inches long, 9 inches wide, and 3 inches deep, should be placed on the floor where the restraining line joins the side at the left for right-handed players, and at the right for left-handed players.

The object of the test is to cause the ball to strike the wall on or above the net line as many times as possible within a thirty-second time limit. To start the test, the subject drops the ball to put it into play. There is no limit to the number of times the ball may bounce before the subject strokes it. Also it is not necessary to allow the ball to bounce on the floor after it has been put into play. All balls must be played from behind the restraining line; however, the subject may cross the line to retrieve the ball. Balls that hit while the subject is over the restraining line do not count. Any number of balls may be used, and if a ball gets out of control the subject should select another from the box placed at either side of the court rather than attempt to retrieve the one that got away. Each new ball is put into play in the same manner as in starting the test.

Scoring.   In scoring the test, each ball striking the wall on or above the net line, before the thirty-second duration is up, counts one point. Each subject is given three trials and the best total score is recorded. Tables containing T-score values to be used with college women appear in the March, 1938, Research Quarterly.

Brady Volleyball Test

The Brady test is to be used with college men for the following purposes: (1) classification; (2) to determine improvement of teaching; (3) as measurement in improvement of skill; and (4) as a basis for grading.

The test consists of repeatedly volleying a ball against a wall for a one-minute period. Reliability of the test was determined by the test-retest method and resulted in a correlation of .925 for 282 subjects.

The validity of the test was determined by correlating the combined subjective judgments of four judges with the scores made on the test. The validity was found to be .86, which is an acceptable level of validity.

Although Brady experimented with several test items in an attempt at arriving at a volleyball skill test he found the wall volley test to be the most valid. He suggests, however, that the test is not as accurate when used with students below college level or for those with very inferior ability.[2]

In giving the test it is necessary to have a smooth wall with a horizontal chalk line 5 feet long and 11½ feet above the floor. Vertical lines should be drawn extending upward toward the ceiling at the ends of the horizontal line.

The subject stands where he wishes and begins the test by throwing the ball against the wall. When the ball returns to the player, he must volley it against the wall and within the boundaries of the chalk lines, as described above. Only legal volleys are counted. If the ball is caught or gets out of control, it is started as at the beginning of the test. The player is timed for one minute, and the number of successful legal volleys that hit within the rectangle on the wall are recorded as his score.

Brady suggests that when the test is used as a method of grading by measuring improvement, the following method was found to be satisfactory: the difference between the scores made on the first test and the last test is added to the last test score. Thus, due credit is given to the poor beginner who learns rapidly as well as to the good beginner who naturally must progress at a slower rate.

The author also indicates that the test, in addition to the uses already mentioned, is functional in that it serves as a drill for developing proficiency in volleyball.

Russell-Lange Volleyball Test

This test was established for use with junior high school girls. In developing an experimental battery the authors first surveyed the literature of volleyball tests and selected those test items that appeared to be practical for use with this particular age level. The final test battery includes two tests, originally used by French and Cooper (with slight modification, however): a serving test; and a repeated volleys test.[22]

Test administration. *Repeated volleys test.* A line 10 feet long is marked on the wall at net height, 7½ feet above the floor; another line, 10 feet long, is marked on the floor, parallel to and 3 feet from the wall.

The player being tested stands behind the 3-foot line, and with an underhand movement tosses the ball to the wall. When the ball returns the player volleys it repeatedly against the wall above the net line for thirty seconds. The ball may be set up as many times as desired or necessary; it may be caught and restarted with a toss as at the beginning of the test. If the ball gets out of control, it must be recovered by the subject and brought back to the 3-foot line to be started over again as at the beginning.

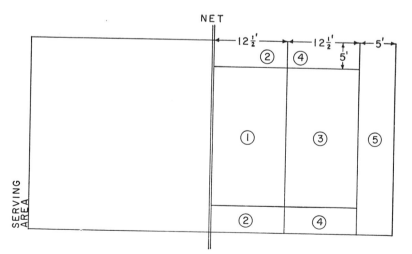

Figure 75. Court markings for Russell-Lange volleyball test.

The score is the number of times the ball is clearly batted (not tossed) from behind the 3-foot line to, on, or above the 7½-foot line on the wall. The total score from the best of three trials is recorded.

Serving test.   A court with special markings, as shown in Figure 75, is prepared. Contained in each of the marked areas are chalked numbers to indicate the score value of the respective areas.

The player being tested stands behind the end line in the serving area and is given ten serves to place the ball into the targets across the net. Any legal service is permitted and a "let" ball is served over.

The score is the point value of the spot on which the served ball lands. A ball landing on a line is scored the higher value of the two areas. Serves in which foot faults occur are scored zero. Two trials of ten serves each are given and the sum of the scores in the areas for the best trial is recorded.

Tables containing scaled scores for the serve and repeated volleys tests appear in reference 22. The sum of the scaled scores for the two tests is used as a measure of volleyball playing ability.

By means of the test-retest method, reliability coefficients ranging from .870 to .915 were obtained. Validity of the test was determined through subjective ratings of the players by seven judges. The resulting coefficients of .677 and .80 for the serving test and the repeated volleys test, respectively, were obtained.

French-Cooper Volleyball Test

The French-Cooper test is designed for use with high school girls and consists of the repeated volleys test and a serving test. The administration of the test items is the same as described in the Russell-Lange volleyball test with the following exception: in the repeated volleys test the subject volleys the ball for fifteen seconds, instead of thirty seconds. Ten trials are given and the score constitutes the sum of the best five trials.

French and Cooper, experimenting with a number of volleyball test items, found that the combination of the repeated volleys test and the serving test yielded a validity coefficient of .811, using the subjective evaluation of three judges.

These authors concluded that, because of the simplicity of administration and scoring, and the economy in time and equipment, these tests may be recommended as teaching devices as well as tests for classifying and diagnosing.[8]

Bassett, Glassow, and Locke[1] recommend a repeated volleys test and a serving test for use with college women. They obtained a validity coefficient of .79 for the serving test and .51 for the volleying test, using the composite ratings of three judges. Reliability coefficients of .84 and .89 were obtained for the serving test and volleying test respectively.

BIBLIOGRAPHY

1. Bassett, Gladys, Glassow, Ruth, and Locke, Mabel: Studies in Testing Volleyball Skills. Research Quart., Vol. 8, No. 4, December, 1937.
2. Brady, George F.: Preliminary Investigations of Volleyball Playing Ability. Research Quart., Vol. 16, No. 1, March, 1945.
3. Broer, Marion R., and Miller, Donna Mae: Achievement Tests for Beginning and Intermediate Tennis. Research Quart., Vol. 21, No. 3, October, 1950.
4. Cornish, Clayton: A Study of Measurement of Ability in Handball. Research Quart., Vol. 20, No. 2, May, 1949.
5. Cozens, Frederick: Ninth Annual Report of the Committee on Curriculum Research of the College Physical Education Association, Report of Subcommittee Four. Research Quart., Vol. 8, No. 2, 1937.
6. Dyer, Joanna Thayer: The Blackboard Test of Tennis Ability. Supplement to Research Quart., March, 1935.
7. Dyer, Joanna Thayer: Revision of Backboard Test of Tennis Ability. Research Quart., Vol. 9, No. 1, March, 1938.
8. French, Esther L., and Cooper, Bernice I.: Achievement Tests in Volleyball for High School Girls. Research Quart., Vol. 8, No. 2, May, 1937.
9. Hyde, Edith I.: An Achievement Scale in Archery. Research Quart., Vol. 8, No. 2, May, 1937.
10. Hyde, Edith I.: National Research Study in Archery. Research Quart., Vol. 7, No. 4, December, 1936.
11. Johnson, L. William.: Objective Test in Basketball for High School Boys. Unpublished Master's Thesis, State University of Iowa, Iowa City, Iowa, 1934.
12. Kelson, Robert E.: Baseball Classification Plan for Boys. Research Quart., Vol 24, No. 3, October, 1953.
13. Knox, Robert Dawson: An Experiment to Determine the Relationship between Performance in Skill Tests and Success in Playing Basketball. Unpublished Master's Thesis, University of Oregon, Eugene, Oregon, June, 1937.
14. Lehsten, Carlson: A Measure of Basketball Skills in High School Boys. The Physical Educator, Vol. 5, No. 5, December, 1948.
15. Leilich, Avis: The Primary Components of Selected Basketball Tests for College Women. Doctoral Dissertation, Indiana University, 1952.
16. Lockhart, Aileene, and McPherson, Francis A.: The Development of a Test of Badminton Playing Ability. Research Quart., Vol. 20, No. 4, December, 1949.
17. McDonald, Lloyd G.: The Construction of a Kicking Skill Test as an Index of General Soccer Ability. Springfield College, Springfield, Mass., Unpublished Master's Thesis, June, 1951.
18. Mathews, Donald K.: Unpublished data, Washington State College, Pullman, Washington.
19. Miller, Frances A.: A Badminton Wall Volley Test. Research Quart., Vol. 22, No. 2, May, 1951.
20. Miller, Wilma K., Chairman: Achievement Levels in Basketball Skills for Women Physical Education Majors. Research Quart., Vol. 25, No. 4, December, 1954.
21. Phillips, Marjorie, and Summers, Dean: Bowling Norms, and Learning Curves for College Women. Research Quart., Vol. 21, No. 4, December, 1950.
22. Russell, Naomi, and Lange, Elizabeth: Achievement Tests in Volleyball for Junior High School Girls. Research Quart., Vol. 2, No. 4, December, 1940.

chapter 8
cardiovascular tests

Researchers have spent a considerable amount of time searching for a single test that would best measure physical fitness. As early as 1884, an Italian by the name of Mosso experimented with the effects of exercising a muscle on an ergometer. He was one of the first physiologists to hypothesize that muscular efficiency was dependent upon circulatory factors. Following Mosso's work, many experiments have been conducted to show certain cardiovascular factors to be related to good physical condition.

Recent studies suggest that physical inactivity may be related to the increasing prominence of ischemic vascular disease, the most significant form being coronary heart disease (CHD). Of particular note is the study of transport workers by Morris and associates,[25] who found a higher incidence of CHD in the less active drivers than in conductors; also, less active postal workers were found to have a much higher incidence of CHD than the postmen.

Fox and Skinner,[18] in summarizing a large number of studies which compared sedentary and active individuals, found a definite trend favoring a lower incidence of CHD among the more active. As a result of these recent studies, much emphasis has been placed upon getting people to exercise and devising new instruments for the evaluation of cardiorespiratory endurance.

In order to achieve some basic understanding of the principles underlying the construction of cardiovascular tests, it seems wise at this point to review briefly the physiological characteristics found to be most generally associated with a highly trained body.

Minute volume. The output of the heart per beat is referred to as the stroke volume, and the output per minute as the minute volume. The stroke volume multiplied by the pulse rate equals the minute volume, and the minute volume divided by the pulse rate equals the stroke volume. It is a common belief that trained athletes usually have a greater stroke volume at rest than do less well-conditioned persons. This development is probably due to the much stronger heart of the athlete. Apparently a graduated program of training not only develops the voluntary muscles, but also increases the muscular power of the heart.

Pulse rate.   The average pulse rate of young men, lying at rest before eating, is 64 beats per minute, with a range from 38 to 110 beats per minute. As Karpovich points out, pulse rate is affected by age, body position, food intake, time of day, emotions, and physical activity.[23] Furthermore, men who are physically fit show a smaller difference between reclining and standing pulse rate than do men in general. A slow pulse rate in the reclining position, with a small increase upon standing, is usually indicative of very good physical condition. The resting pulse rate of highly trained athletes may be 20 or even 30 beats slower than the pulse rate of persons not in training. This seems to indicate that with each heart beat, for the trained person, a greater volume of blood is being ejected from the heart, whereas, in the untrained, the heart does not empty itself as completely. In addition, the trained person probably has a more efficient coronary circulation, that is, as in the development of voluntary muscle, there may be the formation of new capillaries or the opening up of heretofore unused ones.

Pulse rate increases in proportion to the amount of work a person performs, and also shows a linear relationship to the amount of oxygen absorbed during the particular period of work. When the exercise is completed, the pulse rate returns to normal. The time required for this return to normal is dependent upon the intensity of the exercise and the condition of the person. Better physical condition cuts down the time required for return of the pulse rate to normal.

Respiration.   Circulatory efficiency is closely related to respiration, for it is in the alveoli of the lungs that the gaseous exchange of oxygen and carbon dioxide takes place. To work efficiently, muscles are dependent upon oxygen more than upon any other substance. Insufficient amounts of oxygen cause the accumulation of lactic acid in the blood, which impedes the contraction of muscle.

Physical conditioning definitely affects the respiratory mechanism as well as increasing the efficiency of the respiratory function. As a result of training, the expansion of the chest is increased during the growing period, and the depth of breathing is augmented. Furthermore, it has been shown that the person in condition breathes less air and at the same time absorbs a greater percentage of the oxygen from the air he breathes than does the average person.

Karpovich indicates that the trained man ventilates his lungs during rest and under working conditions more economically than does the untrained man.[23] Thus, more oxygen is available to be used during work without an exorbitant increase in respiration.

Finally, the muscular endurance of the respiratory muscles is increased so that the trained person notices few, if any, of the discomforts associated with breathing during strenuous activity that are experienced by the untrained.

Variables in appraising cardiovascular condition. Cardiac function tests are for the most part attempts at measuring certain variables that reflect the condition of the circulatory system in adjusting to work situations. The variables used most generally include pulse rate and blood pressure, which are recorded under various conditions. Extreme care must be exercised in taking these cardiovascular measurements, for such factors as amount of rest before the test, time following last meal, and certain emotional disturbances may greatly affect the results of the evaluation. These factors may cause an unreliably fast "resting" pulse rate as well as an unreliably high systolic blood pressure. For example, Karpovich reports that, during World War II, many applicants for the Air Force frequently had higher pulse rates at the beginning of the medical examination than at the end.[23] Slater-Hammel and Butler found errors in taking normal pulse count by palpation from −12 to +14, and from −33 to +36, for a two-minute period following exercise.[28] These differences are sufficiently large to change the fitness classification of the individual on several physiological tests.

When the test calls for resting pulse rate, the individual should lie on a cot or mat for at least five to ten minutes and the pulse should be taken until two or three successive fifteen-second counts agree before it is recorded. The examiner should also recognize the difference between basal pulse rate and resting pulse rate. The basal pulse rate may best be recorded early in the morning before the subject arises, or when he has had nothing to eat for the previous twelve to fourteen hours.

Although three-quarters of a century have elapsed since the time of Mosso, physiologists have not yet devised a satisfactory test for appraising cardiovascular fitness. Such factors as the variation from one person to another in reacting to the parameters can now be measured. But others, such as variation in the test results of the same subject from day to day, or the difficulty in showing any outward difference between the test results of a highly trained athlete and those of an untrained person when both are at rest, still are obstacles to greater validity and objectivity in the measurement of cardiovascular fitness.

At present, the only way to demonstrate the superiority of the conditioned body is to make the test comparisons during fairly strenuous exercise, when the subject is required to use his physiological reserves. Even though many of the tests in this chapter employ measurements of the return to normal of the pulse rate following a given exercise, there is little if any correlation between an ability to sustain maximal or exhausting work and the return to normal of the pulse rate during recovery. For mild exercise, the return of the heart to normal following work does give some indication of cardiovascular condition. Hence, one must use care in interpreting these test scores.

Aerobic capacity.   Measurement of aerobic capacity, a person's ability to maximally utilize oxygen during exhaustive work, is one of the most valid means of appraising what is commonly referred to as cardiovascular fitness. Measurement requires trained personnel, expensive equipment and a cooperative subject, hence making its use in a school situation impractical. Nevertheless, as a student of tests and measurements you should have some knowledge regarding its meaning since measurements for maximal aerobic capacity tests have been used to validate measures of cardiovascular fitness.

Testing procedure.   The object of the test is to determine a person's oxygen consumption while he is performing maximal or exhaustive work. Bicycles, step benches and treadmills are the usual ergometers employed, the latter being more popular. Running on a treadmill elicits higher values as more muscle mass is used in performing the work. Usually the subject begins by walking on a treadmill set at a 10 per cent grade and at 3.5 miles per hour for three to four minutes. This is considered as the warm-up period which allows the subject to become adjusted to the equipment; essential equipment consists of a mouthpiece, nose-clip and electrocardiogram leads. Following the warm-up he begins running at 6.5 miles per hour on a 2 per cent grade; each two minutes the treadmill is elevated 2 per cent, which increases the work load. Metabolic determinations commence at about the third minute and continue until the subject becomes exhausted and can no longer maintain the pace.

Test results.   Laboratories usually differ in certain specifics regarding aerobic capacity measurements, the above being a general procedure. Hopefully the individual can endure the exercise for at least four minutes so one is assured of obtaining metabolic determinations during maximal exertion. On test-retest studies of objectivity, experienced laboratory personnel find coefficients of correlation in the upper 90's while measurement error is less than 4 per cent.

Maximal oxygen consumption can be expressed in liters of oxygen consumed per minute or in milliliters of oxygen consumed per minute per kilogram of body weight (the latter figure obtained by dividing kilograms of body weight into milliliters of oxygen used per minute). A mean value for college men is about 3.5 liters per minute and for college women 2.7 liters per minute or 46 milliliters per kilogram per minute. These values are primarily dependent upon age, fitness levels and body weight. Individuals who attain large aerobic capacities do so in part by increasing cardiac output and widening the difference between oxygen saturation of the arterial and venous blood (A-V difference).

Characteristics of cardiovascular fitness.   Table 30 contains a summary by Johnson, Brouha, and Darling dealing with characteristics of the fit and unfit man.

Consolazio et al.[12] suggest that a good test should subscribe to the following criteria:

TABLE 30.   *Comparison of the Reaction of a Fit and an Unfit Man of the Same Weight at the Same Rate of Physical Exertion*

Measurement	Fit Man	Unfit Man
Easy work that both can sustain in a steady state*		
Oxygen consumption	Lower	Higher
Pulse rate during work	Lower	Higher
Stroke volume during work	Larger	Smaller
Blood pressure during work (systolic)	Lower	Higher
Blood lactate during work	Lower	Higher
Return of blood pressure to normal after work	Faster	Slower
Exhausting work that neither can sustain in a steady state		
Maximum oxygen consumption	Higher	Lower
Maximum pulse rate during work	Usually lower	Usually higher
Stroke volume	Larger	Smaller
Duration of work before exhaustion	Longer	Shorter
Return of blood pressure to normal after work	Faster	Slower
Return of pulse rate to resting value after work	Faster	Slower

Johnson, R. E., Brouha, L., and Darling, R. C.: Test of Physical Fitness for Strenuous Exertion. Rev. Canad. Biol., 1:491–503, June, 1942.

* It should be emphasized that the lower the metabolic rate, that is, the easier the work, the smaller and less regular the difference between the fit and the unfit.

1. It must place the cardiovascular system under considerable stress by involving large groups of muscles.

2. It should be so intense that at least one-third of all the test subjects will stop from exhaustion within five minutes, but the work intensity should not be so high as to make motivation play a dominant part.

3. It should not demand any unusual type of skill for successful performance.

4. The work load must be carefully determined, reproducible, and fairly easy so that the mechanical efficiency is kept relatively constant.

A number of the tests that follow serve as screening devices for the measurement of cardiovascular condition. For the most part, they separate the extremes of condition: we might say, the men from the boys. They are not, however, definitive measures of cardiovascular condition. Employed wisely, they can be useful in the classroom, in the physician's office, and in the research laboratory.

Blood Pressure Measurement

In tests that include blood pressure measurements, the subject is either placed in a recumbent position or comfortably seated, depending upon the test instructions. Extreme care should be exercised in seeing that

TABLE 31. *Classification of Physical Work by Capacity Test*

Classification of Work	Pulse Rate/Min.	Metabolic Rate O₂, cc./min.	Metabolic Rate Kcal./min.	Ventilation Volume liter/min.	Ventilation Rate liter/min.	R.Q.	Lactic Acid in Multiples of Resting Value	Length of Time Work Can Be Sustained
I. Light								
A. Mild	<100	<750	<4	<20	<14	0.85	Normal	Indefinite
B. Moderate	<120	<1,500	<7.5	<35	<15	0.85	Within normal limits	8 hr. daily on the job
C. Optimal	<140	<2,000	<10	<50	<16	0.9	<1.5X	8 hr. daily for few weeks (seasonal work, military maneuvers, etc.)
II. Heavy								
D. Strenuous	<160	<2,500	<12.5	<60	<20	0.95	<2X	4 hr. two or three times a week for few weeks (special physical training)
E. Maximal	<180	<3,000	<15	<80	<25	<1.0	<5–6X	1 to 2 hr. occasionally (usually in competitive sports)
III. Severe								
F. Exhausting	>180	>3,000	>15	<120	<30	>1.0	6X or more	Few minutes; rarely

Wells, J. G., Balke, B., and Van Fossan, D. D.: Lactic Acid Accumulation during Work. A Suggested Standardization of Work Classification. J. Appl. Physiol., 10:51–55, 1957.

the subject is placed at ease and that time is allowed for recovery from any unusual recent exercise, meals, or apprehension. To take a blood pressure reading, the subject's arm should be completely bared, so as to make certain that clothing does not constrict the blood vessel, as might be the case when the subject is asked to roll up his sleeve. The arm is flexed slightly, abducted, and relaxed. The blood pressure should be taken with the subject in a sitting position, his forearm supported at heart level on a smooth surface. The hand may be either pronated or supinated, depending upon which position yields the clearer sounds. The cuff must be applied evenly and snugly around the arm, with the lower edge approximately 1 inch above the antecubital space. The stethoscope receiver is placed firmly over the artery in the antecubital space, making sure that it is free from contact with the cuff.

As we learn in physiology, blood pressure generally refers to the pressure exerted by the blood on the walls of the vessels. The pressure reaches its highest values during systole in the left ventricle. This systolic pressure rises during activity and falls during sleep. The diastolic blood pressure is the lowest point to which the pressure drops between beats. To record systolic pressure, with the cuff in place, the pressure in the sphygmomanometer is raised rapidly and decreased slowly until a sound is heard with each heart beat; this is recorded as systolic pressure. With continued deflation of the cuff below systolic pressure, the heart sounds undergo changes in intensity and quality. The best index of diastolic pressure is the point at which the heart sounds completely cease.[11]

Balke Treadmill Test

Balke found that a number of discernible physiological changes occur during a given exercise when the heart rate reaches 180 per minute.[2, 3] At this point, the RQ exceeds 1, pulse pressure and oxygen pulse become maximal, and there is a sharp rise in respiratory frequency and minute volume, together with a sudden drop in alveolar carbon dioxide tension. At about this time blood lactate levels begin to rise sharply, indicating the inability of the physiological reserves to keep pace with the increased metabolic needs resulting from exercise.

Balke reports test results in terms of the duration of exercise required to produce a heart rate of 180 per minute (T_{180}). The test consists of having a subject walk at a constant speed on a treadmill, the slope of which is increased each minute, and measuring his heart rate each minute. At the end of one minute the treadmill is raised to a 2 per cent grade and at the end of each succeeding minute the slope is increased by 1 per cent. The test requires a treadmill, a stop watch and an electrocardiograph for measuring the heart rate.

To establish a norm, Balke proposed that the effective work per-

TABLE 32.   *Suggested Rating System for Balke Treadmill Test*

Minutes to T_{180}	Classification	Score in Per Cent of Average Score
12–below	Very poor	74—
13–14	Poor	75–84
15–16	Fair	85–97
17	Average	98–102
18–19	Good	103–115
20–21	Very Good	116–125
22–above	Excellent	126+

formed by the individual during the final minute of the test, W_i, and his body weight, k_i, be compared with the average work of the group studied, during the final minute, W_a, and the group mean weight, k_a, in order to derive a percentage score. This is computed in the following manner:

$$\text{Percentage Score} = \frac{W_i}{W_a} \times \frac{k_a}{k_i} \times 100$$

Table 32 shows a classification of the percentage test scores in terms of minutes of sustained walking required to reach a heart rate of 180 per minute (T_{180}).

Billings and his co-workers, using Balke's test, found the time required to reach a T_{150} reading to be a valid indicator of the subject's capacity for more strenuous work.[5]

The advantage of not requiring exhaustive exercise to appraise cardiovascular condition is obvious. More recent work by Truett, Benson, and Balke,[32] in substantiation of Billings' work, shows that submaximal tests of cardiovascular fitness yield information which is reasonably comparable to that furnished by maximum tests.

Modified Treadmill Test for Children*

Four electrodes are secured by a rubber strap around the chest and placed at a level just below the pectoralis muscles. The two electrodes on the chest are below each nipple, and the two electrodes on the back are just below the inferior angle of the scapula. (See Fig. 76.)

Heart rates are recorded during the middle fifteen seconds of each minute of exercise. At the end of each minute the treadmill is elevated 1 per cent until a maximum of 14 per cent incline is reached. The speed of the treadmill remains constant throughout the test. The subjects in

---

* Developed under support of the Ohio Department of Health and The Ohio State University.

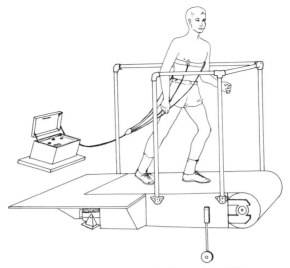

Figure 76. Modified treadmill test for children.

the fourth and fifth grades walk at a rate of 2.8 miles per hour, while those in the eleventh and twelfth grades walk at a rate of 3.5 miles per hour.

The test is terminated when one of the following three criteria is obtained: (1) the subject voluntarily wants to stop as he or she feels too tired to continue, (2) the heart rate increases to 200 beats per minute, or (3) the subject walks a maximum of twenty-five minutes. The incline of the treadmill progresses from 0 to 14 per cent at a 1 per cent increase per minute. Thus, from minutes 14 to 25 the grade remains at 14 per cent. The test is scored by the number of minutes the subject walks.

Alderman[1] studied the reliability of individual responses to graduated exercise on a bicycle ergometer. The data indicated increasing reliability as the heart rate criteria progressively increased from 100 beats to 160 beats per minute. Increasing the criterion beyond 150 or 160 beats per minute produced no further increase in test score reliability; reliability

TABLE 33. *Reliability of Individual Responses to Graduated Exercise Measured by a Bicycle Ergometer*

Reliability Coefficients for Exercise Times								
Heart rate	100	110	120	130	140	150	160	170	180
r	.292	.499	.628	.751	.818	.856	.894	.888	.855

Reliability Coefficients for Recovery Times							
Heart rate	170	160	150	140	130	120	110	100
r	.361	.333	.478	.672	.720	.847	.565	.657

Alderman, Richard B.: Reliability of Individual Differences in the 180 Heart Rate Response Test in Bicycle Ergometer Work. Research Quart., October, 1966, p. 430. (Courtesy American Association for Health, Physical Education, and Recreation.)

is lower at 180 beats per minute than at 160 beats per minute. Table 33 contains reliability coefficients for exercise and recovery heart rates in which scores used were (1) exercise time to reach the required heart rate and (2) time required for subject's rate to return to 100 beats per minute.

Barach Index

Barach,[4] in an attempt to measure the energy of the circulatory system in terms of blood output, developed what he terms "the energy index." This is computed by the following formula:

$$\text{Energy Index} = \frac{(\text{Systolic pressure} + \text{Diastolic pressure}) \times \text{Pulse rate}}{100}$$

Studies show that most healthy persons score between 110 and 160. The upper and lower normal limits are taken as 200 to 90 respectively. Individuals scoring above 200 are noted as hypertensed, while those scoring below 90 are referred to as hypotensed.

Cureton reports 70 to 220 as a normal range of the index, with an average of 140.85 on two hundred Illinois students.[14]

Burger Test

Karpovich reports a test devised by Burger in which the change in systolic pressure as a subject blows against a 40-mm. column of mercury for twenty seconds is employed as a measure of fitness.[23] Blood pressure is recorded at four times: before; at the beginning; immediately after; and at twenty seconds following the exertion. In "normal" people, the pressure drops 20 to 30 mm. during the test; the pressure may drop more than 40 mm. in the unfit; but in highly trained persons, the blood pressure rises.

Carlson Fatigue Curve Test

The Carlson fatigue curve test was designed to place severe stress upon the individual being tested.[10] The author feels that a true physical test of function should be sufficiently demanding to reveal positively as nearly as possible the absolute state of physical condition.

Making use of the general fatigue curve, which is an accepted physiological principle, the physical skill of spot running is used as the medium of exercise. The subject must run as fast as possible in ten-second innings with intervening rest periods of ten seconds. The subject performs ten of these ten-second innings and the following five pulse rates are taken for ten seconds, multiplied by six, and recorded:

1. Before exercise, subject seated on floor or ground.
2. Ten seconds after exercise.
3. Two minutes after exercise.
4. Four minutes after exercise.
5. Six minutes after exercise.

In executing the run, the subject raises and lowers his feet far enough to clear the floor as fast as he can for ten seconds. The subject counts the number of right-foot contacts only, and records them for each inning of the exercise. The total number of right-foot contacts for ten innings is added up to indicate *production*.

Scoring.   The scoring of this test involves counting both the number of right-foot contacts made by the subject during each of the ten innings of exercise, and the pulse rates as indicated above. Fatigue will cause a drop in the number in each succeeding inning if the participant goes "all out." If an inning fails to show fewer repetitions than were recorded for the preceding inning, there is either an error present or a lack of *application* on the part of the pupil. Figure 77 illustrates the plotted

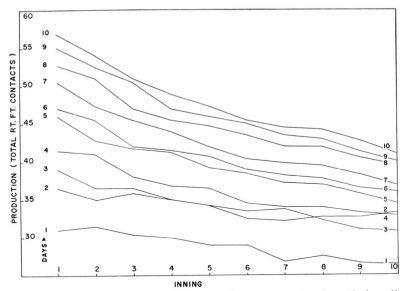

Figure 77. Composite fatigue curves improving for ten consecutive days. (Carlson, H. C.: Fatigue Curve Test. Research Quart., 16: 173, 1945.)

aggregate curves of 200 soldiers. The base line represents the ten innings, while the ordinate shows the number of right-foot contacts. A comparison of the individual curves represents both production and application (in the decreasing number of repetitions of right-foot contacts). In Figure 78 are plotted composite pulse rate curves of condition, corresponding to

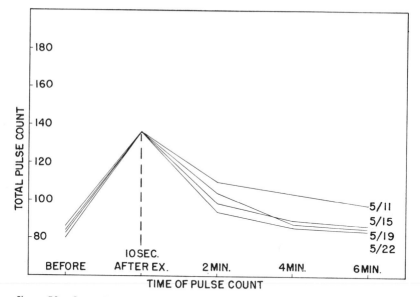

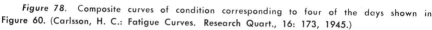

Figure 78. Composite curves of condition corresponding to four of the days shown in Figure 60. (Carlsson, H. C.: Fatigue Curves. Research Quart., 16: 173, 1945.)

four days shown in Figure 77. Apparently the fewer heart beats required for progressively more work are an indication of better conditioning.

Advantages. Among the advantages of the Carlson fatigue curve test are the following:

1. The test can be performed anytime and anywhere with a minimum of equipment.

2. A large number of subjects may be tested in a ten-minute period.

3. The test is a conditioning agent as well as a method of evaluation.

Carlson reports that 200 soldiers cut three seconds from their previous record in the 300-yard shuttle run in two weeks, and that a required 5-mile run became much easier, compared with the discomfort it caused before administration of the series of fatigue-curve tests.

Use. This test may be used with large groups in the regular physical education program in order to keep track objectively of the general condition of the group as well as to locate the extremely deficient. Having the pupils plot their own records affords a good motivating device, and is also a good opportunity to demonstrate the effects of cardiovascular efficiency. Coaches, particularly the basketball coach, might use the test as an exercise for increasing cardiovascular efficiency while obtaining objective evidence as to the condition of the team members. Records kept from year to year would offer an excellent basis for comparison, and hence more meaningful and practical information might be at hand as to the relative condition of the team.

One must remember that this test is a series of tests, administered daily for ten days.

Crampton Blood Ptosis Test

Crampton's blood ptosis test is based on the changes that the vaso-motor control of the splanchnic area undergoes when a subject moves from a reclining to a standing position.[13] Essentially, the test consists of comparing the values of the reclining heart rate and blood pressure to corresponding values in the erect position. Experimenting with high school pupils, Crampton found that a change from the reclining to the erect position results in an increase of heart rate from 0 to 44 beats per minute, and variations in the systolic blood pressure from −10 mm. to +10 mm. of mercury.

Crampton indicates that for vigorous subjects a rise of 8 to 10 mm. of mercury in systolic pressure occurs when the subject stands. On the other hand, for those people in poor condition, the systolic pressure fails to rise, and in fact may fall as much as 10 mm. of mercury. The pulse rate for subjects in good condition failed to increase on standing, whereas in less fit individuals it increased as much as 44 beats. By assigning equal values to the variations in pulse rate and blood pressure, Crampton constructed Table 34 to express the vascular tone of the subject in percentages.

Test administration:

1. The subject is placed in a comfortable reclining position with a low pillow.

2. The resting pulse is recorded for one minute.

3. Systolic pressure is taken.

4. The subject then rises and the standing pulse rate is taken. Care should be exercised to see that the pulse rate has returned to standing normal; that is, that the pulse rates of two fifteen-second counts are identical.

TABLE 34.   *Crampton's Scoring Table*

Heart Rate Increase	Systolic Blood Pressure										
	Increase						Decrease				
	10	8	6	4	2	0	−2	−4	−6	−8	−10
0– 4	100	95	90	85	80	75	70	65	60	55	50
5– 8	95	90	85	80	75	70	65	60	55	50	45
9–12	90	85	80	75	70	65	60	55	50	45	40
13–16	85	80	75	70	65	60	55	50	45	40	35
17–20	80	75	70	65	60	55	50	45	40	35	30
21–24	75	70	65	60	55	50	45	40	35	30	25
25–28	70	65	60	55	50	45	40	35	30	25	20
29–32	65	60	55	50	45	40	35	30	25	20	15
33–36	60	55	50	45	40	35	30	25	20	15	10
37–40	55	50	45	40	35	30	25	20	15	10	5
41–44	50	45	40	35	30	25	20	15	10	5	0

Crampton, C. Ward: A Test of Condition. Medical News, 87:529, 1905.

5. The systolic blood pressure is again taken and recorded in the standing position.

Scoring.   The differences between the lying and standing pulse and between the lying and standing systolic pressures are computed. Table 34 is then consulted to obtain the test score, by reading the value of the difference in systolic blood pressure against the difference in heart rate, found in its appropriate value range. As an illustration, the following hypothetical scores may be used:

PULSE RATE			SYSTOLIC BLOOD PRESSURE		
Reclining	*Standing*	*Difference*	*Reclining*	*Standing*	*Difference*
68	74	+4	100	108	+8

Index score = 95 (Excellent condition)

Crampton asserts that most people in good health will receive a score somewhere between 60 and 100. A person with a score below 50 should be investigated further to determine the cause; and a score below zero is evidence of impaired circulation, a toxic state, or severe physical disturbance.

Foster's Test

Foster's test[17] is based upon the principle that exercise increases the frequency of the heartbeat almost in direct proportion to the intensity of the exercise. If the pulse rate increases out of proportion to the intensity of the exercise, it is concluded the subject is in poor physical condition.

Test administration:

1. The pulse rate per minute is recorded with the subject in the standing position. Care should be taken to make sure that the normal standing pulse is obtained.

2. The subject runs in place for fifteen seconds, at the rate of 180 steps per minute. The pulse rate is taken for five seconds immediately following cessation of exercise and multiplied by twelve to convert to rate per minute.

3. The pulse rate is again taken after forty-five seconds of standing at ease and recorded as rate per minute.

Scoring.   With the data obtained, Table 35 is consulted to determine the score.

The following example will illustrate the method of calculating Foster's efficiency rating from Table 35.

$$
\begin{aligned}
\text{Standing pulse rate} &= 82/\text{min. } (A) &&= &&0 \\
\text{Pulse rate after exercise} &= 100/\text{min. } (B\text{-}A) &&= &&15 \\
\text{Pulse rate after 45 seconds} &= 80/\text{min. } (C\text{-}A) &&= &&-2 \\
&&& \text{Efficiency rating} &&= 13
\end{aligned}
$$

(15 is the maximum score that may be obtained)

TABLE 35. *Foster's Scoring Table*

A Standing Pulse Rate	Points	B Pulse Rate Immediately Following Exercise Minus Standing Pulse Rate (B — A) Difference	Points	C Pulse Rate after 45-Sec. Rest Minus Standing Pulse Rate (C — A) Difference	Points
100 or less	0				
101–105	—1				
106–110	—2	0–20	15		
111–115	—3	21–30	13	5	—1
116–120	—4	31–40	11	6–10	—2
121–125	—5	41–50	9	11–15	—3
126–130	—6	51–60	7	16–20	—4
131–135	—7	61–70	5	21–25	—5

Adapted from Bovard, John F., Cozens, Frederick W., and Hagman, E. Patricia: Tests and Measurements in Physical Education. 3rd ed. Philadelphia, W. B. Saunders Co., 1949, p. 66.

Interpretation of test results. The pulse rate at the beginning of the test should correspond to the average pulse rate. On 2500 boys between the ages of fourteen and eighteen years, Foster reports an average standing pulse rate of 97. The pulse rate following exercise is perhaps the most important factor in this test. Usually the greater differences between the rates before and after exercise accompany the less efficient circulatory systems. Foster claims that in boys between fourteen and nineteen one surely should not find an increase of more than 40 beats per minute for those in *good* condition. In 795 tests of secondary school boys, Foster found an average increase of 25 in pulse rate after fifteen seconds of running in place.

After a forty-five second rest, the pulse rate ought to show a lower rate, which should approach or nearly approach the pulse rate noted immediately before the test.

Gallagher and Brouha Test for High School Boys

The Gallagher and Brouha test is based upon the hypothesis that to evaluate physical fitness (the ability to perform hard work in an efficient manner) the subject should be observed while performing work.[19] The results should measure a boy's dynamic state, for example, his ability to climb a mountain. The test is based upon the principle that the rate at which the heart slows down after it has been accelerated by a standard difficult exercise gives an excellent measure of an individual's physical fitness.

These authors found, in preliminary testing, that, because of the wide range of size in boys between the ages of twelve and eighteen years, it is desirable to divide all boys into two groups on the basis of their computed surface area. This is done by use of the nomographic charts appearing in Figure 79.

Test administration.   The equipment consists of two platforms, one 20 inches high and one 18 inches high, a stop watch, and a nomographic chart (Fig. 79) to calculate surface area.

1. Measure height and weight of each boy and calculate his surface area by means of the nomographic chart (Fig. 79). The subjects are then assigned into two groups; all boys with surface area less than 1.85 square meters are placed in Group I, and all boys with surface area of 1.85 square meters or more are placed in Group II.

2. Group I boys are tested on the 18-inch platform and the boys in Group II are tested on the 20-inch platform.

3. The remaining test administration is the same as in the Harvard step test (p. 247), with the exception that the time limit is four minutes. The full test is as follows:

Time	Command
0 minutes, 0 seconds	"Ready" "Up-2-3-4"
(Exercise continues 4 minutes)	
4 minutes, 0 seconds	"Stop" "Sit down"
5 minutes, 0 seconds	"Start counting"
5 minutes, 30 seconds	"Stop counting"
6 minutes, 0 seconds	"Start counting"
6 minutes, 30 seconds	"Stop counting"
7 minutes, 0 seconds	"Start counting"
7 minutes, 30 seconds	"Stop counting"

Scoring the test.   To score the test, add the three thirty-second pulse counts, and multiply the sum by two to yield rates per minute. The physical fitness score equals the duration of the exercise in seconds times 100, divided by the sum of the pulse rates (which has already been multiplied by two).

$$\text{Physical Fitness Score} = \frac{(\text{Duration of exercise in seconds}) \times 100}{2 \ (\text{Sum of pulse counts})}$$

Following is an example of the scoring procedures:

After four-minute exercise the subject rests for one minute:
Pulse beats during next 30 seconds = 60
Pulse beats 2 minutes after exercise, counted for 30 seconds = 55
Pulse beats 3 minutes after exercise, counted for 30 seconds = 50

$$\text{Physical Fitness Score} = \frac{(240 \text{ seconds}) 100}{2 \ (60 + 55 + 50)} = \frac{24,000}{330} = 73$$

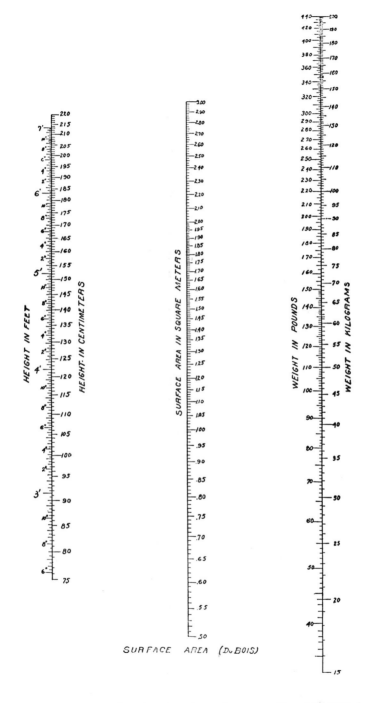

Figure 79. Nomographic chart for computing surface area. (Copyright 1920, by W. M. Boothby and R. B. Sandiford. Courtesy of Mrs. W. M. Boothby.)

If the boy becomes fatigued before the end of the four-minute period the arbitrary score of "45" may be assigned to him. Also, an arbitrary score of "55" may be assigned to all boys who lag behind or show other evidence of doing less work than is demanded by the test.

Tables have been devised to facilitate the calculation of scores, and appear in reference 19. All one has to do to compute the score is to total the actual pulse counts during the three thirty-second periods and read the final score from the table.

The following is a list of standards based upon 600 boys in private school, ranging from twelve to eighteen years of age:

SCORE	CONDITION	PER CENT
50 or less	Very poor	1.5
51 to 60	Poor	18.0
61 to 70	Fair	50.0
71 to 80	Good	25.0
81 to 90	Excellent	4.0
91 or more	Superior	1.0

Gallagher and Brouha Test for Girls

The Gallagher and Brouha test for girls was devised for estimating the dynamic physical fitness of high school girls.[20] The test is based upon the principle that the more fit a girl is, the more rapidly will her heart rate return to normal after exercise. Emphasis is placed on the fact that this test is to be used on persons who are "medically fit," that is, who have no organic defects, such as those of the heart and lungs.

Test administration. The equipment consists of a platform 16 inches high and a stop watch.

The subject stands in front of the platform. When the commands "ready" and "up" are given by the examiner, the subject places one foot on the platform, straightens her legs and back, and immediately steps down again, one foot at a time. The pace, "up-2-3-4, up-2-3-4" (the command "up" coming every two seconds) is given by the examiner. The time is counted from the beginning of the exercise to exactly four minutes, when the exercise is stopped.

At the end of the four-minute exercise the subject sits down immediately and remains quiet. Exactly one minute after cessation of exercise the subject's pulse is counted. The number of beats for the next thirty seconds is counted. Two minutes after exercise the pulse is again counted for thirty seconds, and again at the end of three minutes following exercise.

For keeping the proper cadence the authors suggest use of a drum. Subjects should not wear shoes with slippery soles; preferably, no shoes should be worn. It has been found that it is usually easier for the subject to lead off with the same foot each time and not try to alternate the feet.

However, alternating can be done during the test if one leg becomes tired. The examiner must be sure that the subject steps completely onto the platform during the test. No crouching should be permitted. If the subject falls behind in keeping pace, the observer must stop her after she has been unable to maintain the pace for about fifteen seconds. If a girl becomes overly fatigued before the four minutes have elapsed she should be stopped and the duration of exercise to that point noted.

Calculation of score. The three thirty-second pulse counts are added and the sum is multiplied by two in order to determine rates per minute. The duration of the exercise in seconds times 100 is then divided by the sum of the pulse rates multiplied by two; the result is the physical fitness score.

$$\text{Physical Fitness Score} = \frac{(\text{Duration of exercise in seconds}) \times 100}{2\ (\text{Sum of pulse counts})}$$

Girls who become fatigued may have to be stopped before the four-minute period is completed. Their scores may be calculated on the basis of the original formula, or upon the duration of the exercise (i.e., an arbitrary score of 25 when the subject stops at two minutes, 30 at two and one-half minutes, 35 for three minutes, and 40 for three and one-half minutes). The authors give an arbitrary score of 45 to all girls who complete the test but lag behind, crouch, or show other evidence of doing less work than is demanded by the test.

Harvard Step Test

The Harvard step test was developed by Brouha and associates in the Harvard Fatigue Laboratories during World War II.[7, 8] The test was constructed for purposes of measuring the ability of the body to adapt itself to hard work and to recover from same. The test may prove useful in classifying differences in fitness levels of young men into three groups: least fit, fit, and most fit. On the basis of the test results it then becomes possible to prescribe conditioning programs based upon individual needs.

Original evidence of validity for the Harvard test was based upon endurance in treadmill running, maximum heart rate per minute, and blood lactate level. Studies on Harvard undergraduates showed that athletes scored higher with less variable scores than did non-athletes, and increased their scores with more training, while termination of training resulted in lower scores.

Studies that have incorporated strength and endurance items show low relationships when correlated with the Harvard step test scores. For example, Bookwalter correlated results of the Army physical fitness test and the Harvard step test only to find no significant relationship.[6] Cureton and associates, using some twenty-seven tests of strength, muscular endurance, and running endurance, found low correlations with the Harvard step test.[15]

There are two forms of this test, the long form and the short form.

Long form.   The subject exercises on a 20-inch bench for as long a period as possible up to five minutes. The cadence is thirty steps per minute, which is quite strenuous—the most common criticism of this test. The pulse is counted from one to one and one-half, from two to two and one-half, and from three to three and one-half minutes after cessation of the exercise. The index of physical efficiency is computed by the following formula:

$$\text{Index} = \frac{(\text{Duration of exercise in seconds}) \times 100}{2 \,(\text{Sum of pulse counts in recovery})}$$

Following are standards based upon data obtained from some 8000 college students:

> Below 55 — Poor
> 55 to 64 — Low average
> 65 to 79 — Average
> 80 to 89 — Good
> Above 90 — Excellent

Short form.   In this form the pulse count is made from only one minute to one minute and thirty seconds immediately after the exercise. The scoring formula is as follows:

$$\text{Index} = \frac{(\text{Duration of exercise in seconds}) \times 100}{5.5 \times (\text{Pulse count})}$$

The norms for the short form are as follows:

> Below 50 — Poor
> 50 to 80 — Average
> Above 80 — Good

To facilitate scoring the short form table of the Harvard test, Table 36 may be used.

Karpovich, through a study of several hundred well and convalescing subjects, found the short form of the Harvard test preferable to the long form.[23] He accepted a score of 75 as minimum for "good" condition.

Instructions.   (1) Find the appropriate line for duration of effort; (2) then find the appropriate column for the pulse count; (3) read off the score where the line and column intersect; and (4) interpret according to the scale given for the short form.

TABLE 36.   *Scoring Table for Harvard Step Test (Short Form)*

Duration of Effort	Heart Beats from 1 to 1½ Minutes in Recovery										
	40–44	45–49	50–54	55–59	60–64	65–69	70–74	75–79	80–84	85–89	90–over
0 – 29″	5	5	5	5	5	5	5	5	5	5	5
0′ 30″–0′ 59″	20	15	15	15	15	10	10	10	10	10	10
1′ 0″–1′ 29″	30	30	25	25	20	20	20	20	15	15	15
1′ 30″–1′ 59″	45	40	40	35	30	30	25	25	25	20	20
2′ 0″–2′ 29″	60	50	45	45	40	35	35	30	30	30	25
2′ 30″–2′ 59″	70	65	60	55	50	45	40	40	35	35	35
3′ 0″–3′ 29″	85	75	70	60	55	55	50	45	45	40	40
3′ 30″–3′ 59″	100	85	80	70	65	60	55	55	50	45	45
4′ 0″–4′ 29″	110	100	90	80	75	70	65	60	55	55	50
4′ 30″–4′ 59″	125	110	100	90	85	75	70	65	60	60	55
5′	130	115	105	95	90	80	75	70	65	65	60

Karpovich, Peter V.: Physiology of Muscular Activity. 6th ed. Philadelphia, W. B. Saunders Co., 1965.

Jung[22] modified the Harvard step test in order to obtain a much less strenuous test. Jung's modification differs from the Harvard test in that the steps are taken only half as rapidly. Consequently, nearly everyone could complete the test. Jung refers to the score as the "cardiac recovery index," as it depends on the promptness with which a subject's heart returns to its initial rate after the temporary acceleration caused by the exercise.

Skubic and Hodgkins[27] modified the Harvard step test and found that a three-minute test, using an 18-inch bench and a stepping rate of twenty-four steps per minute, is reliable and valid. The authors claim that it clearly differentiates among females who are highly trained, those who are moderately active, and those who are sedentary. Pulse count is taken for thirty seconds following one minute of rest. Test results correlate .79 with the five-minute test and reliability on a test-retest basis resulted in a correlation of .82.

Johnson, Brouha and Darling Treadmill Test[21]

This test is designed to assess the physical fitness of men for hard muscular work. The subject walks on the treadmill at an 8.6 per cent grade, 3.5 miles per hour for five minutes. Following this warm-up, the subject sits in a chair for five minutes. At a signal he commences to run on the treadmill at a grade of 8.6 per cent and at 7 miles per hour. He runs for five minutes provided exhaustion does not set in. The duration of the run is noted to the nearest second. Radial pulse is recorded during three periods following exercise, in thirty-second periods: one to one and one-half minutes; at two to two and one-half minutes; and at four to four and one-half minutes.

$$\text{Physical fitness} = \frac{(\text{seconds subject ran}) \times 100}{2 \ (\text{sum of the 3 half-minute recovery pulse counts})}$$

Norms:

Below 40 = poor
41-75 = average
76-90 = good
90 and above = superior

Pack Test

To test large groups of men for ability to sustain heavy work, the pack test was developed during World War II.[31]

Test administration:

1. Using an 18-inch bench with a crossbar mounted above the bench, the subject grasps the bar with the left hand and places the left foot on the bench.

2. At the command "go" the subject comes to a vertical position on the bench, and continues the movement with his left foot at a rate of forty steps a minute. Every thirty seconds the subject changes legs without breaking rhythm.

3. The subject starts with a 10-pound weight placed in a pack. Every two minutes an additional 10 pounds is added, until the subject can no longer maintain the cadence.

Scoring. The total exercise time is recorded and used as the score. The pulse rate is counted ten to thirty seconds after the exercise to check whether the subject has put forth maximum effort.

Schneider Test

The Schneider test is an attempt to combine measurement of the effect that standing has on the pulse rate and pulse pressure with measurement of the effect that exercise has on the cardiovascular system.[23] The following measurements are obtained:

1. Reclining pulse rate.
2. Reclining systolic pressure.
3. Standing pulse rate.
4. Standing systolic pressure.
5. Pulse rates at the following times after cessation of exercise: immediately; and then until the rate returns to standing normal, up to two

minutes. The pulse rate is taken for fifteen seconds in each instance and the results are multiplied by four to convert into pulse rate per minute. Tables for scoring the Schneider test appear in reference 23. A perfect score, the sum of the values given to each of the six items, equals 19.

Test administration.   The subject reclines for five minutes, after which the pulse rate is counted for twenty seconds. When two consecutive twenty-second counts are identical, the count is multiplied by three, to convert to pulse rate per minute, and recorded. Next, two or three readings of systolic pressure are taken and the average reading is recorded.

The subject then rises and remains standing for two minutes in order for the pulse to assume a normal rate. When a consistent fifteen-second count is obtained, it is multiplied by four to convert to pulse rate per minute and is recorded as the normal standing rate. The systolic pressure is taken and recorded as before.

The subject next steps upon a chair, 18½ inches high, five times in fifteen seconds. For uniformity, have each subject stand with one foot on the chair at count one. This foot remains on the chair and is not brought to the floor again until after completion of five steps. In other words, the left foot is brought to the chair at the count "up" and lowered at the count "down." At the completion of the fifteen seconds, both feet should be on the floor.

Immediately after the exercise the pulse is counted for fifteen seconds, multiplied by four, and recorded. To facilitate scoring, continue taking the pulse in fifteen-second counts until the rate has returned to the normal standing rate. Note the number of seconds it takes for the pulse rate to return to normal and record this time. In order to make this computation, count from the end of the fifteen seconds of exercise to the beginning of the first normal fifteen-second pulse rate. If the pulse does not return to normal at the end of two minutes, record the number of beats above normal and discontinue counting.

Sloan Test

The Sloan test is a modification of the Harvard step test, suitable for use with women.[29] The subject steps up and down on a 17-inch bench at the rate of 30 steps per minute, for a total exercise period of five minutes or until unable to continue the exercise. The pulse rate is counted three times following exercise, in thirty-second periods: at one to one and one-half minutes; at two to two and one-half minutes; and at three to three and one-half minutes. The Fitness Index (F.I.) is computed as follows:

$$F.I. = \frac{(\text{Duration of exercise in seconds}) \times 100}{2 \ (\text{Sum of pulse counts in recovery})}$$

The standards for interpreting the Fitness Index score are as follows:

Below 55 — Poor
56 to 79 — Average
80 to 89 — Good
Above 90 — Excellent

In more recent studies, Sloan found a "Rapid Fitness Index" based on one pulse count from one to one and one-half minutes following exercise to provide nearly identical results $(r = .996)$.[30] The formula for its computation reads as follows:

$$\text{RFI} = \frac{(\text{Duration of exercise in seconds}) \times 100}{5.5\ (\text{Pulse count from 1 to } 1\tfrac{1}{2} \text{ minutes after exercise})}$$

Tuttle Pulse-Ratio Test

Tuttle's pulse ratio is interpreted as the ratio of the resting pulse rate to the rate after exercise. This ratio is computed by dividing the total number of pulse beats for two minutes after a standard exercise by the number of resting pulse beats counted for one minute. The cardiovascular efficiency of a person is determined by the amount of exercise required to obtain a 2.5 pulse-ratio.[33, 34]

Test administration:

1. The resting pulse with the subject in the sitting position is taken for one minute and recorded.

2. The subject exercises by stepping up and down on a 13-inch bench for one minute. (Twenty steps for males and fifteen steps for females.)

3. The subject, after cessation of exercise, is seated and the pulse counted for two minutes. The total number of pulse beats for two minutes is divided by the resting rate. This is the first pulse-ratio.

4. The subject remains seated until the pulse has returned to normal.

5. Again the subject exercises on the 13-inch bench for one minute. The number of steps should be increased to thirty-five or forty. The number of steps is recorded.

6. After cessation of exercise the pulse is again counted for two minutes. The two-minute total is divided by the resting pulse rate to obtain the second pulse-ratio.

To compute the number of steps required to obtain a 2.5 ratio, Karpovich has suggested use of the following formula:

$$S_0 = S_1 + \frac{(S_2 - S_1)\ (2.5 - r_1)}{r_2 - r_1}$$

Where:

S_0 = number of steps required to produce 2.5 ratio
S_1 = number of steps in first test
S_2 = number of steps in second test
r_1 = pulse-ratio for S_1

obtained by: $\left(\dfrac{\text{Total 2-minute pulse following first exercise}}{\text{Total resting pulse for one minute}} \right)$

r_2 = pulse-ratio for S_2

obtained by: $\left(\dfrac{\text{Total 2-minute pulse following second exercise}}{\text{Total resting pulse for one minute}} \right)$

The following sample values may be substituted in the Karpovich formula to show the method of calculation:

Number of steps in first test = 20
Normal sitting pulse rate = 70
Heart rate after first test = 157

Pulse-ratio for first test = $\dfrac{70}{157}$ = 2.24

Number of steps in second test = 40
Heart rate after second test = 196

Pulse-ratio for second test = $\dfrac{70}{196}$ = 2.8

Calculation:

$$S_0 = 20 + \frac{(40 - 20)\,(2.5 - 2.24)}{2.8 - 2.24} = 20 + \frac{5.2}{0.56} = 20 + 9.3$$

$$S_0 = 29.3$$

Per cent efficiency rating = $\dfrac{29.3 \times 100}{50^*}$ = 58.6%

The norms established for the Tuttle pulse-ratio are: boys, ages ten to twelve years—33 steps; boys, ages thirteen to eighteen years—30 steps; adult males—29 steps; adult females—25 steps.

Validity. Tuttle and his associates found that the pulse-ratio test points out differences in one's ability to perform on the horizontal bar, on parallel bars, and in swimming.[33] Because the test does point out these differences in physical efficiency, Tuttle recommends its use by physical educators, both in the classroom and on the athletic field, as a means for identifying those in need of training programs.

---

* 50 steps for one minute represents the amount of exercise to produce a pulse-ratio of 2.5 in a highly efficient individual. This number was selected to compute percentage of efficiency as it falls far above the requirements for a 2.5 pulse-ratio of the most fit individuals examined in Tuttle's laboratory.

Tuttle and Dickenson, working with pulse-ratio, found as reliable a ratio from a single performance of thirty steps per minute as they did from the exercises used to produce a 2.5 ratio.[34] A correlation of .93 was obtained between the original test and one that consisted of stepping onto a 13-inch bench for one minute (thirty times per minute). When the steps per minute were increased to forty, the correlation became .957.

Phillips and her co-workers found that the Tuttle test had too low a reliability coefficient to justify its use with college women.[26]

Flanagan[16] found a high correlation between the efficiency rating as measured by the pulse-ratio test and endurance in sprint running.

Studies in which the pulse-ratio test has been used show also that the results agree with physicians' judgments in terms of heart abnormalities. On this basis, it seems reasonable to use the Tuttle test as a screening device in schools where a medical examination is not given. Also, in pupils who exhibit symptoms of cardiovascular weakness, the test might be used to gain objective evidence.

The Ohio State University Step Test

The Ohio State University step test is a submaximal cardiovascular test devised to estimate the fitness of men aged eighteen years and above. The test is based on the finding that the time in which the heart rate increases to 150 beats per minute is a valid indicator of a subject's cardiovascular capacity for exhaustive work.[5]

The equipment consists of a split-level bench, 15 inches high at one level and 20 inches high at the other, with an adjustable hand bar; a metronome and a stop watch are required (Fig. 80). The test may be pre-recorded on a tape, which should be timed periodically to ensure accurate replication.

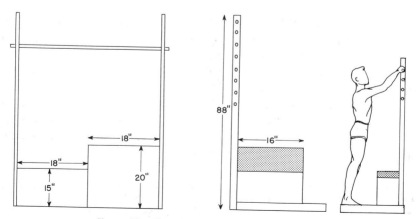

Figure 80. The Ohio State University step test.

The test comprises eighteen innings of fifty seconds' duration (total time, fifteen minutes). Each inning is divided into a thirty-second work period and a twenty-second rest period. During the rest period, a pulse count is taken for ten seconds beginning with second 5 and stopping at second 15. The test is terminated when the pulse rate reaches twenty-five beats (150 beats per minute) or when the subject completes the entire eighteen innings. Scoring is by the number of innings completed. There are three different work loads as follows:

1. Phase I consists of six innings at a cadence of *24 steps* per minute on the 15-inch bench.

2. Phase II consists of six innings at a cadence of *30 steps* per minute on the 15-inch bench.

3. Phase III consists of six innings at a cadence of *30 steps* per minute on the *20-inch* bench. Phases I, II, and III are consecutive.

Test administration.   Adjust the hand bar to the height of the subject and give the following instructions: "Grasp the bar with both hands and step up and down in cadence with the metronome. You will stop at a given command and count your pulse; if you have trouble counting your pulse, I will do it for you. To acquaint you with the procedures, I am going to let you first listen to a complete inning. Be aware of the cadence and instructions as to the exact moment at which you are to begin counting your pulse and the point at which you are to stop. When your pulse count reaches 25 for the ten-second period, the test will be terminated and the number of that inning will be your score."

The subject stands in front of the 15-inch platform and grasps the bar with both hands. When the commands "ready" and "up" are given by the examiner, the subject places one foot and then the other on the platform, straightens his legs and back, and immediately steps down again, one foot at a time. The pace "up" "up" "down" "down" is given every two and one-half seconds. At the end of thirty seconds, the commands "stop" and "find your pulse" are given.

At exactly five seconds into the rest period the examiner commands "count," and at fifteen seconds into the rest period the examiner again commands "stop" and "prepare to exercise." He records the number of beats counted during the ten-second period and continues this procedure for six innings (or until a pulse rate of 150 is reached).

After the ten-second pulse count and prior to the seventh inning, the examiner informs the subject that the cadence will be increased, and continues the same procedure. The 30-step cadence per minute during the seventh through twelfth innings requires that the commands "up" "up" "down" "down" be given every two seconds.

After the ten-second pulse count and prior to the thirteenth inning, the subject is told to move over to the 20-inch platform, where the cadence of 30 steps per minute is continued for the thirteenth through eighteenth innings.

The end point of the test is the eighteenth inning or when the subject's heart rate reaches twenty-five beats in the ten-second pulse count (150 beats per minute), whichever occurs first. The minimum and maximum times for the test are fifty seconds and fifteen minutes respectively. Usually it is easier for the subject to lead off with the same foot each time and not to try to alternate the feet. However, alternating is permissible if one leg becomes tired. The examiner must be sure that the subject steps completely onto the platform during the test. No crouching should be permitted.

Scoring. The subject's score is the inning during which his heart rate reaches 150 beats per minute (twenty-five beats during the ten-second pulse count). The number of subjects, mean age and standard deviation, and mean innings and standard deviation for age groups in the O.S.U. step test were as follows:

TABLE 37.   *Results of the Ohio State University Step Test*

Age Group	Number of Subjects	Mean Age	S.D.	Mean Innings	S.D.
19–29	28	24.0	2.9	12.4	4.7
30–40	30	34.6	2.6	13.0	4.0
41–56	17	47.5	4.2	11.8	3.4

Reliability and validity.   Kurucz[24] measured the energy cost for each of the three phases using the test with and without the hand bar. His results, which appear in Table 38, demonstrate that it is slightly easier to work with the hand bar than without it, and also that innings 10 through 18 are lactate-producing exercises. In a test-retest study, Kurucz showed the reliability to be .94. Using another group of subjects he found that the correlation of the O.S.U. step test results with those of the Balke treadmill test was .94.

The advantages of this test are that:

1. It does not overstrain the individual and yet reflects to a significant degree his cardiovascular capacity for exhaustive work.

2. Since the exercise proceeds gradually, even subjects in poor condition can be evaluated; it builds up to a more strenuous exercise so that the highly fit can be measured.

3. Scoring is simple.

TABLE 38.   *Energy Cost in Liters of O_2 for the Ohio University Step Test*

Test	Number of Subjects	Means of Innings 4, 5, 6	Means of Innings 10, 11, 12	Means of Innings 16, 17, 18
Without bar	7	1.66 L./min.	2.03 L./min.	2.58 L./min.
With bar	7	1.55 L./min.	1.90 L./min.	2.44 L./min.
		$P = <.10$	$P = <.10$	$P = <.10$

Callan Modification for Elementary School.[9] Callan adapted the O.S.U. step test for use with boys in grades four through six. The following modifications were found to result in excellent objectivity and validity:

1. Depth of bench is reduced to 13½ inches from outside of bench to a line dropped perpendicularly from the bar.

2. Pulse rate is determined by the examiner using stethoscope rather than by the subject himself.

3. The test is terminated when pulse rate reaches 29 beats for the ten seconds (174 beats per minute) or the subject completes the entire eighteen innings.

4. A subject completing the eighteen innings is given a score of 19.

5. The three work loads are as follows:
   a. First work load consists of six innings at 24-step cadence/min. on a 15-inch bench;
   b. Second work load comprises six innings at 30-step cadence/min. on a 15-inch bench; and
   c. Third work load requires six innings at 30-step cadence/min. on an 18-inch bench.

The hand bar is adjusted at eye level; instructions (with the above adaptations) are the same as in the O.S.U. step test.

Measuring 153 boys, Callan obtained a test-retest objectivity coefficient of .963. He reported a mean of 13.5 innings and a standard deviation of 4.0 for the three grades. Results showed that the fourth grade boys performed significantly better than the older and larger fifth and sixth grade boys; weight rather than age was found to be the more important factor while height had no significant effect.

Correlating the results of six of his subjects with data obtained using the modified treadmill test (p. 237) Callan obtained a coefficient of .897. He further studied validity through determining the relationship between energy expenditure (ml./kg./min.) and vertical lift calculated by multiplying the weight of the child times the height he lifted himself during the step test (N = 6). A correlation of .955 was found. Average energy expenditures for each of the three innings were found to equal:

Inning	$\dot{V}_{O_2}$ ml./kg.-min.	$\dot{V}_{O_2}$ l./min.
1	23.2 ± 2.6	.836
2	28.5 ± 2.7	1.048
3	31.7 ± 4.1	1.227

Summary and Conclusions

At present the general use of cardiovascular tests in physical education is quite limited. Lack of sufficiently high validity and the difficulty of obtaining reliable test scores are the obvious reasons for their limitation. However, these tests can make a contribution in terms of identifying persons who are extremely low in terms of cardiorespiratory fitness. When the score is extremely low, it is reasonable to refer the person to a physician for diagnosis. If no pathologic process is involved, then a graduated program of individual instruction should be initiated to ameliorate the deficiency.

Cardiovascular tests might also be employed as a screening process when a medical examination is not given. This does not imply, however, that the test is a substitute for a good medical examination.

BIBLIOGRAPHY

1. Alderman, Richard B.: Reliability of Individual Differences in the 180 Heart Rate Response Test in Bicycle Ergometer Work. Research Quart., October, 1966, p. 429.
2. Balke, B.: Arbeitsphysiologie, 15:311, 1954.
3. Balke, B.: J. Appl. Physiol., 7:231, 1954.
4. Barach, J. H.: The Energy Index. J.A.M.A., Vol. 62, February 14, 1914.
5. Billings, Chas. E., Tomashefski, J., Carter, E. T., and Ashe, Wm.: J. Appl. Physiol., 15:1001, 1960.
6. Bookwalter, Karl W.: A Study of the Brouha Step Test. The Physical Educator, Vol. 5, No. 3, May, 1948.
7. Brouha, Lucien: The Step Test: A Simple Method of Measuring Physical Fitness for Muscular Work in Young Men. Research Quart., Vol. 14, No. 1, March, 1943.
8. Brouha, Lucien, Fradd, Norman W., and Savage, Beatrice M.: Studies in Physical Efficiency of College Students. Research Quart., Vol. 15, No. 3, October, 1944.
9. Callan, Donald E.: A Submaximal Cardiovascular Fitness Test for Fourth, Fifth and Sixth Grade Boys. Unpublished Doctoral Dissertation, The Ohio State University, 1968.
10. Carlson, H. C.: Fatigue Curve Test. Research Quart., No. 16, October, 1945.
11. Committee to Revise Standardization of High Blood Pressure Readings, Recommendations for Human Blood Pressure Determinations by Sphygmomanometers. American Heart Association, New York, New York, October, 1951.
12. Consolazio, C. Frank, Johnson, Robert E., and Pecora, Louis J.: Physiological Measurements of Metabolic Functions in Man. New York, McGraw-Hill Book Company, 1963, pp. 341, 373.
13. Crampton, C. Ward: A Test of Condition. Medical News, Vol. 87, September, 1905.
14. Cureton, T. K.: Physical Fitness Appraisal and Guidance. St. Louis, C. V. Mosby Co., 1947.
15. Cureton, T. K., et al.: Endurance of Young Men. Washington, Society for Research in Child Development, Vol. X, No. 1, Serial No. 40, 1945.
16. Flanagan, Kenneth: The Pulse-Ratio Test as a Measure of Athletic Endurance in Sprint Running. Supplement to Research Quart., October, 1935.
17. Foster, W. L.: A Test of Physical Efficiency. American Physical Education Review, Vol. XIX, December, 1914. (See also: Williams, J. F.: The Organization and Administration of Physical Education. New York, The Macmillan Co., 1923, p. 294.)
18. Fox, Samuel M., III, and Skinner, James S.: Physical Activity and Cardiovascular Health. Amer. J. Cardiol., 14:731–746, December, 1964.
19. Gallagher, J., and Brouha, Lucien: A Simple Method of Testing the Physical Fitness of Boys. Research Quart., Vol. 14, No. 1, March, 1943.
20. Gallagher, J. Roswell, and Brouha, Lucien: A Functional Fitness Test for High School Girls. Reprinted from the Journal of Health and Physical Education, December, 1943.

21. Johnson, R. E., Brouha, L., and Darling, R. C.: A Test of Physical Fitness for Strenuous Exercise. Rev. Canad. Biol., 1:491–503, June, 1942.

22. Jung, Frederic T.: The Measurement of Physical Fitness as a Problem in Physical Medicine. Arch. Phys. Med., 32:327, 1951.

23. Karpovich, Peter V., and Synning, W.: Physiology of Muscular Activity. 7th ed. Philadelphia, W. B. Saunders Company, 1965.

24. Kurucz, Robert L.: Construction of The Ohio State University Cardiovascular Fitness Test. Doctoral dissertation, The Ohio State University, September, 1967.

25. Morris, J., Heady, J., Raffle, P., Roberts, C., and Parks, J.: Coronary Heart Disease and Physical Activity of Work. Lancet, 2:1053, 111, November, 1953.

26. Phillips, Marjorie, Redder, Eloise, and Yeakel, Helen: Further Data on the Pulse-Ratio Test. Research Quart., Vol. 14, No. 4, December, 1943.

27. Skubic, Vera, and Hodgkins, Jean: Cardiovascular Efficiency Test for Girls and Women. Research Quart., 34:2, 191, May, 1963.

28. Slater-Hammel, A. T., and Butler, L. K.: Accuracy in Securing Rates by Palpation. Research Quart., Vol. 11, No. 2, May, 1940.

29. Sloan, A. W.: J. Appl. Physiol., 14:985, 1959.

30. Sloan, A. W.: Physical Fitness of College Students in South Africa, United States of America, and England. Research Quart., Vol. 34, No. 2, May, 1963, pp. 244–248.

31. Taylor, Craig: A Maximal Pack Test of Exercise Tolerances. Research Quart., Vol. 15, No. 4, December, 1944.

32. Truett, Jeanne T., Benson, Herbert, and Balke, Bruno: On the Practicability of Submaximal Exercise Testing. J. Chronic Dis., 19:711–715, 1966.

33. Tuttle, W. W.: The Use of the Pulse-Ratio Test for Rating Physical Efficiency. Research Quart., Vol. 2, No. 2, May, 1931.

34. Tuttle, W. W., and Dickerson, R. E.: A Simplification of the Pulse-Ratio Technique for Rating Physical Efficiency and Present Condition. Research Quart., Vol. 11, No. 2, May, 1938.

chapter 9

nutritional measurements and somatotype

Influence on the development of strong, healthy bodies is greatest during the growing years. A primary cause of interruption of the normal growth cycle of children is nutritive deficiency. As a result of the pre-induction physical examination during World War II it was found that one-third of the draftees were unfit for military service directly or indirectly because of nutritional deficiencies.

Furthermore, studies conducted by the National Research Council have revealed that there is widespread prevalence of moderately deficient diets in the United States.[8]

The physical educator is in a vital position to detect and refer cases of possible malnutrition to the health or medical specialist. Because nutrition plays such an important role in the general physical fitness of the child this chapter is devoted to methods of appraising the nutritional status of the public school child.

Nutrition

According to Lusk, nutrition may be defined as the sum processes concerned with growth, maintenance, and repair of the living body as a whole or of its constituent parts.[9] Nutrition deals with the individual cells of the body and the constant exchange of nutrients. Therefore, nutrition is primarily concerned with the supply of essential foodstuffs to all the cells within the body that enable the cells to carry on their proper functions. Actually you might consider that nutrition involves the food supply itself and the entire chain of processes through which the food must go in order to be used properly by the body, whether the essential nutrients go to build or to repair body tissue, to regulate body processes, or to act as fuel for the external and internal work of the body.

Obviously, then, *good nutrition* implies that everything in the chain of processes for nutrition is running smoothly. Food is supplied in the amounts and kinds needed by every individual cell, and the various organs, juices, and enzymes are doing their part in making food available for use by the cells. Each tissue is thus receiving sufficient materials for its proper functioning and for building its structure, as well as being relieved of its waste products.

Poor nutrition implies that some breakdown is occurring in this normal sequence of events. For example, the food supply may be limited in amount, or lacking in particular constituents (protein, carbohydrates, fats, minerals, or vitamins) required by certain of the body cells; or the food supply may be abundant, but the body may be unable to utilize its nutrients because of some defect in the organs or because of abnormal conditions involving some phase of the internal processes of the body.

Whenever a body part is not receiving the kind and amount of the essential nutrients it needs, it is malnourished. Children living under favorable nutritional conditions are frequently reported to be taller, heavier, and better developed in other aspects at a given age than children living under less favorable conditions.

Malnutrition (lack of essential nutrient intake by the body) may be such that retardation of growth will be cumulative to the point that the smallness or frailness of the subject almost appears to be an inherited characteristic, when actually the retardation is the direct result of malnutrition.

In addition to the obvious effects of malnutrition, it is believed that nutrient deficiency causes greater susceptibility to disease than is normal, by lowering body resistance, and is also responsible for slowing down the recovery phase after disease. This is particularly true for such diseases as tuberculosis, rheumatic fever, and diabetes.

It is apparent that nutrition is related to numerous physical manifestations paralleling growth and development of the child. Such related aspects include chronic fatigue, poor or faulty body mechanics, mental health, dental caries, and general all-around organic and neuromuscular development, particularly of the growing child. It behooves all teachers, and especially the trained physical educator, to appraise the nutritional status of the child and to refer those in possible need of medical attention to the proper authorities so that a corrective dietary program may be initiated.

Measuring Nutritional Status

Two general methods for appraising nutritional status are in use today. One method involves subjective judgment. In it the examiner compares the characteristics of the child to a list of characteristics of the well and of the malnourished child. The second method of appraisal is an objective measurement in which the examiner uses special instruments, such as calipers, for making certain anthropometrical measurements. By applying these measurements to specially prepared tables, he is able to determine the nutritional status of the pupil.

SUBJECTIVE EVALUATION

Subjective evaluation should be practiced by teachers continuously. In developing an awareness of characteristics of the poorly nourished child and in practicing observations, the instructor will soon find himself unconsciously appraising the children each day. This is as it should be, because early detection is vital if the condition is to be corrected before harmful effects are sustained by the growing body.

Following is a list of characteristics of children in states of good and bad nutrition as prepared by Bogert.[2]

GOOD NUTRITION	MALNUTRITION
Well-developed body	Body may be undersized, or show poor development or physical defects
About average weight for height	Usually thin (underweight 10 per cent or more), but may be normal or overweight (fat and flabby)
Muscles well developed and firm	Muscles small and flabby
Skin turgid and of healthy color	Skin loose and { pale, waxy, or sallow
Good layer of subcutaneous fat	Subcutaneous fat usually lacking
Mucous membranes of eyelids and mouth reddish pink	Mucous membranes pale
Hair smooth and glossy	Hair often rough and without luster
Eyes clear and without dark circles under them	Dark hollows or circles under eyes
Facial expression alert, but without strain	Facial expression drawn, worried, old; or animated, but strained

GOOD NUTRITION	MALNUTRITION
Posture good $\left\{ \begin{array}{l} \text{head erect} \\ \text{chest up} \\ \text{shoulders flat} \\ \text{abdomen in} \end{array} \right.$	Fatigue posture $\left\{ \begin{array}{l} \text{head thrust forward} \\ \text{chest narrow and flat} \\ \text{shoulders rounded} \\ \text{abdomen protruding} \end{array} \right.$
Good natured and full of life	Irritable, overactive, fatigues easily; or phlegmatic, listless, fails to concentrate
Sleeps soundly	Difficult to get to sleep, or sleeps restlessly
Digestion and elimination good	Subject to $\left\{ \begin{array}{l} \text{nervous indigestion} \\ \text{constipation} \end{array} \right.$
Appetite good	"Finicky" about food
General health excellent	Susceptible to infections; lacks endurance and vigor

To become thoroughly acquainted with this list requires little time. Furthermore, the physical educator, while supervising the shower, will find that he can quickly appraise the youngsters periodically in terms of their nutritional status. It is not necessary to line them up and have a formal inspection, but rather the instructor, without the knowledge of the pupils, may regularly conduct an informal appraisal. As was briefly mentioned earlier, from practice comes proficiency. For the first few children the evaluation may go slowly; however, after inspecting 50 to 100 pupils the process becomes almost automatic.

The inspection method of evaluation alone may be criticized on the grounds of the subjective nature of the test. A great deal of emphasis is placed on the standards of the examiner in terms of what he believes the appearance of a healthy person should be. Franzen, in studying the reliability of physicians' ratings of health status, found considerable differences of opinion.[5] Correlations of reliability between the physicians' ratings ranged from .18 to .82. However, it was found that a physician would consistently agree with himself, that is, if he rated a child as well nourished he was consistent in so doing.

OBJECTIVE MEASUREMENT

To eliminate as much as possible the error that is apt to accompany subjective evaluation, several valid objective tests have been developed. It is wise, when some doubt is cast on the nutritional status of the child, to check him against a more valid measurement than personal inspection.

Age-height-weight tables.   The earliest methods of appraising physical status were tables from which weight could be predicted on the basis of sex, age, and height. In establishing these tables, a large number of people of the same sex, age, and height were weighed. The average weight was computed and recorded as the normal weight for all persons of that same sex, age, and height. The best-known tables of this type are the

Wood-Baldwin Age-Height-Weight Tables. To be sure, one cannot expect a given person to weigh exactly the same as a norm computed on the basis of several thousand people. Hence, the usual interpretation of such norms is that the person should be within 10 to 15 per cent of his own norm.

There are several disadvantages to using age-height-weight tables. In the first place, no consideration is taken into account for differences in body build. That is to say, one youngster may be a tall, slender type while another child of the same age may have inherited a short and stocky build. Because the two youngsters do not conform to the norm does not necessarily imply that one or the other is undernourished.

It is at times an error to accept the average as being normal. The averaging of a large number of weights results in one number. What this average means in terms of health could be anyone's guess. It simply is the best single score for representing the group of scores.

Pryor Width-Weight Tables. Pryor, maintaining that determination of appropriate body weight as an index of nutrition should take into account not only the factors of sex, height, and age, but also the nature of the bony framework and body structure, has devised a test of nutritional status for persons between the ages of one and forty-one.[10]

Following a study of various body measurements that might be used as indexes of body build, the bi-iliac diameter or width of the pelvic crest was selected as the most important and least variable measurement of body width. In addition to this measurement, the thoracic width and the height and weight of the subject are recorded. With these data, specially prepared tables are used to determine the proper weight of the subject. The measurements are made as follows:

1. Record age to the nearest year, height to the nearest inch, and weight to the nearest pound.

2. Thoracic lateral diameter is measured by placing the calipers horizontally at a level with the nipples. No pressure should be applied. The subject should be at rest and measurement taken at the end of normal expiration. Record to nearest tenth of a centimeter.

3. The bi-iliac diameter is measured with caliper held horizontally and with firm pressure against the crest of the ilium. When measuring boys, the arms of the caliper should be tilted slightly downward. Record to the nearest tenth of a centimeter.

In scoring, refer to tables in reference 9. Determine whether the subject has a narrow, medium, or broad chest by referring to the tables for his age and sex. In the proper chest width table, opposite the height measurement and under the bi-iliac diameter measurement, will be found the appropriate weight in pounds for a child of this body build. (If a child's bi-iliac diameter measurement falls between the two columns, interpolate.)

Pelidisi formula. During World War I, in order to keep the spirit up to the highest point, the governments of the Central Powers, particularly Austria, informed their people that the conflict would end in their victory in a few months. As a result, food conservation was practiced very little during the first years of the war. Eventually there was widespread malnutrition, the most outstanding evidence of which was rickets.

Pirquet and staff recognized the situation and went to work to develop a simplified method of locating nutritional deficiency. These investigators demonstrated that the cube of the sitting height in centimeters is approximately ten times the weight in grams of the normal person.[4] Therefore, by knowing the sitting height and weight, the nutritional status of a person may be estimated. This measurement is called the *pelidisi,* a word compounded from the Latin words describing the factors in its calculation. The pelidisi is computed in percentage by the following formula:

$$\text{Pelidisi} = \frac{\sqrt[3]{10 \times (\text{Weight in gm.})}}{(\text{Sitting height in cm.})} = 100 \text{ per cent}$$

In actual practice the pelidisi of a well-nourished child is very close to 100 per cent. An obese child may score up to 110 per cent, while thin children average between 88 and 94 per cent. The thinnest youngster whom Pirquet observed in Austria had a pelidisi of 85 per cent. Generally speaking, a child with a pelidisi between 95 and 100 per cent may be said to be well nourished. An adult, however, with a pelidisi below 100 per cent is undoubtedly undernourished. At 104 or 105 per cent he is overfed and his food intake should be reduced.

Specific gravity. Sloan has stated that weight comparisons among individuals possessing the same stature, age and sex are an unreliable index of obesity.[14] Extra weight may be due not only to obesity but to greater development of bone or muscle. Bone and muscle tissue are more dense, and thus heavier than adipose tissue. Specific gravity, which reflects body density, is a much more reliable measure than weight alone. Density is defined as mass per unit volume:

$$D = \frac{M}{V}$$

D = density
M = mass (weight of body)
V = Volume

Specific gravity of a body may be defined as the ratio of its density to that of an equal volume of water. Body density is commonly determined using the principle of Archimedes which states that when an object is immersed in a fluid it loses an amount of weight equal to the weight of the fluid which is displaced. Consequently, when using the metric system (1 gm. water = 1 cc.) this weight loss is numerically equal to the volume of water displaced. For example, if you were to weigh a solid object in air, then in water, the weight loss in water would equal the weight of the water displaced.

$$\text{Specific Gravity} = \frac{\text{Weight of object in air}}{\text{Weight of water displaced}}$$

or

$$\text{Specific Gravity} = \frac{\text{Weight of object in air}}{\text{Weight in air} - \text{weight in water}}$$

As a simple illustration, what would be the specific gravity of a stone weighing 200 gm. in air and 120 gm. in water? What would its volume equal?

$$\text{Specific Gravity} = \frac{200 \text{ gm.}}{200 \text{ gm.} - 120 \text{ gm.}} = 2.5$$

The stone's volume would equal 80 cc. since the displaced water equals 80 gm. and the volume of 80 gm. of water equals 80 cc. As the stone's density is 2.5 times that of water, the stone would certainly sink.

Measurement of human body density can also be determined through underwater weighing. The subject is immersed up to his neck in a tank of water at a comfortable temperature of around 35° C; he breathes out, and at the end of forced expiration his underwater weight is noted. Pulmonary residual volume is measured and then density of the body (excluding this residual volume) is calculated.

Skinfold measurements (Fig. 81).   Lean body mass is best determined by employing the Archimedean principle by which the individual is weighed both in water and air to obtain his specific gravity. However,

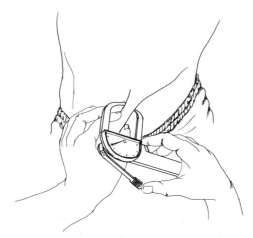

Figure 81.   Use of Lange skin calipers.

because of obvious technical difficulties, studies have been conducted to find a less complex manner of determining body density. It has been found that certain skinfold measurements may be used with considerable accuracy in predicting density.

Among the more popular types of calipers is the Lange, which may be purchased from Cambridge Scientific Instruments in Cambridge, Maryland. Measurements of skinfold may be made in the following regions: chest, abdomen, arm, back, and neck. The right side of the body is usually used; the examiner grasps two thicknesses of skin and subcutaneous fat between his thumb and index finger. Muscle should not be included in the measurement—when in doubt direct the person to perform a movement that will cause a contraction under the tissue being held. In most cases, the folds are taken along a vertical plane with the blades of the calipers held vertically (Fig. 81). Departure from this position is permissible when the natural folds of the skin demand it.

Consolazio et al.[5] feel that a conservative attitude should be taken regarding skinfold measurements. Reproducibility is difficult to achieve even under laboratory conditions. Therefore, the examiner should practice until consistency is obtained. Furthermore, these authors explain the importance of the skin turgor (normal fullness of the blood vessels and capillaries): simple dehydration will increase the skinfold thickness as much as 15 per cent. To obtain valid and reliable results, one experienced examiner should take duplicate measurements early in the morning (to eliminate diurnal variation in state of hydration).

Wilmore and Behnke[16] have proposed several regression equations for estimating body density and lean body weight in young men from anthropometric measures.

$$\text{Lean Body Weight (kg.)} = 44.646 + 1.0817 \ \ (\text{body weight in kg.})$$
$$- \ 0.7396 \ (\text{abdominal circumference in centimeters})$$

The multiple correlation with measured body density equals .938 and the standard error of estimate for the formula is equal to 2.815 kg. Abdominal circumference is measured using a cloth tape at the level of the umbilicus. Fat percentage is calculated from the following equation:

$$\% \ \text{Fat} = 100 - \left(100 \times \frac{\text{LBW}}{\text{Body weight}} \right)$$

An illustration of the calculation follows:

Subject's body weight = 70 kg.
abdominal circumference = 82.5 cm.

$$\text{LBW} = 44.636 + 1.0817 \ (70) - 0.7396 \ (82.5)$$
$$44.636 + 75.719 - 61.017$$
$$120. \ 355 - 61.017$$

$$LBW = 59.338 \text{ kg.}$$

$$\% \text{ Fat} = (100 - 100 \times 59.338/70.000)$$
$$= 100 - 100 \times .848$$
$$= 100 - 84.8$$
$$\% \text{ Fat} = 15.2$$

Wilmore and Behnke studied fifty-four male college men in order to demonstrate how well lean body weight (LBW) could be predicted from various body diameters; their criterion measure was lean body weight estimated by the underwater weighing technique.[17] It was found that the anthropometric predictions of LBW correlated highly with the density–specific gravity estimations of LBW ($r = 0.87$ to 0.92). Means were within $0.09 - 0.59$ kg. of one another and the standard error of estimate was 2.54 kg.

In studies dealing with the calculation of lean body weight (LBW), Behnke has employed several symbols, the definitions being as follows:

W = weight (kilograms)
h = height or stature (decimeters)
c = value of a specific anthropometric diameter for any one individual (centimeters)
$\bar{c}$ = mean value for c of a specific diameter for a given group of people or sample
k = conversion constant which is specific for a given diameter (c) and will be identified later; and
d = c/k.

Behnke had shown in earlier work that LBW could be predicted from the following equation:

$$LBW = 0.204 \times h^2$$

More recently a revised equation has been reported:

$$LBW = D^2 \times h$$

in which D is the average of four d values. The four recommended d values to use are as follows:

1. *Biacromial.* Distance between the most lateral projections of the acromial processes with the elbows next to the body and the hands resting on thighs.
2. *Bitrochanteric.* Distance between the most lateral projections of the greater trochanters.
3. *Wrist.* Distance between the styloid processes of the radius and ulna. Sum of right and left sides.
4. *Ankle.* Distance between the malleoli with the anthropometer pointed upward at a 45° angle. Sum of right and left sides.

Diameters 2 and 4 are measured while the subject stands and diameters 1 and 3 are measured while the subject is seated.

The individual d values are obtained by dividing an individual's measurement (in centimeters) with the conversion factor (c/k). The conversion factor is the average measurement of the group being tested. (For individuals or small groups conversion constants may be taken from Behnke's "reference man."[1])

$$k_i = \frac{\bar{c}_i}{\sqrt{LBW/h}}$$

In which:

$i =$ a single diameter
$\bar{c} =$ mean of specific diameter for any given group
$LBW = 0.204 \times h^2$ (h in decimeters)
$h =$ stature in decimeters

Table 39 contains data from Wilmore and Behnke which will allow us to illustrate the calculations. Referring to the table, column c contains actual measurements of subject THB. Column k was obtained using formula for conversion factor (k_i) and column d is obtained by dividing an individual measurement with its specific conversion factor; that is, by dividing the value in column c by the value in column k. Thus:

$$LBW = D^2 \times h$$
$$D^2 = (1.87)^2$$
$$h = 17.39$$
$$LBW = (3.497)\,(17.39)$$
$$LBW = 60.81$$

$$\% \text{ Fat} = \frac{\text{Body weight} - LBW}{\text{Body weight}} \times 100$$

$$= \frac{76.00 - 60.81}{76.00} \times 100$$

$$= \frac{15.19}{76.00} \times 100 = 19.99\%$$

The lean body weight calculated from actual underwater weighing (61.10 kg.) is not very different from our predicted value (60.81 kg.). The same can be said for lean body fat: actual 19.60% and predicted 19.99%. Attention is drawn to the formula:

$$LBW = 0.204 \times h^2$$
$$LBW = (0.204)\,(17.39^2) = 61.69 \text{ kg}$$

TABLE 39. *Calculation of LBW from Body Diameters*

Subject: THB		Densitometric Analysis	
Age: 27.4 Height: 17.39 dm. Weight: 76.00 kg.		Density: 1.053 % Fat: 19.60 LBW: 61.10 kg.	
Diameter (cm.)	c	k	d
Biacromial	39.3	21.3	1.85
Bitrochanteric	32.5	17.3	1.88
Wrist	10.4	5.9	1.76
Ankle	14.3	7.2	1.99

$$\Sigma d = 7.48$$

$$D = \frac{\Sigma d}{4}$$

$$D = \frac{7.48}{4} = 1.87$$

(Adapted from Wilmore, J. H. and Behnke, A. R.: Predictability of Lean Body Weight Through Anthropometric Assessment in College Men. J. Appl. Physiol., Vol. 25, No. 4, October, 1968, p. 354.)

Employing stature measurement alone, Behnke's formula for LBW results in a value comparable to the actual LBW measurement of 61.10 kg. This value could then be substituted in the formula for a satisfactory estimation of the percentage of body fat.

The ACH Index.   The ACH index is proposed as an aid in sorting out children between the ages of seven and twelve years who should be given a more thorough medical examination by a physician.[7] The index is based upon three measurements: arm girth, chest depth, and hip width. The authors arrived at these measurements as a result of medical judgment coupled with numerous anthropometric data including shoulder breadth, hip width, chest depth and width, height, weight, arm and calf girth, size of deltoid, and thickness of subcutaneous tissue over different areas of arms and legs. The sample consisted of over 10,000 children of varying economic and social backgrounds.

Finally, the measurements regarded as essential to an evaluation of soft tissue for skeletal build were narrowed down to the following: hip width, chest depth, chest width, height, weight, arm girth, and subcutaneous tissue over the upper arm. From these seven measures, arm girth, chest depth, and hip width were selected as the most comprehensive and simple combination to measure in evaluating a large group of persons.

As suggested by the authors, the index may be used as a screening device to select a fourth of the children measured. To this quarter the remaining seven of the anthropometric measures would be applied. Franzen and Palmer assert that this procedure would identify over 90 per cent of the children who would be selected if all seven measures were applied to the entire group. The final group selected should be referred to a physician for examination and diagnosis.

Still another method of using the ACH, particularly in a school situation, would be to set the scale to select only a tenth of the group. This method does cause some extreme defect cases to be overlooked, but Franzen and Palmer feel that the few omissions may be sacrificed in the interest of speed and simplicity of measurement. Its efficiency is still much better than the age-height-weight method. As an illustration, when the ACH index selects three-fifths of extreme defect cases, the age-height-weight method (used in a comparable manner) selects only one-fifth.

In taking the measurements, it is best to have the subjects in their physical education costumes. If this is not possible, heavy outside garments such as jackets and sweaters should be removed.

Girth of the upper arm is measured by means of a gulick tape. If subject is right-handed, measure the right arm; if left-handed, measure the left arm. The subject flexes his arm at the elbow joint. A skin pencil is used to mark the highest point. The subject then places the tips of his fingers on his shoulder at which time the girth of the upper arm in this flexed position is recorded. With the tape in the same position, the subject is asked to drop his arm in a relaxed state at the side of his body. The upper arm is measured in this relaxed state. Readings are recorded to the nearest tenth of a centimeter.

Chest depth is recorded by means of a wooden caliper at both the inspiration and the expiration phase of normal breathing. The caliper is placed just slightly above the nipple line and below the angle of the left scapula; it is held snugly against the chest. The readings for both expiration and inspiration phase are recorded to the nearest tenth of a centimeter.

Width of hips is recorded by placing the caliper on the most lateral portions of the greater trochanters. The width is recorded to the nearest tenth of a centimeter.

Scoring of the ACH is accomplished in the following manner:

1. Add the two chest-depth measurements.
2. Add the two arm-girth measurements.
3. Subtract (2) from (1).
4. From Table 40 determine the difference allowed for a child of this particular hip width.
5. If the difference obtained from measuring is greater than the value found in the table, the child would not be selected for further examination. However, if the obtained difference is less than or equal to the value read from the table, the child should receive a medical examination.

The Wetzel Grid (Fig. 82). The Wetzel Grid is a direct reading control chart on the quality of child growth.[15] The grid is a record of the child's growth as reflected by height and weight, as well as a visual demonstration of whether or not his growth is progressing satisfactorily and the extent to which this is so. The grid provides a means of determining the

TABLE 40. *ACH Index of Nutritional Status (Ages 7 to 12)*

Boys		Girls	
Width of Hips	Minimum Difference between Arm Girth and Chest Depth	Width of Hips	Minimum Difference between Arm Girth and Chest Depth
Below 20.0	0.0	Below 20.0	.5
20.0–20.4	0.0	20.0–20.4	1.0
20.5–20.9	.4	20.5–20.9	1.6
21.0–21.4	1.0	21.0–21.4	2.1
21.5–21.9	1.6	21.5–21.9	2.6
22.0–22.4	2.2	22.0–22.4	3.0
22.5–22.9	2.7	22.5–22.9	3.4
23.0–23.4	3.3	23.0–23.4	3.8
23.5–23.9	3.8	23.5–23.9	4.2
24.0–24.4	4.2	24.0–24.4	4.5
24.5–24.9	4.7	24.5–24.9	4.8
25.0–25.4	5.1	25.0–25.4	5.1
25.5–25.9	5.6	25.5–25.9	5.4
26.0–26.4	6.0	26.0–26.4	5.6
26.5–26.9	6.3	26.5–26.9	5.8
27.0–27.4	6.7	27.0–27.4	6.0
27.5–27.9	7.0	27.5–27.9	6.1
28.0–28.4	7.3	28.0–28.4	6.2
28.5–28.9	7.6	28.5–28.9	6.3
29.0 over	7.9	29.0 over	6.4

Franzen, Raymond, and Palmer, George: The ACH Index of Nutritional Status. New York, American Child Health Association, 1934.

direction of growth and the rate at which growth occurs, from infancy to maturity.

Definition of terms. The following are terms used in the description of the grid.

Level. Each channel is marked off by horizontal cross lines at intervals of five, with accompanying cross lines ranging from 0 to 185. The word *level* refers to the measure of the child's body size, because each level represents a certain value of body surface.

Channel. This is a means of determining a child's physique or body build by plotting height and weight measurements. Wetzel classifies the principal varieties of physiques into nine channels, extending from A4 through B4. All subjects in a given channel have substantially the same body physique regardless of developmental levels: obese subjects have points outside and to the left of channel A4; the stocky, in A3 and A2; those of medium build, in A1-M-B1; the slender, in B2, B3; and the extremely thin, in B4 and below. The purposes of the center grid panel, therefore, are to measure the child's body build by channels and his body size by levels.

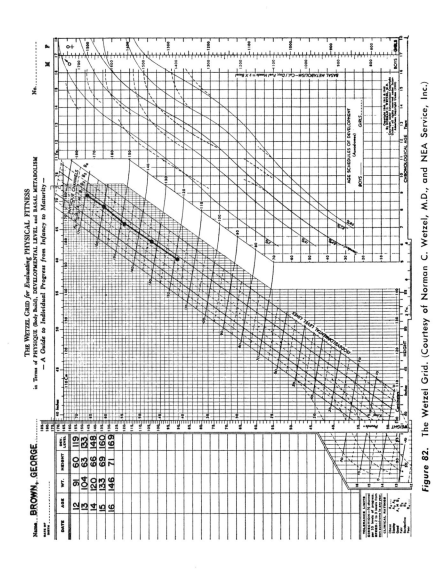

Figure 82. The Wetzel Grid. (Courtesy of Norman C. Wetzel, M.D., and NEA Service, Inc.)

Auxodrome.   By plotting the level a child has reached on the channel system at a given age in the right-hand panel of a grid, one obtains a curve known as the child's auxodrome, which in health parallels one of the five standard auxodromes illustrated. A child's auxodrome is thus an indication of how far the child has traveled along the channel system.

Purposes of grid.   A basic assumption underlying the grid technique is that a child is his own standard of comparison. One of the purposes of the grid is to identify difference in body type, for example, by means of the nine channels designated by Wetzel as A4 through B4. With periodic check-ups a teacher may determine various irregularities in child growth by observing whether or not the pupil remains in his proper growth channel. Without the grid, it may take perhaps a year or more for any nutritional or physiological abnormalities to manifest themselves externally or to disclose what an auxodrome indicates when it shows that growth has slowed down considerably.

Some 2095 children's grid ratings were compared with the clinical appraisals of school physicians. There was an 87.5 per cent agreement between the physician's ratings and the grid. A major portion of the disagreement that did occur was in the evaluation of the physical status of children whose curves and points fell in the B2 channel. Physicians therefore have their greatest difficulty in agreeing on the fitness status of the B2 type children. Omitting these children would have resulted in a 94.5 per cent agreement for the remaining channels.

Wetzel states that the clue to early recognition of malnutrition is invariably found in the evidence that growth and development are retarded or completely stopped. As a rule, growth slows down and developmental lag sets in before a child shows any considerable loss of weight.

Directions for plotting the grid (Fig. 83):

1. At the time of the initial observation, the name, date of birth, age, height, and weight of the child are recorded in the proper places.

2. The center of the grid is made up of a system of coordinates at right angles to each other. The horizontal scales represent height in both centimeters and inches. The vertical scales represent weight in both kilograms and pounds. Locate the child's height at the bottom of the grid. Follow up the vertical line to the point opposite the child's weight. Plot the point corresponding to the height and weight of the subject for the initial observation. (Fig. 83, initial observation: height 60 inches, weight 91 lbs.)

3. Such a point lies within one of the nine channels running diagonally across the grid. (The point just plotted lies in channel B1 at level 119.) Additionally, a channel represents the physique of the subject whose corresponding physical status is classified under the heading "clinical ratings" of the table in the lower left-hand corner.

4. The lines cutting across the channel lines indicate the child's level of development. The child should advance a level line each month along

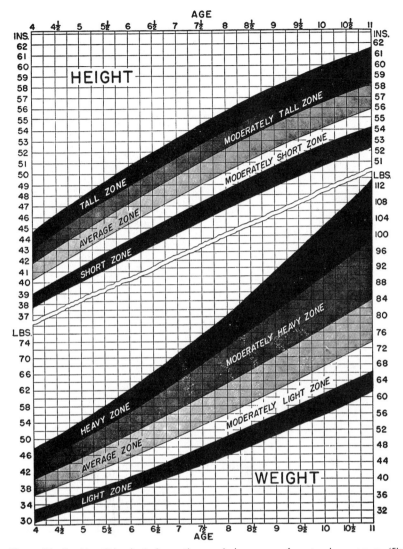

Figure 83, A. Meredith physical growth record: boys, ages four to eleven years. (Figure 66, A-D, reproduced by courtesy of Howard V. Meredith and the Joint Committee on Health Problems in Education of the National Education Association and the American Medical Association.)

his established channel. (Observe that these level lines are in intervals of five.)

5. Referring to the right side of the grid one sees five principal age schedules of development, known as standard auxodromes, which represent the percentage distribution of children reaching the various levels throughout their period of growth. For example, the uppermost curve is the 2 per cent schedule, which indicates that 2 per cent of all children reach, say, level 90 at age seven and one-half years, or earlier, since it crosses level 90 at 7½. By the same token, 15 per cent of the children

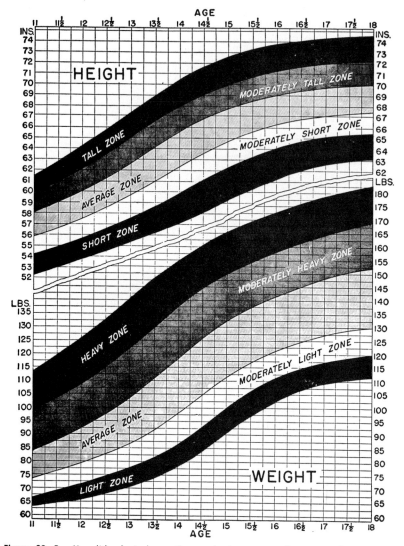

Figure 83, B. Meredith physical growth records: boys, ages eleven to eighteen years.

reach level 90 or above at about nine and one-half years. Hence, all that is needed to draw a child's own auxodrome is the information in columns two and five of the data table, i.e., age and level, the latter having been previously obtained by plotting weight against height in the channel system. By comparing a child's own auxodrome with references to the five standards, a teacher can see whether the child is advanced, normal or retarded with respect to the general population.

6. The two extreme right-hand panels are for determining estimates of basal metabolism and caloric needs. They will not ordinarily concern the physical educator or classroom teacher.

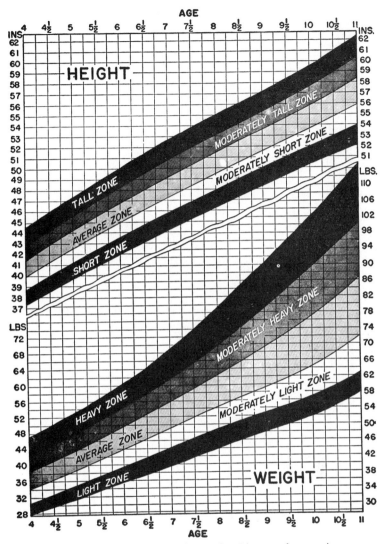

Figure 83, C. Meredith physical growth records: girls, ages four to eleven years.

Interpreting the grid. A child should not depart more than one-half channel per ten levels of advancement from the main direction of the channel system, and even this should not persist if "top quality" growth is to be assured.

As regards speed, a child should not deviate by more than one to two levels, or by three at the very most, from his expected position as determined by projecting this auxodrome forward and parallel to the standards for a distance equivalent to the time interval in question. Failure to keep to his own schedule indicates that the speed of development is not satisfactory. The progress of those youngsters whose positions are in B2 and below or to the right of the 67 per cent auxodrome should be carefully

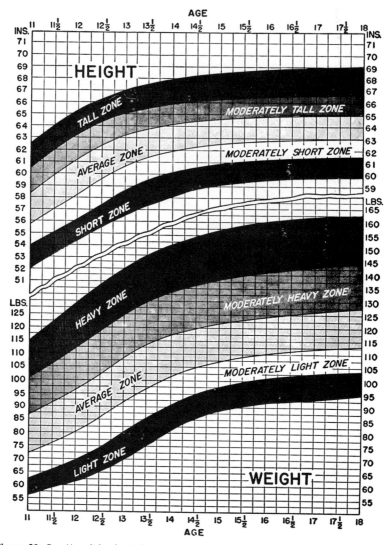

Figure 83, D. Meredith physical growth records: girls, ages eleven to eighteen years.

followed. Obese youngsters (A4 and above) should likewise be closely checked. Any child, however, should be investigated when he manifests clear and persistent deviation from channel-wise progress or from his expected auxodrome.

Meredith Height-Weight Chart. Meredith constructed growth curves by comparing average height and weight at various age levels of a large number of children. These averages were then plotted separately against age, resulting in charts that indicate the average height-age and weight-age curves for boys and girls. Also included on the charts are the normal variations from the computed averages. The charts, appearing as Figure 83, *A* to *D,* show five "normal" zones for height, including tall, moderately tall, average, moderately short, and short; also five "normal" zones for weight, including heavy, moderately heavy, average, moderately light, and light. These normal zones offer a method of identifying those children who deviate from the expected growth pattern.

To use the charts, locate the zone by plotting the particular child's height and weight. If these two points do not fall in the corresponding zones, as tall and heavy, short and light, or if the measures of the child's height and weight, after successive measurements, abruptly jump from one zone to another, the child should be referred to the proper medical authority.

Somatotyping

It is a well-known fact that no two human bodies are exactly alike in physical characteristics. No doubt the variables affecting structure or physique are numerous. In addition to a long history of research studies that have attempted to classify body types, presently referred to as somatotyping, there has been much interest in noting the personality associated with certain body types. For example, we sometimes think of the fat person as being jovial, and of good humor, whereas the lean person often appears high-strung or nervous. Today, the anthropologist studying physiques is able to bring to bear much understanding relative to the classification of physiques as well as to the predominant behavior and growth patterns associated with specific body types or somatotypes.

An understanding of the physical capabilities related to certain somatotypes should be of value to the physical educator in appreciating the individual problems of the pupils with whom he deals. Recognizing the limitations as well as the potentialities of his youngsters enables the physical educator to plan a scientific program that will better serve the needs of his pupils.

Actually, the study of mankind in terms of body physique is generations old. Hippocrates classified the human physique into two fundamental types: *phthisic habitus*, characterized by a long, thin body with emphasis placed on the vertical dimension; and the *apoplectic habitus*, characterized by short, thick body emphasizing the horizontal dimension.[12]

Kretschmer, frequently referred to as the father of modern somatotyping, revived the Greek terms *pyknic*, implying a compact body; and *asthenic*, literally interpreted as "without strength." He added a third component, the *athletic* type, a term first used by the French.

Sheldon's method. In modern times, W. H. Sheldon and his coworkers have made by far the most valuable contributions to the technique of somatotyping.[12] After many years of investigation, Sheldon classified male physiques into three major body types: *endomorphic, mesomorphic,* and *ectomorphic.* Included in these three body components, according to Sheldon, are the following physical characteristics:

Endomorphy (the first component) is characterized by roundness and softness of body. The anteroposterior diameters as well as the lateral diameters tend toward equality in the head, neck, trunk, and limbs. Also features of this type are predominance of abdomen over thorax, high square shoulders, and short neck. There is a smoothness of contours throughout, with no muscle relief. The breasts are always developed, usually as a result of fatty deposit. As Sheldon so aptly states, the entire trunk gives the impression of being under moderate pneumatic pressure. The buttocks have a round fullness and no noticeable dimpling. The skin is soft and smooth, and rarely is there a great deal of chest hair.

Mesomorphy (the second component) is characterized by a square body with hard, rugged, and prominent musculation. The bones are large and covered with thick muscle. Legs, trunks, and arms are usually massive in bone and heavily muscled throughout. An outstanding characteristic of this type is the forearm thickness and heavy wrist, hand, and fingers. The thorax is large and there is a relatively slender waist. Shoulders are broad, and the trunk is usually upright with trapezius and deltoid muscles quite massive.

The abdominal muscles are prominent and thick, and are characterized by rippling musculature at Poupart's ligament. The buttocks almost always exhibit a muscular dimpling. The skin appears coarse and takes a deep tan readily, holding it for a long time.

Ectomorphy (the third component) includes, as predominant characteristics, linearity, fragility, and delicacy of body. The bones are small and the muscles thin.

Shoulder droop is a constant in the ectomorph. The limbs are relatively long and the trunk short; however, this does not mean that the individual must be tall. The abdomen and the lumbar curve are flat, while the thoracic curve is relatively sharp and elevated. The shoulders are mostly narrow and lacking in muscle relief. There is no bulging of muscle at any point on the physique. As the shoulder girdle lacks muscular support and padding, the scapulae tend to wing out posteriorly.

Sheldon's choice of the three body types was made because they exhibit the characteristics of the extreme variants found in the population. Once the components were classified, 4000 males were photographed and classified in accordance with the characteristics of the three basic components. On the basis of this analysis, it was determined that the pure type does not exist, but rather that each person is made up in part of all three components. That is, each one exhibits somewhere in his body make-up some trace of all three components.

In order to develop a system whereby each person could be classified more precisely on the basis of the three components, the body was divided into five regions for closer scrutiny and measurement. The head, face, and neck made up the first region, while the second was the thoracic trunk. The third region consisted of the arms, shoulders, and hands. The fourth region was the abdominal trunk, and the fifth region included the legs and feet.

After considerable study of numerous anthropometric measurements in the five regions of the body, a scaling technique for the somatotype was finally developed. The somatotype of a given subject is made up of three numbers, each designating the degree of the three components. The numeral one stands for the lowest observed amount of the component, while seven indicates its maximal dominance. Thus a somatotype of 711 would indicate extreme endomorphy; 171, extreme mesomorphy; and 117, extreme ectomorphy. A 444 indicates a physique falling at the mid-point of the three components.

Today the technique of Sheldon's somatotyping procedure has become considerably refined. First, photographs of the subject showing front, rear, and side views are taken. Next, an *exact* weight and height history of the subject is recorded. Emphasis is placed on the maximal weights achieved by the subject before the age of 20 and for each five-year period following 20. Present height and weight are measured, the former by having the individual stretch to his full extension against a wall stadiometer or wall scale graduated to tenths of an inch. Two indices are derived: the somatotyping ponderal index (height divided by the cube root of the weight) and the trunk index (TI). The somatotyping ponderal index (SPI) is a measure of the person's maximal achieved mass over his surface area, which may be reached at any age. This is why it is extremely important to obtain as accurate a weight history of the subject as possible.

The trunk index is a most important advance, for it permits quite objective means of obtaining the somatotype. It is the photographic area of the thoracic trunk over that of the abdominal trunk, both measured from the frontal or dorsal photograph with a planimeter (an engineering instrument used for measuring the area of any plane figure by passing a tracer around its perimeter). According to Sheldon, it has been found to remain constant throughout adult life, regardless of weight changes. The TI is a measure of the relative strength of endomorphy and mesomorphy, whereas the SPI is a measure of the relative strength of ectomorphy against the sum of the other two components.

The somatotype is obtained by consulting a table containing two parameters, the SPI on the vertical axis and the TI on the horizontal axis. The crossing of these two parameters approximately determines the somatotype within the limits of two to five different possibilities. A second table to which one must refer is a stature table, containing the distribution of the somatotypes plotted against the height or maximal stature. Somatotypes that are virtually identical with reference to SPI and TI will be found to vary sharply in size, and the stature table offers a final step in pinpointing the somatotype. At present these tables have not been published, but they may be obtained by contacting Dr. W. H. Sheldon at the University of California, Berkeley, California.

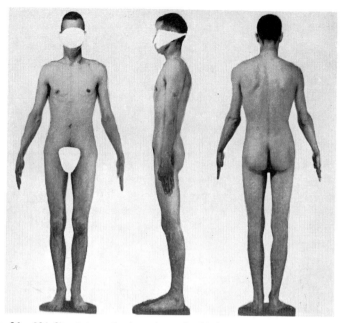

Figure 84. 136 Somatotype: Tends to be agile, likely competent in long-distance walking or hiking, occasionally able to compete at cross-country running. Far too light and brittle for athletic games involving rough bodily contact. Like the 127, children of this type tend to involve themselves in athletic ambitions which may lead to serious frustration: In other words, their obtainable achievement lies far outside their natural potentialities. (Sheldon, William H.: Atlas of Men. New York, Harper & Brothers, 1954, p. 46.)

Sheldon has reported the identification of eighty-eight somatotypes from what he holds to be 343 theoretical possibilities.[12]

The application of somatotyping to physical education may result in better understanding of the pupil, particularly in terms of the activity program. Figures 84 through 89 depict a selected number of somatotypes. In the legends appear descriptions by Sheldon relative to the characteristics of the particular body types.

Heath-Carter Anthropometric Somatotype. Recently Heath and Carter have contributed extensively to the field of somatotyping. They suggest that there are essentially three ways of obtaining a somatotype rating: (1) an anthropometric rating may be made without a somatotype photograph; (2) experienced somatotypers may make reliable photoscopic or inspectional ratings when age, height and weight and a standard somatotype photograph are available; and (3) a combination of these two methods, which is the procedure used by Heath and Carter. The measurement techniques and instructions for determining the Heath-Carter Somatotype which follow were prepared by Dr. Carter and are reproduced here with his kind permission.

Anthropometric measurement techniques
Height.
Instruments.   Wall scale and Broca plane.

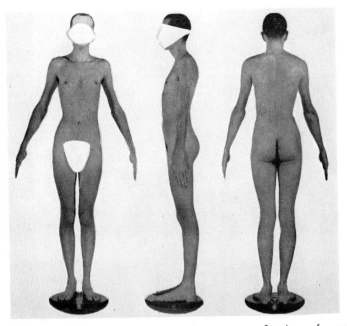

Figure 85. 217 Somatotype: A languid flaccidity or even a floppiness of movement and a looseness at the joints which might cause a young physical educator to bite his nails. Even the best of postural training will not correct the difficulty. There is little in organized athletics to which this type is adapted. He can learn to swim and has great buoyancy: (Sheldon, William H.: Atlas of Men. New York, Harper & Brothers, 1954, p. 75.)

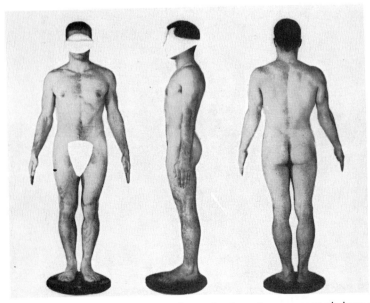

Figure 86. 171 Somatotype: Being mostly muscle, the extreme mesomorph loves acitivity and welcomes a strenuous way of life. Apt to gain considerable weight from age thirty to fifty, which of course is not healthy. Should be cautioned about overeating and encouraged to exercise. (Sheldon, William H.: Atlas of Men: New York, Harper & Brothers, 1954, p. 65.)

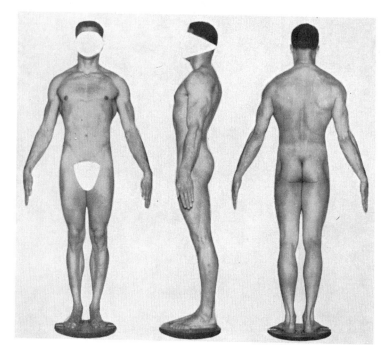

Figure 87.   172 Somatotype: Maximal muscularity and sufficient linearity and length of limb for great striking power. Often heroes of the comic strip, e.g., Smilin' Jack, Dick Tracy, and Li'l Abner, are very close to the 172. Even though of massive musculature, the most durable fighters and players of hard games are cushioned and rendered elastic by a 2, 3, or even 4 in endomorphy. (Sheldon, William H.: Atlas of Men. New York, Harper & Brothers, 1954, p. 71.)

Definition of Measurement.   Erect body length from the soles of the feet to the vertex.

Landmark.   Vertex—the most superior part of the head when the head is held with the visual plane horizontal.

Posture.   The subject stands erect, feet together, with heels, buttocks, upper back, and rear of head in contact with wall scale.

Technique.   As the observer brings the square onto the subject's vertex, the subject is instructed to take a deep breath and to stretch up to his full height. (This brings out the subject's maximal height and eliminates the "diurnal variation" that has often been reported.) Height is recorded to the nearest 0.1 inch.

Weight.

Instrument.   Accurate scales, balance type if possible.

Technique.   The subject stands in the center of the scale platform, nude except for minimal clothing. Weight is recorded to the nearest 0.5 pound with an allowance deducted for the clothing.

Subcutaneous fat: General instructions.

Instrument.   Harpenden skinfold caliper.

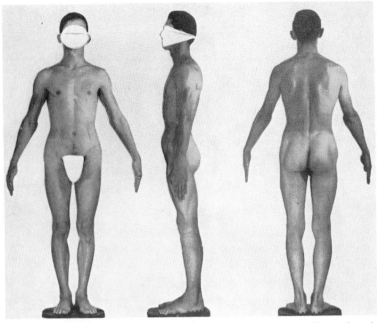

Figure 88. 154 Somatotype: Possesses agility and may have the makings of a champion at such athletic competition not requiring resilient bounce or the ability to prosper and take severe punishment. Probably many long-distance runners have been close to this somatotype, as was Tilden, a great tennis player. (Sheldon, William H.: Atlas of Men. New York, Harper & Brothers, 1954, p. 53.)

Technique. The objective is to measure the thickness of a complete double layer of skin and subcutaneous tissue without including any underlying muscle tissue. A double layer of skin and subcutaneous tissue is grasped with the thumb and forefinger, the fold being large enough to get a complete double layer, but not so large as to get so much skin and fat as may cause excessive amounts of tension beyond the fingertips. The fold of skin and fat is held somewhat loosely while the centers of caliper faces are 1 cm. from the edges of the thumb and forefinger.

The reading on the dial of the caliper is taken after applying the full spring pressure of the instrument for all measurements. The examiner must allow time for the full pressure of the caliper to take effect, but not so long that the fat is being "squeezed out" of the skinfold. Considerable practice is required to make this judgment for skinfolds of varying sizes and degrees of compressibility. (Firmer pressure of the fingers on the skinfold will normally arrest the movement of the indicator if the movement is excessive.) The measurement is recorded to the nearest 0.1 mm.

TRICEPS

Posture. The subject stands with the arm by the side and the elbow extended but relaxed. (Muscle fibers are excluded, if necessary, by locking the elbow joint momentarily in full extension.)

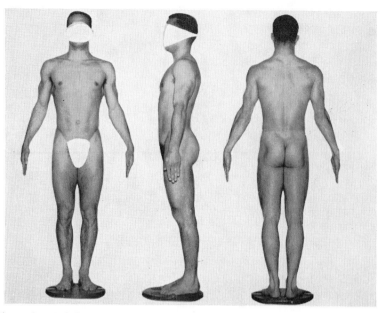

Figure 89. 262 Somatotype: When you watch a baseball game between the Yankees and the Red Sox, with possibly thirty players appearing on the field in the course of the afternoon, you can approximately somatotype most of them merely by playing the averages. Probably two-thirds of the players are 262's, 263's, or 462's. If it were professional football, the same somatotypes would almost surely predominate, but there would be more 7's in mesomorphy, and in the lines would be six or eight of the heavier extremes like 371, 471, and even 561 (a heavyweight wrestler somatotype). (Sheldon, William H.: Atlas of Men. New York, Harper & Brothers, 1954, p. 120.)

Technique. The skinfold is raised with the thumb and forefinger of the left hand over the triceps muscle on the back of the right arm, halfway between the acromion and the elbow. The skinfold runs parallel to the long axis of the arm.

SUBSCAPULAR

Posture. The subject stands with shoulders erect but relaxed and arms by the sides.

Technique. The skinfold is raised with the thumb and forefinger of the left hand lateral to the inferior angle of the right scapula, the skinfold running downward and outward in the direction of the ribs.

SUPRAILIAC

Posture. The subject stands in normal erect posture.

Technique. The subject is instructed to draw in a medium breath and hold it. The skinfold is raised with the thumb and forefinger of the left hand in a position one to two inches above the right anterior superior iliac spine so that the fold runs forward and slightly downward.

CALF

Posture. The subject sits on a chair with his foot on the floor and the leg vertical.

Technique. The skinfold is raised with the thumb and forefinger of the left hand on the medial side of the right calf just above the level of the maximum calf girth so that the fold runs vertically.

Bone diameters: General instructions.

Instrument.   Modified sliding steel caliper. (3-inch branches, ½-inch discs at extremity.)

Definition of measurement.   Bi-epicondylar diameter of the distal extremity of the humerus and femur.

Landmarks.   The points on either epicondyle of the distal extremity of the humerus or femur most lateral to the medial plane of the bone.

Technique.   The discs on the branches of the caliper are applied against the epicondyles in such a manner as to bisect the angle of the joint and to lie in the same plane as the limb. Firm pressure is applied and the measurement is recorded to the nearest .05 cm. Measurements are taken on both limbs, and the larger measurements are recorded.

HUMERUS

Posture.   The arm of the subject is raised forward to approximately the level of the shoulder and the forearm is flexed upward at a right angle to the arm.

Technique.   The discs are applied to the epicondyles, bisecting the angle of the elbow, and lying in the same plane as the arm and forearm.

FEMUR

Posture.   The subject sits on a chair with his foot on the floor and the leg vertical.

Technique.   The observer kneels in front of the subject and applies the discs to the epicondyles, bisecting the knee angle and keeping the caliper branches in a plane parallel to the thigh and the leg.

Muscle girths: General instructions.

Instrument.   Flexible steel or linen tape.

Definition of measurement.   The maximum girth of the muscle when measured at right angles to its long axis.

Technique.   The tape is passed around the limb and the region of the muscle explored with the tape always at right angles to the long axis of the bone, until the largest reading is obtained. The tape is in light contact with the skin, and maximum girth is recorded to the nearest 0.1 cm. Measurements are taken on both limbs, and the larger girths are recorded.

BICEPS

Posture.   The arm of the subject is horizontal, the forearm is supinated and the elbow fully flexed. The subject is instructed to clench his fist and contract his biceps as strongly as possible.

Technique.   The tape is passed around the arm approximately midway between the acromion and the elbow, at right angles to the long axis of the arm.

CALF

Posture.   The subject stands on a table with his feet six to nine inches apart, with his weight equally distributed through both lower limbs.

Technique.   The tape is passed around the leg near the top of the calf muscle and lowered until the greatest girth is located, at right angles to the long axis of the leg.

Procedures for calculating Heath-Carter Somatotype.   When comparing the distributions of two independent measures on the same subjects, the means should not differ significantly, and the correlation coefficient should be above .90. Specifically, height and weight should have test-retest values of $r \geq .98$; the girths and diameters should have r's between .92 and .98; and for the skinfolds, r's between .90 and .96 are reasonable. Because skinfolds tend to be the least reliable measures and because the sum of three skinfolds is used for calculating endomorphy, the following procedures are recommended for use with all subjects:

1. Skinfolds, diameters, and girths are taken in this order.
2. The four skinfolds are repeated and recorded.
3. After the second series, the following rules are applied:
    a. If the second measure is not within 5 per cent of the first measure, a third measure is taken. The recorder simply says, "Repeat triceps and suprailiac," without informing the measurer of his "scores."
    b. The two closest measures are averaged and entered on the rating form.
4. Either of the following procedures may be used to calculate reliability, depending on the investigator's purpose, but in both cases the r for the sums of the skinfolds should be at least .95.
    a. Sum three skinfolds (triceps, subscapular, suprailiac) for the first and second series and calculate the significance of the mean difference.
    b. Sum all four skinfolds and determine the significance of D, and r.

The rating form (Fig. 90)

1. Record pertinent identification data at top of form.

First component (endomorphy) rating (Steps 2–5)

2. Record the measurements from each of the four skinfolds.

3. Sum the triceps, subscapular, and suprailiac skinfolds and record in the box opposite Total Skinfolds.

4. Circle the closest value in the Total Skinfolds scale to the right. (Note: The scale reads vertically from low to high in columns, and horizontally left to right in rows. The rows, "lower limit" and "upper limit," are to provide exact boundaries for each column and these values should only be circled when the Total Skinfolds are within a few millimeters of the limit. In most cases the value in the row "mid-point" is circled.)

5. Circle the value in the row First Component which is directly under the column circled in number 4 above.

Second component (mesomorphy) rating (Steps 6–12)

6. Record the height (in inches) and the humerus and femur diameters in the boxes. Before recording the biceps and calf girths in their

HEATH-CARTER SOMATOTYPE RATING FORM

NAME: D.C.
OCCUPATION: Phys. Ed. student   AGE: 23.6   SEX: M Ⓔ   NO: 96
PROJECT: A.T.P.   ETHNIC GROUP: Cauc.   DATE: May, 1966
MEASURED BY: L.C.

TOTAL SKINFOLDS (mm)

	½	1	1½	2	2½	3	3½	4	4½	5	5½	6	6½	7	7½	8	8½	9	9½	10	10½	11	11½	12
Upper Limit	10.9	14.9	18.9	22.9	26.9	31.2	35.8	40.7	46.2	52.2	58.7	65.7	73.2	81.2	89.7	98.9	108.9	119.7	131.2	143.7	157.2	171.9	187.9	204.0
Mid-point	9.0	13.0	17.0	21.0	25.0	29.0	33.5	38.0	43.5	49.0	55.5	62.0	69.5	77.0	85.5	94.0	104.0	114.0	125.5	137.0	150.5	164.0	180.0	196.0
Lower Limit	7.0	11.0	15.0	19.0	23.0	27.0	31.3	35.9	40.8	46.3	52.3	58.8	65.8	73.3	81.3	89.8	99.0	109.0	119.8	131.3	143.8	157.3	172.0	188.0
FIRST COMPONENT	½	1	1½	2	2½	3	3½	4	4½	5	5½	6	6½	7	7½	8	8½	9	9½	10	10½	11	11½	12

	½	1	1½	2	2½	3	3½	4	4½	5	5½	6	6½	7	7½	8	8½	9
Height (in.)	55.0	56.5	58.0	59.5	61.0	62.5	64.0	65.5	67.0	68.5	70.0	71.5	73.0	74.5	76.0	77.5	79.0	80.5
Bone: Humerus (cm)	5.19	5.34	5.49	5.64	5.78	5.93	6.07	6.22	6.37	6.51	6.65	6.80	6.95	7.09	7.24	7.38	7.53	7.67
Femur	7.41	7.62	7.83	8.04	8.24	8.45	8.66	8.87	9.08	9.29	9.49	9.70	9.91	10.12	10.33	10.53	10.74	10.95
Muscle: Biceps	23.7	24.4	25.0	25.7	26.3	27.0	27.7	28.3	29.0	29.7	30.3	31.0	31.6	32.2	33.0	33.6	34.3	35.0
Calf	27.7	28.5	29.3	30.1	30.8	31.6	32.4	33.2	33.9	34.7	35.5	36.3	37.1	37.8	38.6	39.4	40.2	41.0
SECOND COMPONENT	½	1	1½	2	2½	3	3½	4	4½	5	5½	6	6½	7	7½	8	8½	9

(continued)

	9½	10	10½	11	11½	12
Height (in.)	82.0	83.5	85.0	86.5	88.0	89.5
Humerus	7.82	7.97	8.11	8.25	8.40	8.55
Femur	11.16	11.37	11.58	11.79	12.00	12.21
Biceps	35.6	36.3	37.1	37.8	38.5	39.3
Calf	41.8	42.6	43.4	44.2	45.0	45.8

	½	1	1½	2	2½	3	3½	4	4½	5	5½	6	6½	7	7½	8	8½	9
Upper limit	11.99	12.32	12.53	12.74	12.95	13.15	13.36	13.56	13.77	13.98	14.19	14.39	14.59	14.80	15.01	15.22	15.42	15.63
Mid-point	and	12.16	12.43	12.64	12.85	13.05	13.26	13.46	13.67	13.88	14.01	14.29	14.50	14.70	14.91	15.12	15.33	15.53
Lower limit	below	12.00	12.33	12.54	12.75	12.96	13.16	13.37	13.56	13.78	13.99	14.20	14.40	14.60	14.81	15.02	15.23	15.43
THIRD COMPONENT	½	1	1½	2	2½	3	3½	4	4½	5	5½	6	6½	7	7½	8	8½	9

Skinfolds (mm):
Triceps = 24.0
Subscapular = 10.4
Suprailiac = 8.9
TOTAL SKINFOLDS = 43.4
Calf = 17.1

Height (in.) = 67.8
Bone: Humerus (cm) = 6.03
Femur = 9.35
Muscle: Biceps (cm) 29.8 − 2.4 = 27.4
− (triceps skinfold)*
Calf* = 36.4
− (calf skinfold)
*38.1 − 1.7 =

Weight (lb.) = 137.0
Ht./∛Wt. = 12.36

	FIRST COMPONENT	SECOND COMPONENT	THIRD COMPONENT
Anthropometric Somatotype	4½	4½	2
Anthropometric plus Photoscopic Somatotype			

BY: L.C.
RATER:

Figure 90. Heath-Carter Somatotype Rating Form.

respective boxes, the corrections for skinfolds must be made. To do this, subtract the triceps skinfold (convert to cm. first by dividing by 10) from the biceps girth, and subtract the calf skinfold (convert to cm.) from the calf girth.

7. Mark the point of the subject's height on the height scale which is directly to the right. (Note: Regard the height row as a continuous scale).

8. For each bone diameter and girth, circle the figure in the proper row which is nearest the measurement. (Note: If the measurement falls exactly mid-way between two values, circle the lower value. Because the largest girths and diameters have been recorded the conservative procedure is used.)

9. Now, *deal only with columns,* not with numerical values. Find the column, or space between the columns, that is the average of the column deviations for the diameters and girths only (not height). To do this:

  a. Consider as the zero column the left-most column containing a circled figure.
  b. From this zero column, add the total number of columns you must travel horizontally to reach each of the other three circled numbers.
  c. Divide this total by 4.
  d. Take the number obtained by this division and, starting at the zero column, count this number of columns to the right and place a mark (e.g., asterisk) at that point (whether the point be in the middle of a column or a fraction of the way between one column and the next).

10. Still considering columns only, count horizontally the number of columns you must travel from the asterisk to the marked height (or vice versa).

11. From the number 4 in the row marked Second Component move this number of columns to the right or left, depending upon the direction of the asterisk from the height marker. If the asterisk is to the right of the height marker, move that number of columns to the right of number 4, and if the asterisk is to the left, move left. Because the columns in this row are in half-unit increments, the number of columns and half-unit increments (or decrements) are equivalent.

12. Circle the closest Second Component value determined in number 11 above. (If the point is exactly mid-way between two rating points, circle the value closest to the 4 on the scale. This regression toward the 4 is the conservative approach, and is less likely to produce spuriously extreme ratings.)

Third component (ectomorphy) rating (Steps 13–16)
13. Record the weight (in pounds).

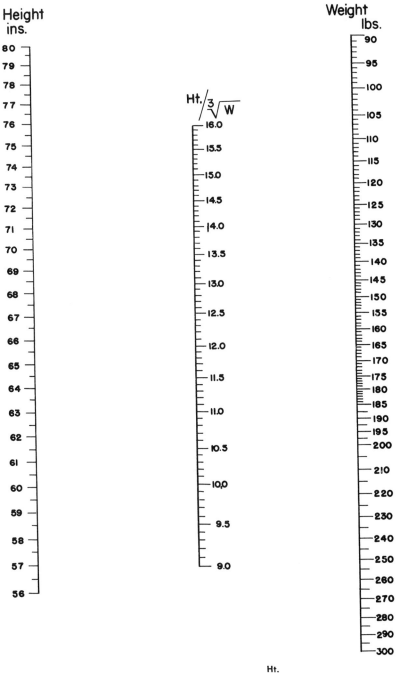

Height ins.

80
79
78
77
76
75
74
73
72
71
70
69
68
67
66
65
64
63
62
61
60
59
58
57
56

$$Ht.\Big/\sqrt[3]{W}$$

16.0
15.5
15.0
14.5
14.0
13.5
13.0
12.5
12.0
11.5
11.0
10.5
10.0
9.5
9.0

Weight lbs.

90
95
100
105
110
115
120
125
130
135
140
145
150
155
160
165
170
175
180
185
190
195
200
210
220
230
240
250
260
270
280
290
300

Figure 91.   Ponderal index: $\dfrac{Ht.}{\sqrt[3]{W}}$

14. Refer to the nomograph (Fig. 91) to find the height: weight ratio (H.W.R., or height/cube foot of weight). Record the H.W.R. in the box.

15. Circle the closest value in the.H.W.R. scale. (See Note in number 4 above).

16. Locate the Third Component value below the column of the circled H.W.R. and circle it.

The Heath-Carter Anthropometric Somatotype

17. Record the circled values obtained above in the appropriate columns in the row Anthropometric Somatotype.

18. The person calculating the rating should sign to the right.

Table 41 is a scale to be used in appraising boys and girls less than 55 inches tall; it is particularly useful in growth studies. Figure 92 contains a somatotype distribution of thirty-five San Diego football players.

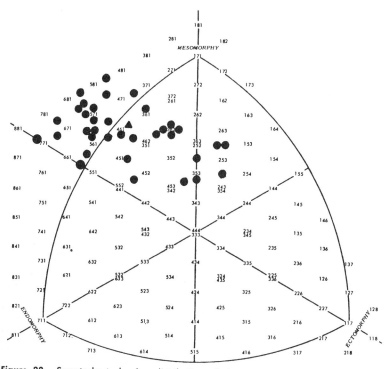

Figure 92. Somatochart showing distribution of the somatotypes of 35 San Diego State College football lettermen. Somatotype ratings were made using the Heath-Carter anthropometric somatotype method. The mean somatotype (triangle) is 4.2-6.3-1.4. (Carter, J. E., and Heath, Barbara: Somatotype Methodology and Kinesiology Research. Kinesiology Review. AAHPER, 1971, p. 10.)

Sloan-Weir nomograms for predicting body density and total body fat. Sloan and Weir, using measurements from two skinfold thicknesses, derived formulas for predicting body density in young men eighteen to twenty-six years and women seventeen to twenty-five years. In young men, the best predictions were found to come from a vertical skinfold in the

TABLE 41. *An Extended Scale of the Second Component (Mesomorphy) for Use in the Heath-Carter Anthropometric Somatotype.* The scale as presented is for heights less than 55.0 inches and is particularly useful in growth studies. It is used for both sexes.

Height	31.0	32.5	34.0	35.5	37.0	38.5	40.0	41.5	43.0	44.5	46.0	47.5	49.0	50.5	52.0	53.5
Humerus	2.87	3.01	3.16	3.30	3.45	3.59	3.74	3.89	4.03	4.18	4.32	4.47	4.61	4.76	4.91	5.05
Femur	4.09	4.30	4.50	4.71	4.92	5.13	5.34	5.54	5.75	5.96	6.17	6.37	6.58	6.79	7.00	7.21
Biceps	13.1	13.7	14.4	15.1	15.7	16.4	17.1	17.7	18.4	19.0	19.7	20.4	21.0	21.7	22.4	23.0
Calf	15.3	16.1	16.9	17.6	18.4	19.2	20.0	20.7	21.5	22.3	23.1	23.9	24.6	25.4	26.2	27.0
Second Component			½	1	1½	2	2½	3	3½	4	4½	5	5½	6	6½	7

Heath, B. H., and Carter, J. E. L.: A modified somatotype method. *Am. J. Phys. Anthrop.*, 27:57–74, 1967.

anterior midline of the thigh, halfway between the inguinal ligament and the top of the patella, and a subscapular skinfold running downward and laterally in the natural fold of the skin from the inferior angle of the scapula. In young women, the best predictions were found to come from a vertical skinfold over the iliac crest in the mid-axillary line and from a vertical skinfold on the back of the arm halfway between the acromion and olecranon processes (measured with the elbow extended).

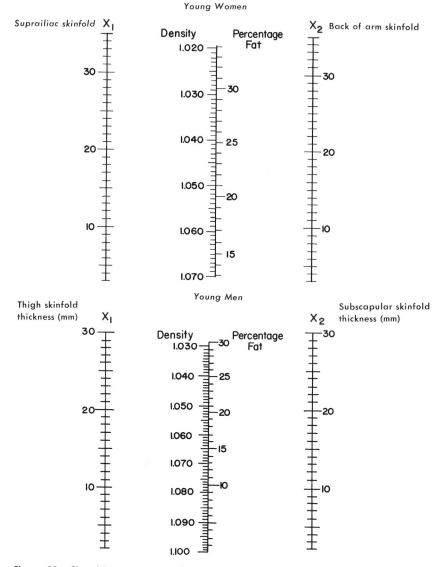

Figure 93. Sloan-Weir nomograms for prediction of body density and total body fat from skinfold measurements. (J. Appl. Physiol., Vol. 28, No. 2, February, 1970, p. 221.)

TABLE 42. *Sloan-Weir Formulas for Predicting Body Density and Total Body Fat**

	Female	Male
Height	174 cm.	178 cm.
Weight	59 kg.	75.9 kg.
Thigh skinfold	—	18 mm.
Subscapular skinfold	—	—
Suprailiac skinfold	19 mm.	—
Triceps skinfold	15 mm.	9.5 mm.
Actual density	1.0524 gm./ml.	1.0678 gm./ml.
(measured by underwater weighing)		
Predicted density	1.0478 gm./ml.	1.0693 gm./ml.
Fat	21.9%	13.1%

Men: $1.1043 - 0.00133$ (Thigh skinfold) $- 0.00131$ (subscapular skinfold)
$1.1043 - .0350 = 1.0693$ gm./ml. (Standard error of estimate $= 0.0069$ gm./ml.)

Women: $1.0764 - 0.00081$ (suprailiac skinfold) $- 0.00088$ (triceps skinfold)
$1.0764 - .0286 = 1.0478$ gm./ml. (Standard error of estimate $= 0.0082$ gm./ml.)

Fat Percentage $= 4.570/$Body density $- 4.142 \times 100$.

*Data by Sloan and Weir and recalculated by L. Laubach of Webb Associates, Yellow Springs, Ohio.

Sloan, A. W. and Weir, J. B. de V.: Nomograms for Prediction of Body Density and Total Body Fat from Skinfold Measurements. J. App. Physiol., Vol. 28, No. 2, February, 1970, p. 221.

By using the formula developed by Brozek et al., Sloan and Weir[14] could relate total body fat to body density and thus predict body fat from these two skinfold measurements. The formulas and an example of computation appear in Table 42 while Figure 93 contains the nomograms.

BIBLIOGRAPHY

1. Behnke, A. R.: Quantitative Assessment of Body Build. J. Appl. Physiol., Vol. 16, No. 6, 1961, pp. 960–968.
2. Bogert, L. Jean: Nutrition and Physical Fitness. 6th ed. Philadelphia, W. B. Saunders Company, 1954.
3. Brozek, J., and Keys, A.: The Evaluation of Leanness-Fitness in Man: Norms and Interrelationships. Brit. J. Nutr., 5:194–206, 1951.
4. Carter, William E.: The Pirquet System of Nutrition and Its Applicability to American Conditions. J.A.M.A., Vol. 77, No. 20, November 12, 1921.
5. Consolazio, C. Frank, Johnson, Robert E., and Pecora, Louis J.: Physiological Measurements of Metabolic Functions in Man. New York, McGraw-Hill Book Company, 1963, p. 303.
6. Franzen, Raymond: Physical Measures of Growth and Nutrition. New York, American Child Health Association, 1929.
7. Franzen, Raymond, and Palmer, George: The ACH Index of Nutritional Status. New York, American Child Health Association, 1934.

8. Inadequate Diets and Nutritional Deficiencies in the United States. Bulletin of the National Research Council, Washington, National Academy of Science, Bulletin Number 109, November, 1942.

9. Lusk, Graham: The Elements of the Science of Nutrition. 4th ed. Philadelphia, W. B. Saunders Company, 1931.

10. Pryor, Helen B.: Width-Weight Tables. Stanford University, California, Stanford University Press, 1940.

11. Rathbun, E. N., and Pace, N.: Studies on Body Composition Showing the Determination of Total Body Fat by Means of the Body's Specific Gravity. J. Biol. Chem., 158:667–676, 1945.

12. Sheldon, William Herbert: Atlas of Men. New York, Harper & Brothers, 1954.

13. Sheldon, William Herbert, Stevens, S. S., and Tucker, W. B.: The Varieties of Human Physique. 2nd ed. New York, Harper & Brothers, 1940.

14. Sloan, A. W., and Weir, J. B. de V.: Nomograms for Prediction of Body Density and Total Body Fat from Skinfold Measurements. J. Appl. Physiol., Vol. 28, No. 2, February, 1970.

15. Wetzel, Norman C.: The Treatment of Growth Failure in Children. Cleveland, NEA Service, Inc., 1948.

16. Wilmore, Jack H., and Behnke, Albert R.: An Anthropometric Estimation of Body Density and Lean Body Weight in Young Men. J. Appl. Physiol., Vol. 27, No. 1, July, 1969, pp. 25-31.

17. Wilmore, J. H., and Behnke, A. R.: Predictability of Lean Body Weight through Anthropometric Assessment in College Men. J. Appl. Physiol., Vol. 25, No. 4, October, 1968, p. 354.

chapter 10

evaluation of body mechanics

Introduction

"The person with poor posture is ungainly, awkward and unesthetic. . . ."[25]
"Erect posture enhances the feeling of well-being. There is in the ability to consciously stand well the same joy which comes with any skill. To know that you know how to stand well, that you can and are standing well, gives a feeling of self-confidence and poise. . . ."[12]

No one can deny the validity of the above statements. Yet, how many of us had the privilege of good postural training in our formative years? Do *you* stand and move gracefully? Are you proud of your carriage?

Look around at your elders and select someone whom you would like to emulate in terms of physical appearance. In most cases your choice from individuals in your immediate environment limits the selection to a few. On the other hand, if you were to make this choice from a group of people who recognize that their success depends to a large extent upon their physical appearance, your problem would be simplified. For example, movie actors and actresses, dancers, and most theatrical people realize the necessity for maintaining grace and poise of stature and movement. They understand the values of such skills, and work hard to accomplish excellence in basic movement. In addition, schools of charm spend considerable time in teaching their students how to move. It goes without saying that the key to good appearance lies in a well-trained body. Then too, age seems to be kind to those who practice and perfect the fundamentals of movement.

How disheartening it is to see a girl dressed in a pretty party dress, but possessing such poor postural characteristics as a rounded upper back, a poked head, or a protruding abdomen. Poor posture is also detrimental to the appearance of a young man. The next time you are at a dance take careful note of the carriage of those present. Then remember this: most of those people with poor posture will become *progressively worse* as they grow older.

Teaching efficient use of the body in skills of standing, walking, and sitting is a very valuable part of the physical education program, particularly on the elementary and junior high school level. When this phase of the curriculum is neglected a grave injustice is done to the pupils. We know that a body characterized by firm musculature and esthetic movement *can* be acquired through physical training. How proud we should be, knowing that physical education can offer this gift to children.

Recognition and appreciation of good body mechanics in the early years of schooling will significantly reduce the number of pupils in corrective classes. Howland, an outstanding leader in the field of body mechanics, brings our attention to the fact that grownups move in patterns of body movement developed early in childhood.[14] Many of them slump and slouch without knowing it. Then, in most instances, when poor alignment and inefficient body mechanics are recognized, it is difficult to ameliorate the deficiency. The adage "as the twig is bent so grows the tree" is an age-old truth. It is during childhood that attention must be given to the development of fundamental motor movements to insure lifelong benefits of efficient body mechanics.

Purpose of good posture. No one will argue the value of good posture as it contributes to the appearance of an individual. Thus a primary purpose for teaching body mechanics is for an esthetic reason. However, some authorities extol the health values associated with good posture. A great deal of controversial material on this point appears in the literature, some authorities supporting a positive relationship and others stating that no relationship whatsoever exists. To illustrate a few of these differences, some of the statements and studies relative to this problem are given below:

Klein and Thomas,[17] in summary of the Chelsea, Massachusetts, study, report the following effects upon health and efficiency of teaching good body mechanics to 1708 grammar school children:

1. Improvement of body mechanics was associated with improvement of health and efficiency.

2. Improvement of body mechanics was associated with improvement in school work.

3. Improvement in retraction ability of the lower abdomen resulted in elevation of the stomach and intestines.

Carnett, using x-ray techniques and administering barium or bismuth to adult subjects, found that the stomach commonly elevated 3 to 4 inches when the individual changed from a slumped to an erect posture.[4]

The effect of drooped chest on the action of the diaphragm was studied by Goldthwait and associates, using fluoroscopic tracings.[13] The results of the study showed that in the correct standing position with the chest held up, the diaphragm is also held up in its fullest possible motion.

The Baruch Committee on Physical Medicine reports that many ailments and disabilities, including severe and crippling pain, may have abnormal posture as their causative factor—perhaps many more than is currently realized—and they therefore may be susceptible of benefit when this functional abnormality is corrected.[20]

The studies reported above fail to show *specific* relationships as to the manner in which improvement of posture objectively affects *physiological* function. In most cases the statements made are generalizations and hence quite vague in terms of specifically correlating posture and health.

Karpovich tells us that lordosis may be associated with orthostatic albuminuria (slight loss of protein in the urine); however, there is no scientific proof that improvement in posture leads to definite improvements in physiological functions of the body.[16] In commenting on the claims that visceroptosis (sagging of the bowel) depends upon posture, Karpovich asserts that this has yet to be proved.

In summary then, Howland, in a comprehensive search of the literature relative to the relationship between posture and health, has concluded that no writer seems to disclaim the health values of posture in their entirety.[14] Some reject the health claims because scientific proof is lacking, yet all writers appear to claim that some correlation between posture and health does exist. It remains a problem to prove or disprove this correlation scientifically, and to ascertain in what aspects of health and in which pattern of posture the correlation significantly exists. Writers, on the whole, are in accord (though expressed empirically) with the opinion that faulty posture is conducive to some inefficiency in body functioning and organic fitness.

Regardless of the relationship between health and posture, the esthetic as well as functional values resulting from teaching fundamental patterns of movement warrant the inclusion of good posture training as a vital part of the physical education program. Through the use of scientific measuring devices, youngsters needing extra work in body mechanics can be discovered and steps may be taken to ameliorate the condition.

What is good posture? Obviously, before measurement can take place, what is going to be measured must be defined. The definition or, better yet, the description of what good posture is, actually becomes the criterion for the measurement. That is to say, the description indicates the norm or standard upon which we base our measurements. In terms of posture evaluation this is not easy. Each person is unique unto himself; this makes it difficult to establish an *objective* standard. For example, some people have a more pronounced lumbosacral curve than others, but this is quite normal. Because of this uniqueness of body structure, it not only becomes difficult to establish definitive standards, but it may actually be against the best interest of the individual to do so. As an illustration, when I first commenced to study physical education, my teacher stressed a flat lower back for *every* student. The class worked hard to obtain this flat lower back, which is contrary to the normal structure of the spinal column in most persons. To further illustrate the uniqueness of body structure, McCloy reports that the shapes of vertebrae vary from ones that necessitate an unusually straight vertebral column to ones that necessitate a fairly great degree of curvature in the vertebral column.[24]

Other studies discuss individual differences in the structure of the pelvis and lumbar spine as they are related to body mechanics.[2, 15] Thus we may conclude that individual structural differences must be recognized in any definition of "good posture." Concerning its definition, Massey, in a comprehensive analysis of the literature, came to the conclusion that there seemed to be a general argreement in the choice of criteria used to describe the conditions of "good posture." From this analysis, Massey concluded that postural definitions fell into two categories, those that were descriptive and those that were anatomical.[21]

Descriptive definition. The principal segments of the body should be balanced evenly over the base of support. The feet are slightly separated, the toes point straight forward or slightly outward, the weight of the body is borne mainly over the middle of the foot. There is easy extension of the knee and hips. There should be such position of the pelvic bones as will balance the weight directly over the acetabula, the spine functioning as a poised column with the weight distributed about it. This involves the preservation of a moderate curve in the lumbar region and an easy backward position of the shoulders, to bring the weight upon the spine rather than upon the chest. In this position the shoulder blades are approximately flat, the chest is carried moderately high but not thrust forward, and there is normal tonus of the abdominal muscles. The erect head also balances easily without backward tension or forward stretch. The position is alert and the individual capable of movement in any direction. The position does not represent an artificial, arbitrary, or complex combination of postural adjustments, but the most natural, comfortable, and perfectly poised position that the body can assume in standing.

Anatomical definition. The standards for normal anteroposterior posture are defined by Steindler in the following manner.[31] Beginning approximately at the mastoid process, the line of gravity passes downward posteriorly to the vertebrae of the neck, intersecting the spine near the seventh cervical vertebra, passes anteriorly to the dorsal vertebrae, touches the spine again at the lumbosacral junction, passes behind the lumbar spine, passes in front of the sacro-iliac junction to the center of the hip joint, then passes in front of the knee joint and drops to the base of support at the feet directly in front of the ankle joint. Balanced in this way, with the shoulders retracted, minimum moments of force are said to be in effect for bending the body segments out of the line of balance.

These definitions are the basis for postural appraisal. Thus, before proceeding further into the evaluation of posture, the reader should have two definite facts in mind: posture is unique to the individual; and regardless of whether a posture test is classified as subjective or objective, in the final analysis the criterion must be derived from expert opinion.

Early Posture Tests

For the most part, early attempts at evaluating posture were based upon the reasoning that each body segment, the head, trunk, the lower limbs, has its own center of gravity, and that when the centers of gravity of all segments are perfectly aligned over one another, the gravitational forces acting upon the body are in equilibrium. That is to say, as gravity is a constant force that must be offset in the upright position, it becomes necessary to describe body alignment in such a way that the moments of force tending to bend the body segments out of line must be brought into equilibrium. Authorities claim that the body is in good balance when a perpendicular line may be passed through the following five landmarks: (1) lobe of ear; (2) middle of tip of shoulder; (3) middle of greater trochanter; (4) just back of patella; and (5) in front of outer malleolus.

As might be expected there are some differences of opinion as to the exact points through which this line passes. For example, Steindler[31] places the line of gravity 4 cm. in front of the ankle joint, whereas Fox and Young[11] experimentally determined this line to lie just anterior to the center of the ankle joint, or to be exact, 0.95 cm. in front of the anterior border of the tibia.

Early posture tests made use of the gravital line by having the examiner hang a plumb line, or stand a pole, beside the subject. In this manner the traditional five body landmarks, as well as exaggerated spinal curvatures, might be described in terms of deviations from that which was accepted by the examiner as normal.

Bancroft's vertical-line test and triple-line test[1] as well as the Crampton wall test[6] and Lowman's[20] method of examination were a few of the initial endeavors making use of the gravital line in measuring posture. This type of evaluation may be criticized because of its highly subjective nature. The test in essence becomes as good as the examiner's ability to determine deviations from normal. The plumb line, however, may serve as a useful instrument in teaching body alignment, for it is simple to make and is tangible evidence of the gravital line for the pupil.

Following the plumb line tests, a great deal of interest was exhibited in using silhouettes for posture appraisal. In this type of evaluation, silhouettes were taken for a large number of subjects, then judges graded the silhouettes, thus permitting the experimenter to establish a scale or letter classification for posture.

Recent Posture Tests

Recent development of postural appraisal techniques has been in the direction of more precise and specific measurement. Precision instruments are used in measuring such factors as segmental angulation relative to the gravital line and the longitudinal axis for photographs, silhouettes, and x-rays. Even though considerable progress has been made, it appears that the true validity of these tests must rest, in the final analysis, with the skill of the examiner. We shall see, as we study the tests to follow, that perhaps in no other area of physical education is the instructor asked to bring to focus and apply his knowledge of such courses of physiology, kinesiology, and anatomy as in the evaluation of body mechanics. It is here that the physical educator truly demonstrates his ability in appraising human body structure so that deficiencies may be noted and the proper steps taken to ameliorate them.

The application of evaluation of body mechanics to the physical education program may be classified into four categories:

1. *Static anteroposterior posture tests,* which include appraisal methods designed to measure deviations associated with the lateral or side view of the child in a standing position. Such deficiencies as poked head, kyphosis, lordosis, shoulder overhang, and protruding abdomen may be evaluated in these tests.

2. *Functional appraisal methods,* dealing with the subjective evaluation that accompanies the classroom instructional unit of body mechanics. For example, the ability of the child to stand, walk, sit, climb and descend stairs, raise and lower weights, and walk in high heels are examples of skills that may be taught during the body mechanics unit. Here the instructor may subjectively evaluate these specific activities as the program progresses, making functional appraisal and teaching a continuous and interdependent process.

3. *Screening tests,* which are rapid forms of posture appraisal used to select subjectively those children with marked mechanical deficiencies. Such tests are usually administered at the beginning or during the first few weeks of school in order to select those children who are in need of additional, individual attention.

4. *Refined posture appraisal,* which deals more with quantitative measurement and evaluation, such as angle of pelvic tilt, amount of spinal curvature, and differences in leg lengths. This type of evaluation

is used on those children selected, from the results of screening test, as markedly deficient. Refined appraisal is more definitive and time-consuming, hence it is logical that such measurement be used only on those youngsters who have been referred for it as a result of the screening test.

STATIC ANTEROPOSTERIOR POSTURE TESTS

Static anteroposterior tests may be further divided into two groups. The first group consists of silhouettes or shadow prints for lateral standing posture. This method of evaluation generally begins with taking a silhouette of the pupil and subjectively comparing it with a standardized set of prints. The second group might be called objective anteroposterior tests, in which photographs are taken and various landmarks on the prints are measured. The term "objective" is used in that the measurements are quite precise, requiring the use of protractors, calipers, and certain other specially designed instruments.

Silhouettes. *Brownell Test.* Brownell made use of judges who arranged, in order of merit, 100 silhouettes of pupils' postures.[3] Through appropriate statistical treatment of these data, a scale of thirteen silhouettes was finally developed. This scale is arranged in order of rank with numerical units ranging from 20 to 120 assigned to each picture.

To use the scale, the teacher compares the pupil's silhouette with each type of posture appearing on the scale. The procedure is first to start at the bottom of the scale with the silhouette in question and work toward the top; then start at the top and work toward the bottom. By averaging the two comparisons a posture grade for the pupil may be obtained.

Objective anteroposterior tests. *Cureton-Gunby Conformateur.* Cureton, seeking the answers to effects of corrective exercises upon the spine, recognized the need for valid and reliable instruments to measure anteroposterior spinal curvature.[9] The conformateur (Fig. 94), the spinograph (Fig. 95), and the silhouette were studied in terms of reliability and validity.[69]

The conformateur consists of a wooden upright erected from a base, having a number of spindles that slide horizontally through holes bored in the upright. The spindles are locked into position by a system of springs attached to cords woven in and out between the spindles. The subject stands with his back toward the rods so that when the rods are gently tapped in place, the tips of the rods just touch the spinous processes of the vertebrae.

The spinograph uses a pointer that lightly traces the subjects spine and simultaneously records the spinal contour on a blackboard.

As a result of this investigation, Cureton found that the conformateur and spinograph gave comparable results, whereas the silhouette measure-

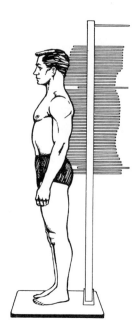

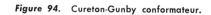

Figure 94.   Cureton-Gunby conformateur.

Figure 95.   The spinograph.

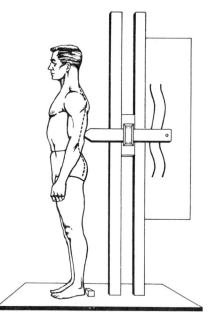

ments were in error. The data taken from the silhouettes showed exaggerated thoracic curvature, smaller lumbar curve than actually existed, and exaggerated displacement of the posterior spine of the sacrum.

In commenting on the profile error of the silhouette, Cureton says that the individual differences in development of the posterior back muscles becloud true measurement. Furthermore, the position of the hands has much to do with the profile view. In the event that an error of just a few millimeters is made in measuring the picture, a much larger error results if the measurements are multiplied by the enlargement ratio.

To eliminate error resulting from inconsistencies of subjects assuming exact positions in a series of trials, a manikin was measured with the various instruments. On the basis of these results, the Cureton-Gunby conformateur was devised. It is a combination conformateur, spinograph, and stadiometer with the following features:

1. Metal rods, precisely machined to uniform length and proper diameter, plated with cadmium to prevent rusting, and having tapered ends.

2. Locking device that permits the rods to be clamped into position as they are adjusted to the subject standing in a normal position.

3. Clamps to aid in certain studies.

4. Rods at the bottom to allow the location of the internal malleoli.

5. A plumb bob and line to allow the curve obtained to be related to the internal malleoli as a point in the base of support. The adjustable plumb line allows a vertical to be erected to any portion of the curve.

6. A levelling attachment to guarantee that the instrument is true vertically in relationship to the plumb line for anteroposterior measurements.

7. Holes are placed the entire length of the column to permit measuring a person of any size or measurement in the sitting posture.

Cureton recommends a combination of the conformateur and the silhouette for best results. Deviations of the spine can be measured with an experimental error as small as 1 per cent. The complete measurement can be made, including the picture, in four minutes.

Massey Posture Test. Massey has devised a usable and accurate method of measuring standing anteroposterior posture.[21] In the construction of this test, silhouettes were taken of 200 male students. A criterion was developed through the combined ratings of three qualified judges and through the further use of the methods of paired comparisons. A number of angles and indices were scaled and measured from the silhouettes, which were then correlated with the criterion. Elimination of certain of the variables was on the basis of low correlations with the criterion and in favor of convenience and precision of measurement. The remaining variables were combined statistically, and a posture formula expressed in regression form was devised. However, since the sum of the final test variables correlated .97 with the criterion and since the weighted items in the regression equation raised the correlation only slightly (.985), the extra work of computing the grade from the posture formula does not make it worth while.

The following are the instructions for obtaining the posture angle measurements from Figure 96.

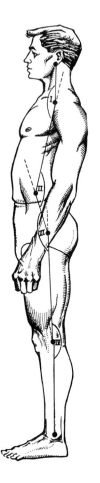

Figure 96. Posture angle measurements for Massey posture test.

Angle I: Lines connecting the tragus to a midpoint bisecting a horizontal line drawn from the suprasternal notch to the spine, and to a midpoint bisecting the horizontal lumbar-anterior abdomen line.

Angle II: Lines connecting the midpoint of the suprasternal spine line to the midpoint of the lumbar-abdominal line and to the greater trochanter.

Angle III: Lines connecting the midpoint of the lumbar-abdominal line to the greater trochanter and to the styloid process of the fibula (midpoint of the knee joint).

Angle IV: Lines connecting the greater trochanter to the midpoint of the knee and to the lowest point of the external malleolus.

The angles are recorded in terms of deviation in degrees from a straight line. That is, if angle I is 170 degrees, it would lack 10 degrees of being a straight line. Therefore, the reading of 10 degrees is recorded. Direct recording of the angles may be made by extending the drawn lines as indicated by the broken extensions in Figure 96.

To obtain the posture grade, compute the sum of the angles and find the appropriate grade in Table 43.

As a basis of comparison, Massey correlated several postural tests with his final criterion. The obtained coefficient of correlation with the Goldthwait test was .71; with the MacEwan and Howe, .560, and with the Kellog test ("head angle," "chest ratio," and angle of "pelvic obliquity") , .855. On the basis of this analysis one may conclude that the Kellog test and the Massey test measure approximately the same thing, and either could be used as an accurate measure in the appraisal of anteroposterior posture.

Howland Alignometer. Howland developed a technique for measuring and teaching structural balance of the body trunk in standing.[14] This was accomplished by determining the balanced relationship between the tilt of the pelvis and the upper trunk indicated by two anatomical landmarks: the center of the sternum and the superior border of the symphysis pubis.

It was found that when the sternopubic landmarks formed a perpendicular line parallel to the long axes of the separate parts of the body, as they approximate the vertical balance line (line of gravity) , structural alignment of the trunk occurred. The technique was validated by use of radiographs, photographs, and a constructed measuring instrument, called the alignometer (Fig. 97) .

TABLE 43. *Posture Grades Based upon Approximate Steps of One Standard Deviation Above and Below the Mean*

Total Degrees Angulation and Equivalent Posture Grades	
Sum of Angles I, II, III, IV	Posture Grade
8°–22°	A
23°–36°	B
37°–51°	C
52°–65°	D
66°–78°	E
79°–93°	F

Massey, Wayne W.: A Critical Study of Objectives Methods for Measuring Anterior-Posterior Posture With a Simplified Technique. Research Quart., Vol. 14, No. 1, 1943.

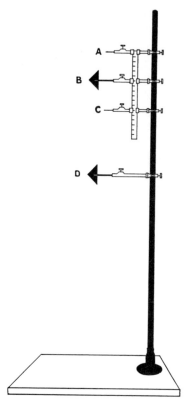

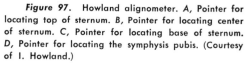

Figure 97. Howland alignometer. A, Pointer for locating top of sternum. B, Pointer for locating center of sternum. C, Pointer for locating base of sternum. D, Pointer for locating the symphysis pubis. (Courtesy of I. Howland.)

Study of the radiographs of experimental subjects revealed the following items.

1. Disalignment of the body trunk:
   a. The sternopubic landmarks were disaligned.
   b. The spinal column assumed exaggerated curvatures.
   c. The pelvic tilt presented a forward-upward direction at the symphysis pubis with a flattening of the lower back.
   d. The thorax lowered, the head and neck inclined forward, and the upper back rounded.
   e. The knee joints appeared disaligned, either in hyperflexion or hyperextension.
   f. The weight distribution line appeared to fall anterior or posterior to the supporting base between the feet (midway between the naviculars).

2. Assumed alignment of the body trunk:
   a. The sternopubic landmarks were aligned (vertically), and by linear measurement a rectangular parallelogram was constructed between these landmarks and the plumb line (line of balance).
   b. The spinal column appeared to assume its natural curvatures.

c. The head, thorax, and upper back appeared balanced over the pelvis.

d. The pelvic tilt appeared to assume its midway position at a normal angle with the horizontal plane of the pelvis.

e. The knee joints appeared to assume a closer proximity to the 180-degree angle between the articulating segments.

The alignometer (Fig. 97) was designed by Howland for the purpose of measuring objectively the ability of a person to assume trunk alignment in accordance with the developed technique. It is used, also, as a teaching device through which the technique may be more readily interpreted and practiced. The instrument consists of a simple arrangement of two sliding, calibrated pointers attached to a perpendicular steel rod. The rod is firmly supported on a wooden plank. The two sliding pointers used to locate the center of the sternum and the superior border of the symphysis pubis have a calibrated extension from their supporting arms, and the arms slide along the perpendicular rod to meet the varying heights of tested subjects. Additional similar, but non-calibrated, sliding pointers are located above and below the sliding pointer indicating the center of the sternum. A vertical calibrated rod connects these two additional pointers; it is used in determining the exact center between the upper pointer, which locates the superior border of the sternum, and the lower pointer, which locates the base of the sternum. The sternal center is found by measuring the half distance between the upper and lower pointers on the sternum. The central sliding pointer is then set at the center of the sternum.

When the subject is in balanced trunk alignment (center of sternum directly over the symphysis pubis) the difference in readings, between the calibrated pointers at the sternal center and the superior border of the symphysis pubis, should be zero.

The objectivity of the instrument was determined by the test-retest method that resulted in a correlation of .923. The relationship between the sternopubic line and this criterion (traditional lateral landmarks) was determined by computing the linear distances between them and correlating the line lengths. A high relationship was found between the sternopubic line and the distance between the acromion process of the scapula and the greater trochanter of the femur, $r = .889$. This is interpreted as meaning that when the center of the sternum and the center of the symphysis pubis are aligned, the upper and lower portions of the body trunk are considered aligned to a high degree.

The Howland technique, as taught and as measured by the alignometer, appears to represent the most encouraging scientific advancement in the appraisal and teaching of standing structural balance that has been proposed for some time. The following advantages of this method seem to overcome many problems characteristic of testing:

1. The alignometer is a teaching as well as a testing device.

2. The instrument is simple to construct and its technique is quickly and easily mastered.

3. The technique takes into consideration the uniqueness of body structure regardless of age, size, or sex.

4. The test is valid in terms of the criteria as well as being objective.

Center of gravity test. Cureton and his associates investigated the center of gravity in subjects as related to posture, fitness, and athletic ability.[8] Cureton's center of gravity test, adapted from Reynolds and Lovett's original work, indicates the distance that the center of gravity of a subject is being in front of the internal malleoli.[27]

The test (Fig. 98) is administered in the following manner:

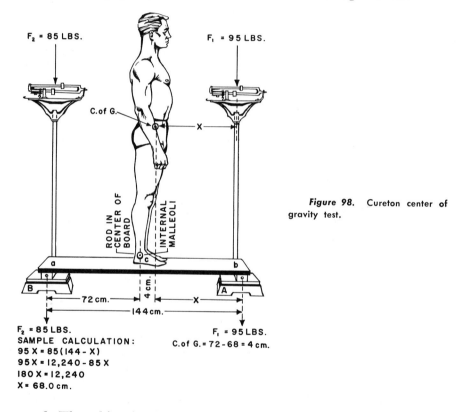

$F_2 = 85$ LBS.

$F_1 = 95$ LBS.

C. of G.

X

ROD IN CENTER OF BOARD

INTERNAL MALLEOLI

a

B   c   4 cm.   A   b

72 cm.   X

144 cm.

Figure 98. Cureton center of gravity test.

$F_2 = 85$ LBS.
SAMPLE CALCULATION:
$95 X = 85(144 - X)$
$95 X = 12,240 - 85 X$
$180 X = 12,240$
$X = 68.0$ cm.

$F_1 = 95$ LBS.
C. of G. $= 72 - 68 = 4$ cm.

1. The subject is asked to step upon the balance board, facing in the direction of the length of the board.

2. The internal malleoli are lined up even with a vertical pin located in the exact center of the board. The board is supported at both ends from the center of each scale.

3. The scales are balanced—first the forward one then the rear scale —until both have their lever arms swinging freely between the guide stops. (Toledo scales facilitate this measurement.) The subject is then instructed to step down from the balance board. The scales are read and

both readings recorded. One-half the weight of the board is deducted from each reading.

4. The calculation is made in accordance with the procedures appearing in the illustration, the result being the distance that the center of gravity is being balanced in front of the internal malleoli.

With expert examiners, the objectivity of the Cureton center of gravity test is .91 as reported on seventy-four subjects.

In order to determine the significance of the test the outcome was correlated with a number of measurements of posture, physical fitness, organic condition, and athletic ability. The results of these experiments are as follows:

1. There is a definite trend for men who habitually stand with their weight more forward to have straighter upper backs than do those who hold their weight less forward.

2. There is a slight indication that men who stand with their center of gravity relatively more forward tend to have lower arches. This seems to bear out Cureton's original observation that stronger men have slightly flatter footprints.

3. Of interest are the correlations with the Rogers strength index and PFI. A correlation of .506 was obtained between the SI and the center of gravity test, while correlations of .75, .59, and .505 were obtained between the center of gravity test and the PFI. It appears that men in better condition as indicated by the strength tests stand habitually with their weight carried relatively farther forward of the vertical line erected through the malleoli.

4. The correlation between the center of gravity test and the Sargent vertical jump was .490, indicating that the men who stood with their center of gravity relatively more forward are better athletes as measured by the Sargent test.

Cureton suggests that this simple center of gravity test opens up the way for many possible studies, including:

a. The effect of high-heel shoes on the carriage of body weight with relation to the base of support.

b. Typical weight balance of extremely fat persons, hunchbacks, pregnant women, old men bent with age, persons with foot trouble, and others with special postural conditions.

c. Norms for erect standing balance for all ages and both sexes.

d. The relationship between weight balance and foot defects.

The center of gravity may also be measured through the use of one scale instead of two. In this case the subject stands at the center of the board, which is balanced at the point of two triangular blocks 1 meter apart. One block rests on the platform scale while the other block rests on a support standing at the same height as the platform scale. The following formula is applied to determine the distance in centimeters (D) that the center of gravity is in front of the point resting on the block:

$$D = \frac{\text{(Weight of subject on board)} - \text{(Weight of board on scale)}}{\text{Weight of subject}} \times 100$$

Since the distances that the heel and toe are from the center of the board can be measured, the relationship of the center of gravity to the foot may be determined.

SCREENING TESTS

Washington State University Screening Test. The posture screening test is used to select those subjects from the total group whose body statics indicate a need for a more detailed examination. Subjective ratings are made by the examiner of anteroposterior and lateral balance, and alignment of the feet and legs in the standing position. In addition to static balance the efficiency of the gait is evaluated, the subject being observed from the side, back, and front positions.[29]

General procedure. In order to screen a group of students in a minimum period of time, a series of numbers should be placed on the floor in a single line. Each student writes his name on a card and then assumes his position immediately back of a number, from 1 to 40 or 50. The examiner and a recorder write the number on the student-held card and collect all cards.

The recorder is provided with a master card for the total group. On this card a series of numbers from 1 to 40 or 50 has been placed under each of the following categories:

1. Anteroposterior. Combinations of obvious deviations such as marked fatigue slump, shoulder overhang, and imbalance of the segments such as the head, shoulders, back, and legs are observed from the side view of the subject.

2. Lateral deviations. The subjects are observed with either face or back toward the examiner.
   a. Head tilt to one side.
   b. Shoulder height (one shoulder higher).
   c. Hip prominence (one hip more prominent).
   d. Rib prominence (one side of rib cage more prominent).
   e. Leg alignment (knock knee, bow leg, tibial torsion, or inward rotation of thighs).
   f. Feet (pronation, supination; short heel cord, hammer toes, hallux valgus).

Throughout the static balance screening test, the frequent change of position from side view to front view to back view will be noted. These changes of position are intentional to enable the student to change positions frequently in order to facilitate circulation, and minimize fatigue.

Specific procedure:

1. The students, facing the examiner and standing behind a number, make a quarter turn indicated as right or left by the examiner. The recorder and examiner then move along the line about 6 feet from the subjects, and, as noticeable imbalance is detected, the correct number is circled under AP by the recorder.

2. The students turn and face the examiner. Again the same procedure is used. Head tilt right or left, and shoulder high right or left are recorded when observed.

3. Each subject stands with his back toward the examiner, who moves down the line and observes if the hip line is symmetrical. An R or L is placed on the appropriate number if one hip appears to be more prominent than the other.

4. Assuming the same position as in No. 3, the feet are separated approximately 2 inches with the heels in horizontal alignment (one foot should not be in advance of the other). As each number is called the subject curls the trunk forward with the head, shoulders, and arms relaxed forward, the finger tips reaching midway between the knees and feet; he then returns slowly to the erect standing position. The examiner keeps his eyes on a level with the back, noting any protrusion of one side of the rib cage. The recorder indicates R or L on the number if asymmetrical rib prominence is present.

5. The subjects face the examiner and knock knees, bow legs, tibial torsion, inward rotation of thigh, or other imbalance in the transmission of body weight to the base of support are noted.

6. The subjects stand with the back toward the examiner, with the feet separated slightly. Observations are made for deviations of the heel cord from a straight line, and if the weight thrust is greater to the medial or lateral side of the foot. Pronation or supination of the foot is noted and if present R, L, or bilateral (Bil.) is recorded, and, if the condition is severe, marked (mkd.) is added.

Observation of gaits. A right-angle triangle is marked by placing two objects on the floor at two of the angles while the examiner stands at the right angle. The distance of the two sides of the right angle is approximately 20 feet in length. This arrangement will enable the moving subject to be viewed from the back, side, and front.

Efficiency of gait is noted on the following points:

1. Functional foot use—heel, ball, toe action.
2. Flat feet or marked pronation.
3. Increased pelvic oscillation.
4. AP balance while walking on the diagonal.
5. Repeat of 1, 2, 3 observation as the subject walks toward the examiner.

With efficient organization of the procedure, approximately forty subjects may be screened in a forty-five minute period.

Name					Age	Height	Weight	
Standing	Slight	Marked		Walking			Slight	Marked
AP Imbalance				Lateral Balance				
Lat. Imbalance				AP Balance				
Hip Prominence				Pelvic Oscillation				
Left								
Right				Func. Use of Foot				
Rib Prominence								
Left				Pronation of Feet				
Right				Remarks:				
Leg Imbalance								
Foot Imbalance								

Figure 99. Individual body mechanics screening card used at Washington State University for all incoming freshman girls.

After the screening the findings may be recorded on the student's card (Fig. 99) from the master sheet. The students in need of a more thorough evaluation are thus identified at the beginning of their physical education class work.

FUNCTIONAL BODY MECHANICS APPRAISAL

Functional body mechanics appraisal employs a check list comprised of selected criteria used in evaluating the body subjectively, both in a static and a dynamic state. The tests are referred to as functional because the pupil is appraised on specific skills that are taught and practiced in the classroom.

Figure 100 shows a score card that may be used in making such an appraisal. Figure 101 depicts a suggested floor plan for conducting the functional test. This particular method of evaluation was worked out over a period of several years and was found to be quite efficient, in that with it eight to ten pupils may be carefully evaluated in thirty minutes.

The following outline gives the order in which the evaluation is made as well as notations of the more important mechanical factors that should be observed.

1. In the standing posture, the examiner from the side view looks for such traits as are listed on the card appearing in Figure 100 under "Standing AP Posture."

2. The subject makes a quarter turn and the examiner then evaluates lateral balance in accordance with the items appearing in Figure 100.

3. The pupil is now asked to walk to the chair (Fig. 101) and be seated. The examiner looks for control of the weight over the rear foot and segmental alignment of the body as the subject lowers himself to the

Name	Score				Age	Height Score				Weight
Standing AP Posture					Leg imbalance					
Shoulder overhang					Foot imbalance					
Forward head					Mechanics of Sitting					
Round back					Down					
Hollow back					Up					
Hyper knees					Walking AP Posture					
Pron. ft.					Lateral balance					
Lateral Balance					Pelvic control					
Shoulder height Lt.					Foot position Heel-ball-toe					
Rt.					Reaching Mechanics					
Hip Prominence Lt.					Stair Climbing Up					Rating Scale: 1—Excellent
Rt.					Down					2—Good 3—Fair
Rib Prominence Lt.					Lifting Mechanics Lowering weight					4—Poor
Rt.					Raising weight					
					Rope Skipping					

Figure 100.   Functional body mechanics appraisal scoring card.

sitting position. One foot should be to the rear of the other; hands and arms should remain relaxed and comfortable.

4. In the "up movement," once again the examiner makes note of transfer of body weight from the rear or supporting foot as the body is moved forward and up.

5. The tester now moves to position himself so as to observe the child from the rear as he walks the length of the room. The observer should note and record whether there is hip oscillation, whether the foot follows through in the heel-ball-toe movement, and whether the weight is thrust to the inside of the foot.

6. As the subject nears the end of the room he turns to his right and walks three-quarters of the distance across the room. This permits the examiner to check walking mechanics from the side or AP position. Segmental balance and general carriage of the body are noted.

7. At approximately three-quarters the distance across the room, the pupil is asked to stop and reach upward and slightly forward toward the ceiling. The examiner notes control of the pelvis, and its relationship to the upper extremity, in order to determine mechanical efficiency of the body in this extended position.

8. The child is then asked to continue walking across the room and

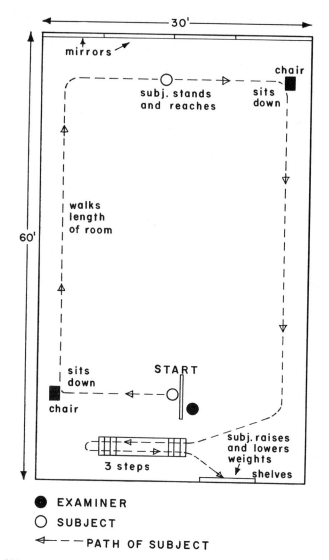

Figure 101. Diagram of floor plan for administering functional body mechanics test.

to be seated in the chair (Fig. 101). Once again the examiner checks for weight transfer and body position as in steps 3 and 4, for sitting, and for rising from the chair. (While the subject remains seated the examiner may take this opportunity to recheck his recording of deficiencies noted up to this point.)

9. The examiner then asks the pupil to rise from the chair and walk toward him. This permits observation of performance of the foot and leg function in walking, hip oscillation, erectness of carriage, and head tilt.

10. The pupil is now asked to climb and descend the stairs while the examiner watches for the proper transfer of body weight and align-

ment of the body parts. This is repeated in order that the examiner may observe the subject from the side, front, and back view. In the up movement, first the ball of the foot and then the heel make contact; there is an easy extension of the body weight over the supporting foot as the next step upward is made. In the down movement the observer notes particularly the pelvic control and whether the pupil bends the supporting leg adequately as the toe touches in order to allow the foot to be lowered with a minimum hip oscillation.

11. The child is then tested on lowering a weight of approximately 5 to 8 pounds from a shelf above his head to the floor and returning it to its original position. A series of shelves arranged from the floor to a height of about 7 feet facilitates this evaluation. Particular notation is made of segmental balance, the manner in which the legs are used in moving the weight, and whether or not the pupil holds the weight to the gravital line of the body.

12. The final test consists of having the pupil skip rope. The examiner observes segmental alignment and the control and coordination that the pupil exhibits in this activity. A quiet landing, as the youngster skips, is indicative of good control.

REFINED POSTURE APPRAISAL

Refined posture appraisal tests are generally given to children who, from the results of a rapid screening process, have been referred to a special class in body mechanics. It now becomes the duty of the instructor to investigate thoroughly the underlying causes of the deficiency. For example, you have discovered that little Mary Jones in the fourth grade has a scoliosis. Certainly, before you begin a training program for her, you must determine if this curvature is structural or whether it is the result of bad posture habits. It is possible, if the cause of a deficiency is not completely understood, to do more harm than good. Hence, all structural deviations or conditions that you are doubtful about must be referred for medical or orthopedic diagnosis. When referral is made, you, as a physical educator, should determine through a conference with the nurse, doctor, and parent if you might assist the child in an individual program under the supervision of the physician. In such cases more refined and specific instruments of evaluation may be employed to determine status and measure progress. Also such objective evidence as gained through the use of measurement will be a valuable motivator for the child and the instructor.

Kraus-Weber Refined Posture Test. During twenty years of existence of the Posture and Corrective Exercise Clinic of Babies Hospital and the Vanderbilt Clinic,[18] it was found that systematic evaluation of body mechanics must satisfy the following requirements:

1. Sufficient morphologic (body form and structure) information.
2. Sufficient functional data (physiological tests).
3. A clear picture of the condition.
4. Simple procedures, economical to administer.
5. Only simple instruments to save expenses and to adhere to the above four steps.
6. Only necessary tests.

In an effort to work out a scientific evaluation of posture, the structural and functional measurements made according to the following outline have been found to be successful.

A. *Directions:*

1. Measurements are taken with the subject in the standing position unless otherwise noted.
2. The subject stands with feet 1 to 2 inches apart.
3. The weight of the subject's body is evenly distributed on both feet; the knees are straight.
4. The subject looks straight ahead at a mark on the wall opposite to him, at eye level.
5. The subject's body is relaxed and inactive, his arms are hanging at his side.
6. The subject stands in the above position for two minutes to allow him to sink into habitual alignment before starting the test.
7. The examiner marks anatomical points on the subject in order to test with facility. (Skin pencil or lipstick may be used.)

B. *Structural measurements* (using body landmarks):

1. *Chest expansion* (in inches over xyphoid bone):
   a. In neutral or midway position.
   b. On extreme inspiration.
   c. On extreme expiration.

2. *Scapulae-spine distance* (in inches using caliper and ruler):
   a. From posterior process of the dorsal vertebrae, at level of the inferior medial angle of the scapula, to the inferior medial angle of the same scapula.
   b. The above measurement is repeated for the other scapula.
   c. The caliper is used to find the distance; the distance is measured with the ruler.

3. *Level of the scapulae* (caliper and water-level ruler):
   a. The water-level ruler is placed horizontally so that it touches the inferior angles of the scapulae.
   b. If not on a horizontal level, the level is held horizontal at the *lower* scapula and extended across the back *beneath* the other scapula. The caliper is used to measure the distance from the water-level ruler held at the lower scapula to the bottom of the highest scapula.

4. *Level of the anterior superior spine of the ilium:*
   a. The water-level ruler is placed at the level of the anterior superior spines of the iliac bones.
   b. If it is not level, the same procedure is used as in the scapulae test.
5. *Length of legs* (use steel tape to measure) :
   a. The subject is supine on the table.
   b. The distance from the anterior superior spine of the ilium to internal malleolus (medial) is measured.
6. *Angle of pelvic tilt* (protractor measurement) :
   a. The protractor is held against the lateral aspect of the hip joint so that the straight line (0 to 180 degrees) is parallel to the long axis of the femur. The knees are kept straight. The protractor is adjusted so that it is parallel with the sacrum. The obtuse angle between the 0- and 180-degree line and the arm of the protractor is then read. (Normal reading: 160 to 165 degrees.)
7. *Dorsal kyphosis and lumbar lordosis* (plumb line and calibrated water level) :
   a. The subject is placed with his back to the plumb line, which is suspended from the ceiling.
   b. The distances from the plumb line to each of the following points is measured, using the calibrated water-level ruler:
      1. Posterior process of several cervical vertebra.
      2. Posterior process of vertebra at the apex of kyphosis.
      3. Posterior processes of fifth lumbar vertebra.
   c. Dorsal kyphosis and lumbar lordosis degrees are computed by taking the apex of the kyphosis as reference 0 reading and subtracting its distance to the plumb line from other distances.

Example:

READINGS OF RULE	SUBTRACT KYPHOTIC APEX	REFERRED TO APEX 0
7th cervical 8½"	1½"	7"
Kyphosis apex 1½"		
5th lumbar 5½"	1½"	4"

C. *Functional measurements* (muscle tests of elasticity and strength) : The length of the muscles, measured by the maximum degree of active joint range, indicates muscle elasticity.
1. *Total elasticity of the pectoral muscle* (protractor) :
   a. This is indicated by the angle formed by the arm when the fully raised arm is parallel with the long axis of the thorax.
   b. The subject raises his arm in the forward direction as high as possible.

    c. The protractor is held laterally against the subject's shoulder joint with the straight line of 0 to 180 degrees parallel to the long axis of the thorax.

    d. The arm of the protractor is adjusted parallel to the length of the axis of the humerus, and the obtuse angle read.

    e. The above steps are repeated on other shoulder joint.

    f. Normal muscle reading: 170 to 180 degrees.

2. *Total elasticity of hamstring muscles:*

    a. This is measured by the angle to which the legs may be lifted from the supine position without causing a motion in the fourth and fifth lumbar vertebrae.

    b. The subject lies completely relaxed in the supine position on the table.

    c. The protractor is placed with the straight line of 0 to 180 degrees on the table next to subject's hip joint.

    d. The examiner places his fingers lightly on the posterior spinous processes of the fourth and fifth lumbar vertebrae under the subject's back.

    e. The assistant slowly lifts the subject's legs, holding them at the heels (preferably one at a time).

    f. The instant that the examiner feels motion in fourth and fifth vertebrae, the full length of hamstrings has been reached. Further movement of the legs upward causes movement of the lumbar region in a posterior direction.

    g. When the examiner feels motion, the assistant stops lifting and holds the angle.

    h. The arm of the protractor is adjusted parallel to the length of the axis of the femur and the acute angle between the table level and the femur is read; 30 degrees is a normal reading.

3. *Total elasticity of erector spinae and hamstring muscles:*

    a. The subject bends forward and touches the floor with his fingertips.

    b. The knees are straight.

    c. The distance from the fingertips to the floor is measured with a ruler.

    d. Normally proportioned subjects will touch the floor with their fingertips.

Muscle Power and Holding Power Measurements

Muscle power (strength) is tested according to its ability to overcome gravity by assuming a test position. The holding ability of the muscle is measured by the time the subject can hold a position. The first five Kraus-

Weber tests of minimal muscular fitness, appearing in Chapter 4 are used in this area of evaluation.

Interpretation of measurements taken:

A. *Structural measurements* (using body landmarks) :

1. The chest expansion measurement. This is of value in determining the relative expansion and breathing capacity.
2. The scapulae-spine distance. If this is unequal a lateral curvature of the dorsal spine is a possibility.
3. Level of scapulae. If this is uneven there is a lateral curvature of the spine or a disturbance of tension in the muscles of the shoulder girdle.
4. Level of the anterosuperior spine of the ilium. If this is not horizontal there is a lateral tilt of the pelvis, possibly due to scoliosis in the lumbar region.
5. Comparison of leg lengths. One leg shorter than the other may indicate a lateral tilt of the pelvis and a curvature in the lumbar spine with the apex of the curve on the side of the shorter leg.
6. Measurements of the angle of the forward pelvic tilt. If the angle is less than 160 degrees, increased lumbar lordosis is a possibility; if it is more than 170 degrees, this is indicative of a flat back.
7. Measurements for dorsal kyphosis and lumbar lordosis. These show an increase of the curves in direct proportion to the increase in distance between the seventh cervical and fifth lumbar vertebrae, to the apex of the curve marked 0, and a corresponding decrease if these distances decrease.

B. *Functional measurement* (muscle tests of elasticity and strength) :

1. Pectorals. If the angle is less than 170 to 180 degrees, there is a possibility of shortened pectoralis muscle group, which is associated with anterior displacement of the shoulder, a narrow chest, restricted range of motion in the shoulder joint, and possible dorsal kyphosis.
2. Hamstrings. If the angle measured is less than 30 degrees this indicates a shortness of the muscle group of hamstrings.
3. Erector spinae and hamstrings. In the bending test the distance from the fingertips to the floor gives an indication of the length of both muscle groups. Comparison with 2 above indicates whether the erectors or the hamstrings are contracted.

Evaluation of the Feet

Too frequently, little attention is given to the feet until they begin to cause pain. Many shoes worn by women are particularly harmful to the health of the feet. There is a minimum of scientific construction evident in the present shoe design; beauty and personal appeal essentially dictate the form of the shoe. The most glaring example of foot abuse is the spike heel on women's shoes. Such construction causes the weight of the body to be shifted forward over the balls of the feet, resulting in restricted movement of the Achilles tendon, perhaps eventually causing it to shorten. Then, too, high heels frequently are the cause of hard calluses appearing on the soles of women's feet as a result of the body's compensating for this unnatural weight placement. As a matter of fact, data from the American Foot Care Institute indicate that about 85 per cent of all foot troubles come from faulty footwear.

Bancroft states that from 57 to 61 per cent of all cases of flat feet are serious enough to be discovered between the ages of ten and twenty-five years, indicating a need for special training in hygiene of the feet during this time of neuromuscular development and rapidly increasing weight.[1] Stafford found, in examinations of school groups and army recruits, that 6 to 13 per cent of those examined had true flat feet or sunken arches and 73 to 78 per cent had weak feet.[30]

Footprint. One of the early methods of evaluating feet was by means of the footprint. The most convenient method for recording the footprint is by use of the pedograph. Directions for the use of this instrument are as follows:

1. The subject should be in his bare feet.

2. The machine should be properly inked so that the print is clear. It will be necessary to re-ink the machine for approximately every fifty pupils.

3. The stamping cover is pulled over clean paper. The subject is instructed to place his bare heel against the steel plate of the pedograph and then stand firmly on the stamping cover. There should be no unnecessary movement of the foot, which might result in an inaccurate print. The opposite foot should be removed from the floor so that the full weight of the subject is brought to bear over the foot being tested.

4. The subject is instructed to step off the stamping cover. The sheet is then removed. The subject's name and the date of print are recorded.

5. The procedure is repeated with the subject's other foot.

Clarke Footprint Angle. Schwartz originated the footprint angle, which is a measure of the height of the longitudinal arch.[28] Clarke made slight modification of Schwartz' original work, with a resulting 968 objectivity coefficient.[5] Figure 102 illustrates the Clarke footprint angle, which is scored in the following manner:

1. Line A is drawn to represent the medial border of the footprint between the imprint of the head of the first metatarsal bone and the imprint of the calcaneus.

2. Line B is drawn from a point where line A first touches the imprint of the inner side of the big toe to the point just touching the edge

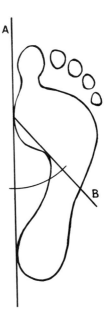

Figure 102. Clarke footprint angle.

of the print on the inside of the arch. This line represents the slope of the metatarsal border of the longitudinal arch. No white paper should show between this line and the print.

3. The angle at junction of lines A and B is measured with a protractor.

The average for college freshmen, according to Clarke's data, may be considered as 42 degrees. Clarke claims that individuals with angles below 30 degrees may definitely be considered as proper subjects for individual foot corrections. Students with angles between 30 and 35 degrees may be considered as borderline subjects, and should be given a re-examination to determine the possible need for corrective treatment.

Objectivity and validity of footprint angle. Cureton studied the validity of the footprint angle method of measuring the height of the longitudinal arch by comparing the vertical depth of the arch imprint in moist sand (sand box method) to the Clarke footprint angle.[7] The correlations between the arch angle and the arch height on two separate sets of data were .857 ± .016 and .958 ± .007.

In order to determine the validity of footprints as a measure of the functional efficiency of the foot, Cureton selected such events as running, jumping, weight bearing, shot putting, lifting, and balancing on the balance beam to correlate against the height of the arch. These types of events were selected because it was felt the foot is used vigorously in their execution.

Twenty-one correlations of the longitudinal arch with the selected skills showed that there was some positive correlation with 440-yard running. This might indicate that the men with the flatter prints have a tendency to fatigue more quickly, which Cureton feels may be true of most big muscled-men.

Of the 600 men tested, Cureton reported that 150 had arch angles under 21 degrees and only four or five men complained of pain. Apparently the height of the longitudinal arch does not represent either strong or weak feet. Actually, on the basis of Cureton's findings, the footprint angle serves no other purpose than to motivate the pupil in directing attention to the feet.

The pedorule.   The pedorule was devised to measure the position of the foot in relation to the leg, as contrasted to the footprint angle, which measures the height of the arch.[10] By use of the pedorule those subjects with abnormally low arches would not be given a misdiagnosis of weak feet, thus negating an obvious weakness in the footprint angle test.

The pedorule is a rectangle of heavy plate glass, 7 inches wide and 9 inches high, with the surface scored in parallel lines $\frac{1}{10}$ inch apart. It measures the amount of deflection that the Achilles tendon makes from a straight line. In weak feet the lower portion of the tendon appears to be deflected outward.

Directions for measuring with the pedorule are as follows:

1. The pedorule is placed immediately behind the foot being measured, and two points are established by ink marks: the midpoint of the Achilles tendon as high on the calf of the leg as possible, and the midpoint of the back of the heel.

2. The center line of the pedorule (which for convenience should be colored) should then bisect these two ink marks, on the normal foot.

3. In making observations one eye should be closed; the examiner should be in such a position that the open eye will be approximately 24 inches directly behind the center of the pedorule.

4. From this position (above) three readings can be made: (1) the distance from the extreme tip of the external malleolus to the center of the tendon; (2) the distance from the internal malleolus to the center of the tendon; and (3) the distance from the center of the tendon to the center of the pedorule. (The center line of the pedorule will coincide with the center line of the tendon of Achilles if the arch is neither flat nor weak.)

A second method of determination of flat-footedness by the pedorule is as follows:

1. Place the center line of the pedorule directly behind the center of the tendon at the point where it is bowed inward the farthest.

2. Count the number of lines from this point to the tips of the malleoli and subtract the distance from the tendon to the internal malleolus from the distance from the center of the bowed-in tendon to the external malleolus. The distance that the tendon of Achilles deviates from the perpendicular will thus be found.

Danford recommends this latter method for it is less confusing and more efficient than the one first described. The perfect foot would be "zero," thus showing the tendon to be equidistant between the malleoli throughout its entire length. The objectivity coefficient was found to be .94.

Validity of the pedorule. Danford intercorrelated three methods of evaluating the feet: between two subjective examiners; between the pedograph and the pedorule; and between each of the instruments and the examiners.

The relatively high correlation that was shown between the subjective examiners and the pedograph (.54 and .50) is attributed to the fact that, in judging subjectively, an examiner notes the portion of the foot not touching the floor, and the pedograph print merely shows the ground plan of the foot. Thus, in both examinations, to a great extent, the ground plan of the foot is studied without taking into consideration whether or not the foot is normal, or has become flattened.

The correlation between subjective examiner number one and the pedorule was .38, while that between the subjective examiner two and the pedorule was four points lower. This may be explained by the fact that subjective examiner one had included in his records the position of the tendon Achilles in relation to the foot.

The low correlation of .30 between the pedograph and the pedorule indicates that these instruments are not measuring the same thing. The pedograph measures the footprint angle, while the pedorule is measuring the distance that the tendon has departed from its normal position, which indicates how much the arch has flattened.

Two extreme cases of disagreement between the pedograph and the pedorule tests were selected for more careful analysis. A subject with a footprint angle of 11 degrees and pedorule reading of zero for both feet was questioned as to any discomforts that might be caused by his feet. It was learned that the subject believed that he had fallen arches because of information given him. However, he never suffered any pains in his feet, legs, or back that could be attributed to flat feet.

In another extreme, where the pedograph had recorded a footprint angle of 42 degrees, which is supposedly average, the pedorule score was "five-tenths" for the right foot and "four-tenths" for the left. Because of this sharp discrepancy the subject was asked if he had ever had any trouble with his feet, whereupon it was found that he could not take hikes, or play basketball, or stand on his feet very long at a time, because of severe pains in his feet, legs, and back. He also reported frequent headaches.

These two cases, of course, are not sufficient to validate the pedorule completely. However, implications that measurement of deflection of the Achilles tendon is a better method of evaluating feet than merely recording the footprint has been supported. This study clearly illustrates that the greater bowing-in of the tendon, the flatter the arch, although arches were often recorded as flat by the pedograph when the tendons were not bowed in.

When either the pedograph or pedorule is used, both feet should be measured, for in some subjects the right foot might be markedly pronated or flat while the left foot is apparently normal. Rogers reports a correlation of only .28 between the right and left feet using the footprint angle.

Truslow Foot Ratio. Truslow has found, through clinical experience, that the ratio of the height of the arch to the length of the foot is a valid determinant in regard to the functional efficiency of the foot.[32] From numerous foot measurements, Truslow found a normal mean ratio between the height of the arch and length of the foot to range from 7.7 to 8.3 per cent. The computation is simply the height of the arch in centimeters divided by the length of the foot in centimeters multiplied by one hundred.

The equipment used for the measurements consists of a small draftsman's triangle (about $12 \times 12 \times 18$ cm.) measured off, on one of its shorter sides, into half centimeters; and a shoe dealer's foot-measuring rod, rescaled from the heel post forward into half centimeters.

The measurements taken are as follows:

1. Height of arch with subject standing. The subject stands with feet parallel and about 12 inches apart. The examiner places the measured side of the triangle against the inner side of the foot, at the position of the scaphoid (navicular) bone; then places his pencil point beneath the bone and reads the height on the triangle. He records this for the right foot, and then measures the left.

2. The height of the arch for both right and left feet is also measured with the subject in a sitting position.

3. The length of the foot is measured with the subject in a sitting position. The reading at the tip of the great toe is noted and recorded for both the right and left feet.

The measured height of the right foot with the subject standing is divided by the measured right-foot length and the quotient recorded. The same calculations are made for the left foot (using the left-foot length, if it differs from that of the right foot), and also for both right and left foot with the measurements made while the subject was sitting.

Objectivity and reliability of this method have not been recorded. The validity of the test rests with the clinical validation obtained from numerous measurements made on men, women, and children.

The interpretation of results, according to Truslow, are as follows:

1. A standing ratio of 8 per cent is a fair average for efficient feet. Lacking other harmful factors, a standing range of 7 per cent to 9 per cent may safely be considered as constituting military or civilian efficiency.

2. The higher the figure of standing ratio (above 8 per cent) the

more is it an expression of existing "hollow foot" (pes cavus), a condition that may become quite as disabling as flat foot.

3. The lower the figure of standing ratio (below 8 per cent) the greater is the indication of the existence of flat foot (pes planus).

4. A fairly low standing ratio compared with a high sitting ratio indicates a temporary muscular weakness.

5. A standing ratio, at whatever low level, compared with a sitting ratio that is but little, if any, higher than the standing ratio points to spasticity of the feet, which may be correctable by prolonged treatment.

6. Marked discrepancy between the right- and the left-foot lengths, or between the right and the left ratios, calls for more careful study on the part of the examiner, who may expect to find antedating pathologic or traumatic causes for such discrepancy.

Truslow takes note of the importance of other factors in foot efficiency, but insists that the use of this form of foot measurement can be an important aid in the evaluation of the effectiveness of military registrants as well as individuals in civilian life.

Evaluation of Flexibility

Flexibility has long been recognized as an important factor in athletic proficiency. The definition of this term is most frequently given as "the range of movement about a joint." However, one must not fail to recognize that the degree of joint flexibility is dependent upon physiological characteristics underlying the extensibility of the muscles and ligaments surrounding the joint. In addition to noting that flexibility is significant in performing skills, the recent advancements in physical medicine and rehabilitation have indicated the importance of flexibility as it is related to general physical fitness. Particularly, if a person maintains a satisfactory degree of flexibility, he is less susceptible to certain muscular injuries.

Exactly how much flexibility an individual should possess has not, as yet, been scientifically demonstrated. In the Kraus-Weber floor touch test, which involves the extensibility of the erector spinae, gluteal, hamstring, and gastrocnemius muscles, a passing grade is the ability to touch the floor. The only reported validity for this test is the evidence gained from examination of numerous patients by the medical people who have assisted Kraus.

Mathews and his co-workers studied hip flexibility of college women and elementary school boys as related to length of body segments.[22, 23] In each instance no significant relationship was found between flexibility of the hip joint and length of body segments. Examination of the extremes of the distribution of lower limb length seems to support the hypothesis that flexibility is independent of lower limb length.

Leighton Flexometer Tests.   Leighton has contributed the most comprehensive technique for measuring objectively the flexibility of thirty joint movements.[19]

The instrument employed in making the measurements is called the Leighton flexometer (Fig. 103). It has a weighted 360-degree dial and a

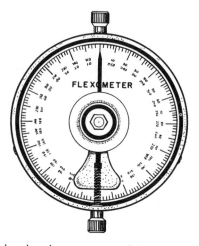

Figure 103.   Leighton   flexometer.

weighted pointer mounted in a case. The dial and pointer operate freely and independently; the movement of each is controlled by gravity. The instrument will record movement while in any position which is 20 degrees or more off the horizontal. The zero mark on the dial and the tip of the pointer move freely to a position of rest and coincide when the instrument is placed in any position off the horizontal, as indicated. Independent locking devices are provided for the pointer and the dial, which stop all movement of either, at any given position. While in use the flexometer is strapped to the segment being tested. When the dial is locked at one extreme position (e.g., full extension of the elbow) the direct reading of the pointer on the dial is the arc through which the movement has taken place. In addition to the flexometer a projecting wall corner, a long bench or table, and a low-backed armchair are also required.

Validity of these tests is based upon the now clearly recognized and defined segmental joint movements of the body. Reliability was determined by the test-retest method, using 120 boys. Coefficients of correlation ranged from .913 to .996.

Measurement technique Neck. Flexion and Extension. Starting position—Supine position on bench, head and neck projecting over end, shoulders touching edge, arms at sides. Instrument fastened to either side of head over ear.

Movement—Count (1) head raised and moved to position as near chest as possible, dial locked, (2) head lowered and moved to position as near end of bench as possible, pointer locked, (3) subject relaxes, reading taken.

Caution—Shoulders may not be raised from bench during flexion, nor back unduly arched during extension. Buttocks and shoulders must remain on bench during movement.

Lateral Flexion. Starting position—Sitting position in low-backed armchair, back straight, hands grasping chair arms, upper arms hooked over back of chair. Instrument fastened to back of head.

Movement—Count (1) head moved in arc sideward to the left as far as possible, dial locked, (2) head moved in arc sideward to the right as far as possible, pointer locked, (3) subject relaxes, reading taken.

Caution—Position in chair may not be changed during movement. Shoulders may not be raised or lowered.

Rotation. Starting position—Supine position on bench, head and neck projecting over, shoulders touching edge and arms at sides of bench. Instrument fastened to top of head.

Movement—Count (1) head turned left as far as possible, dial locked, (2) head turned right as far as possible, pointer locked, (3) subject relaxes, reading taken.

Caution—Shoulders may not be raised from bench.

Shoulder. Flexion and Extension. Starting position—Standing position at projecting corner of wall, arm to be measured extending just beyond projecting corner, arms at sides, back to wall; shoulder blades, buttocks, and heels touching wall. Instrument fastened to side of upper arm.

Movement—Count (1) arm moved forward and upward in an arc as far as possible, palm of hand sliding against wall, dial locked, (2) arm moved downward and backward in an arc as far as possible, palm of hand sliding against wall, pointer locked, (3) subject relaxes, reading taken.

Caution—Heels, buttocks, and shoulders must touch wall at all times during movement. Elbow of arm being measured must be kept straight. Palm of hand of arm being measured must be against wall when dial and pointer are locked.

Adduction and Abduction: Starting position—Standing position with arms at sides, left (right) side of body toward wall, shoulder touching same, left (right) fist doubled with knuckles forward, thumbside of fist touching hip and opposite side of fist touching wall, feet together, knees and elbows straight. Instrument fastened to back of right (left) upper arm.

Movement—Count (1) palm of right (left) hand pressed against side of leg, dial locked, (2) arm moved sideward, outward, and upward in an arc as far as possible, pointer locked, (3) subject relaxes, reading taken.

Caution—Left (right) wrist must be kept in contact with the body and wall at all times. Knees, body, and elbows must be kept straight throughout movement. Arm must be raised directly sideward, not forward or backward. Heels of feet may not be raised from floor.

Rotation: Starting position—Standing position at projecting corner of wall, arm to be measured extended sideward and bent to right angle at elbow, shoulder extended just beyond projecting corner, opposite arm at side of body, back to wall; shoulder blades, buttocks, and heels touching wall. Instrument fastened to side of forearm.

Movement—Count (1) forearm moved downward and backward in an arc as far as possible, dial locked. (2) forearm moved forward, upward, and backward in arc as far as possible, pointer locked, (3) subject relaxes, reading taken.

Caution—Upper arm being measured must be held directly sideward and parallel with the floor during movement. Heels, buttocks, and shoulders must touch wall at all times.

Elbow. Flexion and Extension. Starting position—squatting or sitting position facing table or bench with upper portion of arm being measured resting back down across nearest table corner so that the elbow extends just beyond one edge and the armpit is resting against the adjacent edge. Instrument fastened to back of wrist.

Movement—Count (1) wrist moved upward and backward in an arc to position as near shoulder as possible, dial locked, (2) wrist moved forward and downward until arm is forcibly extended, pointer locked, (3) subject relaxes, reading taken.

Caution—Upper arm may not be tilted or moved during measurement.

Radial-ulnar. Supination and Pronation. Starting position—Sitting position in standard armchair, back straight, forearms resting on chair arms, fists doubled and extended beyond ends of chair arms, wrist of arm to be measured held straight. Strap is grasped in hand, fastening instrument to front of fist. (Common chair and table of suitable height may be substituted for armchair.)

Movement—Count (1) thumb-side of fist turned outward and downward as far as possible, dial locked, (2) thumb-side of fist turned upward, downward, and inward as far as possible, pointer locked, (3) subject relaxes, reading taken.

Caution—Body and forearm must remain stationary, except for specified movement, throughout measurement. No leaning of the body may be permitted.

Wrist. Flexion and Extension. Starting position—Sitting position in standard armchair, back straight, forearms resting on chair arms, fists doubled and extended beyond ends of chair arms, palm of hand to be measured turned up. Instrument fastened to thumb-side of fist. (Common chair and table of suitable height may be substituted for armchair.)

Movement—Count (1) fist moved upward and backward in an arc as far as possible, dial locked, (2) fist moved forward, downward, and backward in an arc as far as possible, pointer locked, (3) subject relaxes, reading taken.

Caution—Forearm may not be raised from chair arm during movement.

Ulnar and Radial Flexion: Starting position—Sitting position in standard armchair, back straight, forearms resting on chair arms, fists doubled and extended beyond ends of chair arms, thumb-side of hand to be measured turned up. Instrument fastened to back of hand. (Common chair and table of suitable height may be substituted for armchair.)

Movement—Count (1) fist moved upward and backward in an arc as far as possible, dial locked, (2) fist moved downward and backward as far as possible, pointer locked, (3) subject relaxes, reading taken.

Caution—Forearm may not be raised from chair arm during movement. Fist may not be turned inward or outward during measurement.

Hip. Extension and Flexion. Starting position—Standing position, feet together, knees stiff, arms extended above head, hands clasped with palms up. Instrument fastened to either side of hip at height of umbilicus.

Movement—Count (1) bend backward as far as possible, dial locked, (2) bend forward as far as possible, pointer locked (3) subject relaxes, reading taken.

Caution—Knees may not be bent but must remain straight throughout movement. Feet may not be shifted. Toes and heels may not be raised.

Adduction and Abduction. Starting position—Standing position, feet together, knees straight, arms at sides. Instrument fastened to back of either leg.

Movement—Count (1) starting position, dial locked, (2) leg to which instrument is not attached is moved sideward as far as possible, pointer locked, (3) subject relaxes, reading taken.

Caution—Body must remain in upright position throughout movement. Knees must be kept straight with the feet assuming a position on line and parallel.

Rotation. Starting position—Sitting position on bench with left (right) leg resting on and foot projecting over end of bench, knee straight, right (left) leg extending downward, foot resting on floor. Instrument fastened to bottom of left (right) foot.

Movement—Count (1) left (right) foot turned outward as far as possible, dial locked, (2) left (right) foot turned inward as far as possible, pointer locked, (3) subject relaxes, reading taken.

Caution—Knee and ankle joints must remain locked throughout movement. Position of hips may not be changed during measurement.

Knee. Flexion and Extension. Starting position—Prone position on box or bench with knees at end of bench and lower legs extending beyond end of bench, arms at sides of bench and hands grasping edges of bench. Instrument fastened to outside of either ankle.

Movement—Count (1) foot moved upward and backward in an arc to position as near buttocks as possible, dial locked, (2) foot moved forward and downward until leg is forcibly extended, pointer locked, (3) subject relaxes, reading taken.

Caution—Position of upper leg may not be changed during movement.

Ankle. Flexion and Extension. Starting position—Sitting position on bench with left (right) leg resting on and foot projecting over end of bench, knee straight, right (left) leg extending downward, foot resting on floor. Instrument fastened to inside of left (right) foot.

Movement—Count (1) left (right) foot turned downward as far as possible, dial locked, (2) left (right) foot turned upward and toward the knee as far as possible, pointer locked, (3) subject relaxes, reading taken.

Caution—Knee of leg being measured must be kept straight throughout movement. No sideward turning of the foot may be allowed.

Inversion and Eversion. Starting position—Sitting on end of bench, knees projecting over and lower legs downward with calves resting against end board. Shoes (low cut) should be worn. Instrument fastened to front of foot.

Movement—Count (1) foot turned inward as far as possible, dial locked, (2) foot turned outward as far as possible, pointer locked, (3) subject relaxes, reading taken.

Caution—Position of lower leg may not be changed during measurement.

Trunk. Extension and Flexion. Starting position—Standing position, feet together, knees straight, arms extended above head, hands clasped with palms up. Instrument fastened to either side of chest just below armpit at nipple height.

Movement—Count (1) bend backward as far as possible, dial locked (2) bend forward as far as possible, pointer locked, (3) subject relaxes, reading taken.

Caution—Knees must be kept straight throughout movement. Feet may not be shifted. Toes and heels may not be raised from floor.

Note—This movement involves trunk and hip extension and flexion. To obtain the measure for trunk extension and flexion alone, the measure for hip extension and flexion must be subtracted from the score obtained above.

Lateral Flexion. Starting position—Standing position, feet together, knees straight, arms at sides. Instrument fastened to middle of back at nipple height.

Movement—Count (1) bend sideward to the left as far as possible, dial locked, (2) bend sideward to the right as far as possible, pointer locked, (3) subject relaxes, reading taken:

Caution—Both feet must remain flat on floor, heels may not be raised during measurement. Knees must be kept straight throughout movement. Subject may bend sideward and backward, but must not be allowed to bend forward.

Rotation. Starting position—Supine position on bench, legs together, knees raised above hips, lower legs parallel to bench and body. Assistant holds subject's shoulders. Instrument fastened to middle rear of upper legs, strap going around both legs.

Movement—Count (1) knees lowered to the left as far as possible, dial locked, (2) knees brought back to starting position and lowered to the right as far as possible, pointer locked, (3) subject relaxes, reading taken.

Caution—Subject's shoulders must not be permitted to rise from the bench during movement. Knees must be moved directly sideward at the height of the hips, not above or below.

Table 44 contains means and standard deviations for the thirty flexibility measures recorded from a group of fifty sixteen-year-old California boys.

TABLE 44. *Flexibility Means and Standard Deviations for a Group of Fifty Sixteen-Year-Old California Boys**

Test	M	σ
1. Neck flexion-extension	123.40	11.82
2. Neck lateral flexion	88.40	10.66
3. Neck rotation	158.40	12.43
4. Right shoulder flexion-extension	257.50	10.60
5. Left shoulder flexion-extension	257.70	10.19
6. Right shoulder adduction-abduction	173.20	8.83
7. Left shoulder adduction-abduction	173.20	9.76
8. Right shoulder rotation	170.40	15.65
9. Left shoulder rotation	170.90	12.82
10. Right elbow flexion-extension	141.10	7.70
11. Left elbow flexion-extension	142.70	6.32
12. Right radial-ulnar supination-pronation	161.90	11.64
13. Left radial-ulnar supination-pronation	161.50	10.53
14. Right wrist flexion-extension	130.10	14.03
15. Left wrist flexion-extension	131.70	13.69
16. Right wrist ulnar-radial flexion	75.50	9.59
17. Left wrist ulnar-radial flexion	75.90	10.31
18. Hip extension-flexion	55.50	13.37
19. Hip adduction-abduction	63.30	14.00
20. Right hip rotation	68.60	12.73
21. Left hip rotation	70.00	13.50
22. Right knee flexion-extension	136.00	13.17
23. Left knee flexion-extension	135.90	11.25
24. Right ankle flexion-extension	62.70	10.67
25. Left ankle flexion-extension	62.80	9.87
26. Right ankle inversion-eversion	43.12	7.97
27. Left ankle inversion-eversion	43.60	8.57
28. Trunk extension-flexion	78.50	21.38
29. Trunk lateral flexion	95.80	15.43
30. Trunk rotation	128.60	9.60

* Note: All means and standard deviations are computed in degrees and fractions of degrees. The symbol for degree is omitted since no other unit of measure is used. (Courtesy of Professor Jack Leighton, Eastern Washington College, Cheney, Washington, 1957.)

Wells Sit and Reach Test. The Wells Test was devised to take the place of the flexibility test that required the subject to stand on a gymnasium bench. In this "bench test," the arms and trunk are relaxed forward, with hands in front of a vertical scale attached to the front of the bench. The subject bobs downward four times, keeping the knees straight, and on the fourth reach holds the position of maximum forward and downward flexibility. Because many students had feelings of insecurity and apprehension while performing this test, Wells and Dillon decided that it would be wiser to perform the tests, if at all possible, from a sitting position.[33]

The equipment consists of a 24- $\times$ 8-inch piece of plywood, with lines drawn horizontally at half-inch intervals. The center line is marked 0, the inch lines on one side are numbered from 1 up, and those on the opposite side are numbered from —1 up. The support for the scale is in the form of a plus sign made of 11-inch boards resting on their edges. These are referred to as the cross board and the stem board. Footprints are outlined on one surface of the cross board one on either side of the stem board. The scale is attached to the upper edges of the support in

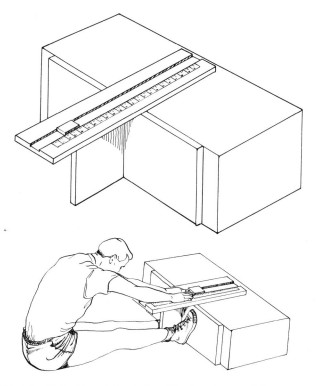

Figure 104. The Wells Sit and Reach Test. The Camaione modification of the instrument permits both sitting and standing flexibility measures. Administration of the standing test can be observed by rotating the picture 90 degrees clockwise. (Mathews, D. K., Kruse, R., and Shaw, V.: The Science of Physical Education for Handicapped Children. New York, Harper & Brothers, 1962, p. 209.)

such a way that when the subject is seated on the floor with feet against the footprints, the zero line coincides with the near surface of the cross board and the minus values are toward the subject (Fig. 104). Another method of constructing the number scale is to countersink a portion of a yardstick into the plywood surface.

With the feet placed in the footprints on the cross board, the subject reaches forward, palms down, along the scale. The maximum distance reached is recorded as the measure of flexibility. The authors report the reliability of this test as .98, when the subjects are permitted three preliminary bobs.

Summary and Conclusions

Body mechanics should be taught and evaluated, particularly in the elementary and junior high schools. Here youngsters are in the formative stages of development and much can be done to diminish the number requiring remedial or adapted classes as they grow older.

There is no objective evidence which shows specific relationships between posture and physiological function, thus the reasons for teaching body mechanics are functional, esthetic, and a preventive measure for the chronic orthopedic difficulties encountered in later years.

The basic criterion for evaluating body mechanics is expert opinion, and the experts do agree in general as to what constitutes good posture.

The posture screening and functional evaluation tests as well as the refined posture appraisal are the most practical tests. Once skill, gained through experience, is acquired, objective and valid results of postural appraisal can be obtained. The screening test aids in selecting those most seriously deficient for further attention in remedial classes.

From the information gained through screening, an individual program may be initiated, provided the physical educator clearly understands the underlying cause of the postural deficiency. If the cause of the deficiency is not clearly understood, referral should be made to a physician. All subjects with serious lateral imbalances are examples of persons who should be referred. The physical educator should follow up on the referral in order to determine what aid he may render. It is quite possible, when therapeutic services are non-existent or limited, that the physician may prescribe an exercise program to be conducted by the physical educator. In situations such as this, refined postural measurements such as those in the Kraus-Weber test will prove of value in determining progress as well as for motivating the child. This is another important phase of developmental and remedial work in which the cooperation of the physician and physical educator can result in marked contributions to the normal growth and development of our youngsters.

The evaluation of body mechanics applies to three phases of the physical education program: (1) the screening phase, the primary purpose of which is to locate the seriously deficient requiring individual attention; and (2) the general instructional phase, the primary purpose of which is twofold: to allow practice of such specific skills as standing, walking, and sitting, and, at the same time, to assign a mark of proficiency in each of the events; and (3) the more definitive measurement, which is used with those pupils seriously deficient—the ones who have been placed in an individual program on the basis of the screening test.

BIBLIOGRAPHY

1. Bancroft, Jesse H.: The Posture of School Children. New York, The Macmillan Co., 1913.
2. Boynton, Bernice: Individual Differences in the Structure of Pelvis and Lumbar Spine as a Factor in Body Mechanics. M.A. Thesis, State University of Iowa, 1933.
3. Brownell, C. L.: A Scale for Measuring Anterior-Posterior Posture of Ninth Grade Boys. New York, Bureau of Publications, Teachers College, Columbia University, 1928.
4. Carnett, J. B.: Extracts from Discussion. White House Conference on Child Health and Protection, Body Mechanics: Education and Practice. New York, The Century Co., 1932.
5. Clarke, H. Harrison: An Objective Method of Measuring the Height of the Longitudinal Arch in Foot Examinations. Research Quart., Vol. 4, No. 3, October, 1933.
6. Crampton, C. W.: Work-a-Day Tests of Good Posture. American Physical Education Review, Vol. 30, November, 1925.
7. Cureton, Thomas K.: The Validity of Footprints as a Measure of Vertical Height of the Arch and Functional Efficiency of the Foot. Research Quart., Vol. 6, No. 2, May, 1935.
8. Cureton, Thomas K., and Wickens, J. Stuart: The Center of Gravity of the Human Body in the Antero-posterior Plane and Its Relation to Posture, Physical Fitness, and Athletic Ability. Supplement to Research Quart., Vol. 6, No. 2, May, 1935.
9. Cureton, Thomas K., Wickens, J. Stuart, and Elder, Haskel P.: Reliability and Objectivity of Springfield Postural Measurements. Supplement to Research Quart., Vol. 6, No. 2, May, 1935.
10. Danford, Harold R.: A Comparative Study of Three Methods of Measuring Flat and Weak Feet. Supplement to Research Quart., Vol. 6, No. 1, March, 1935.
11. Fox, M. S., and Young, O. S.: Placement of Gravital Line in Antero-posterior Standing Posture. Research Quart., Vol. 25, No. 3, October, 1954.
12. Glassow, Ruth: Fundamentals in Physical Education. Philadelphia, Lea & Febiger, 1932.
13. Goldthwait, J. E., Brown, L. T., Swaim, L. T., and Kuhns, J. G.: Body Mechanics in the Study and Treatment of Disease. Philadelphia, Lea & Febiger, 1930.
14. Howland, Ivalclare Sprow: Body Alignment in Fundamental Motor Skills. New York, Exposition Press, 1953.
15. Howland, Ivalclare S.: A Study of the Position of the Sacrum in the Adult Female Pelvis and Its Relationship to Body Mechanics. M.A. Thesis, State University of Iowa, 1933.
16. Karpovich, Peter V., and Sinning, Wayne E.: Physiology of Muscular Activity. 7th ed. Philadelphia & London, W. B. Saunders Co., 1971.
17. Klein, A., and Thomas, L. C.: Posture and Physical Fitness. Children's Bureau, Publication No. 205, Washington, D. C., Government Printing Office, 1931.
18. Kraus, Hans, and Weber, S.: Evaluation of Posture Based on Structural and Functional Measurements. Physiotherapy Rev., Vol. 26, No. 6, 1945.

19. Leighton, Jack: An Instrument and Technic for the Measurement of Range of Joint Motion. Arch. Phys. Med., September, 1955.

20. Lowman, Charles L., Colestock, Claire, and Cooper, Hazel: Corrective Physical Education for Groups. New York, A. S. Barnes & Co., 1928.

21. Massey, Wayne W.: A Critical Study of Objective Methods for Measuring Anterior-Posterior Posture with a Simplified Technique. Research Quart., Vol. 14, No. 1, March, 1943.

22. Mathews, D. K., Shaw, V., and Bohnen, M.: Hip Flexibility of College Women as Related to Length of Body Segments. Research. Quart. 28:352–356, Dec., 1957.

23. Mathews, D. K., Shaw, V., and Woods, J.: Hip Flexibility of Elementary School Boys as Related to Body Segments. Research Quart., 30:297–302, October, 1959.

24. McCloy, Charles H.: X-ray Studies of Innate Differences in Straight and Curved Spines. Research Quart., Vol. 9, No. 2, May, 1938.

25. Rathbone, Josephine L.: Good Postures, the Expression of Good Development. Symposium on Posture, Phi Delta Pi, March, 1938.

26. Report of the Baruch Committee on Physical Medicine (Chairman, Ray L. Wilbur). New York, 597 Madison Avenue, April 1, 1945.

27. Reynolds, E., and Lovett, R. W.: Method of Determining the Position of the Center of Gravity in Its Relation to Certain Body Landmarks in the Erect Position. Am. J. Physiol., May, 1909.

28. Schwartz, L., Britten, R. H., and Thompson, L. R.: Studies in Physical Development and Posture. U. S. Public Health Bulletin, No. 179, 1928.

29. Shaw, Virginia: Unpublished data. Washington State College, Pullman, Washington, 1957.

30. Stafford, George T.: Preventive and Corrective Physical Education. Revised ed. New York, A. S. Barnes & Co., 1950.

31. Steindler, Arthur: Kinesiology of the Human Body under Normal and Pathological Conditions. Springfield, Ill., Charles C Thomas, 1955.

32. Truslow, W.: Body Poise. Baltimore, Williams & Wilkins Co., 1943.

33. Wells, Katharine F., and Dillon, Evelyn K.: The Sit and Reach—A Test of Back and Leg Flexibility. Research Quart., 23:115–118, March, 1952.

chapter 11

evaluation
of social
development

We socialize our pupils or contribute to their social learnings when they learn the ways of the group, become functioning members of it, act according to its standards, accept its rules, and in turn become accepted by the group. We socialize youth by helping them acquire social experiences, social habits, and social relationships. Our interest is in the development of the social phases of personality, attitudes, and values by means of games, sports and related activities.[6]
Charles C. Cowell

Social development implies the degree of ability that a youngster has in getting along with others. Such traits as sportsmanship, attitudes, and appreciations are a part of the child's total personality and character, and they contribute to his social effectiveness; ". . . personality is the most inclusive frame of reference in which an individual can be judged. It includes the sum of all his characteristics and his behavior—his intelligence, knowledge, attitudes, interests, and his responses to and interaction with his environment." Personality deals with the total adjustment of an individual to his environment. Good adjustment manifests itself in a happy, healthy outlook on life. The well-adjusted individual gets along with others and has an inner feeling of well-being, contentment, and satisfaction.

Abundant evidence verifies the vital role that physical education plays in aiding children to develop socially. Prominent educators recognize the inherent potential yet to be realized fully by our profession in this important area. For example, at a research conference in California, a group of 1000 educators, in reply to a questionnaire presented by E. L. Thorndike, gave to the games in the physical education program the largest number of first rankings as the school activity having the greatest influence on character. Consequently, you and I as physical educators must be cognizant of the part that physical education plays in developing an individual socially. To be truly effective in structuring our programs so that such an important objective as social efficiency is realized, we must study and then use the evaluative measures that apply.

Counseling responsibilities of the physical educator. Physical educators, because of their excellent relationship with pupils, frequently are involved with counseling responsibilities. Recognizing this as an important aspect of the physical educator's work, Jaeger and Slocum prepared a study to determine: (1) what general problems the pupils brought to the physical educator for help in solving, ranked by frequency of occurrence; (2) what specific problems were encountered within these areas; (3) what the frequency of occurrence of these specific problems was; and (4) to what extent the physical education teacher participated in more formal guidance services.[7]

Sampling a total of 691 men and women teaching physical education, either as a major or minor field in the secondary schools of Minnesota, these investigators concluded:

1. Students do come to their physical education instructor with a great variety of personal problems.

2. Problems involving health and physical development; personal, social, and emotional development; and social and recreational life constitute the most important areas of concern.

3. The size of school and the grade level taught appear to be of minor importance in determining the rank of the problem areas.

4. A large percentage of physical education teachers are called upon to confer with classroom teachers, serve as participants in individual case conferences, serve as members of special committees, and carry advisory functions. About one-third to one-half of the physical education teachers carry some responsibility with regard to homeroom and class advising. A small few assume responsibility for some part of the psychological testing program.

As a result of this study, the authors, among other recommendations, suggest that professional students of physical education should clearly understand their function in helping boys and girls with their problems. Perhaps the most important function is to recognize when the teacher of physical education needs the service of the guidance specialist in the school, and when and how to direct pupils in need of expert counseling.

Contribution of physical education to social adjustment. One might say that the activity program in physical education is actually a laboratory situation in which pupils may learn and practice desirable standards of conduct. For example, in the coeducational dancing program the pupils are not only taught the skills of dancing, but the boys are instructed how to ask a young lady for a dance, to escort her back to her chair, and to thank the young lady for the dance. Such social graces are valuable outcomes of the dancing unit.

The sports program offers an excellent opportunity for the instructor to teach basic principles of democracy. It is here that rules of the game must be followed; each individual is taught to recognize the need for cooperative effort if the team is to be successful; and even though the competition is keen and the game close, the coach exemplifies desirable modes of conduct in his dealings with the officials and opposing team. Because of the strong influence that the coach has over his team, such actions become tangible evidence for the team as well as spectators to observe and practice.

The influence of such fine attributes was recently affirmed in a letter sent from Captain George Herring of the United States Marines to Coach Odus Mitchell at a homecoming game upon the coach's recent retirement from North Texas State University. Writing from the battlefield, where he was wounded before the letter was finished, the former co-captain wrote:

> If it were any way possible, I would attend the ball game, just to let you know how much I think of you and what contributed to making me become a man. . . . We've been in the field for 45 days and casualties have been pretty bad. In this constant rain and terrible terrain, leadership is sometimes critical. . . . My company's spirits always remain high and [we have been able to] attain our mission of destroying the enemy. I was taught the traits of leadership by the finest man and leader of men that I have ever known, you, Coach Mitchell. . . . I only wish I could express to you what an honor it was and still is to have been one of your boys. . . . I only hope that I can leave a small fraction of your type [of] influence [with] my men . . . [to] help them all their lives.

A number of scientific studies have been conducted to show the value of the physical education program as it contributes to the all-around social development of the child. As an illustration, Jones, in a longitudinal study of growth in adolescence, arrived at some very interesting conclusions relative to the social efficiency of boys related to their status on a strength test. (The strength test consisted of right and left grip strength, plus push and pull strength, which was measured by means of a special attachment to the grip manuometer.) Jones measured eighty-nine boys and eighty-seven girls from the time they were eleven years old until they reached the age of seventeen and one-half years.[9] Concerning the boys, he concluded that:

1. Boys scoring in the top 10 per cent on the strength test exhibited

a nice-looking physique; matured earlier; were high in social prestige; and possessed an apparently satisfactory level of social adjustment.

2. Boys scoring in the lower 10 per cent on the strength test appeared to have an asthenic physique; matured later; had a poor health record; encountered social difficulties; suffered lack of status within the group; and experienced some feelings of inferiority was well as personal maladjustments in other areas.

In another study, Kuhlen and Lee set up an experiment in which they studied social acceptance and personality characteristics of 700 sixth, ninth, and twelfth grade boys and girls.[11] These investigators found that, among boys in the adolescent period, social acceptance within a group was significantly related to the ability to perform in sports. Similar conclusions were reported by Tryon, who found that the seventh grade boy poor in skills ability and who rejects participation in organized sports is shunned and ridiculed by the group. Furthermore, Tryon found that outstanding ability in athletics for the twelfth grade boy is a valuable prestige factor for the boy in gaining acceptance to the group.[20] Interestingly enough this was found to be true even though the boy had few other desirable social assets.

Skubic, in a questionnaire study that included an analysis of attitudes of parents and players toward "little league" and "middle league" competitive baseball, found that boys chosen on teams show greater achievement in school subjects, possess greater motor ability, and are better adjusted socially and emotionally than boys who are not members of teams.[16]

Other studies also report that, even as low as the third grade, youngsters high in motor proficiency appear to be more socially accepted than do their contemporaries. However, Tryon points out that skills ability for girls, although of some importance in gaining acceptance to a group, is not valued as highly as it is by boys judging their peers.[20]

We must conclude from a host of studies so well summarized by Cowell[6] that physical education without question contributes significantly to the social development of youth.

We find evidence of our profession's contribution not only to healthy children, but also to those who are mentally retarded or disturbed by psychological problems. Play apparently offers an opportunity to rid oneself of factors contributing to antisocial behavior. It is here that the physical educator must be aware of structuring his activities to permit the satisfaction of social and emotional needs. Our tremendous challenge lies in developing instruments for more objective evaluation, to result in better programing and hence more effective teaching of our pupils.

There is little doubt as to the tremendous contributions that the physical educator can make to a child's growth and development through a good program, as evidenced by the findings reported above. To do a complete job of recognizing the social factors and planning for desirable social outcomes in the program, the teacher obviously must measure. As a result of the numerous variables and complex factors comprising the area of social efficiency, it is a most difficult objective to measure and evaluate. Although the psychologist has at his command many tests of personality and character, they become for the most part useless in the hands of the physical educator, because he does not have the background and training to interpret the test results. However, there are certain instruments available from which a selection can be made to help the instructor to gain insight into individual and group behavior patterns, and to become more cognizant of the need for *planning* for desirable social outcomes.

Approach to the measurement of an individual's total personality involves two quite general areas of measurement. In one situation, the person responds to questions regarding himself; in the other, a neutral person, or examiner, observes and records the individual's behavior.

Such instruments as personality inventories, tests of attitudes and interests, and projective techniques, which usually result in a score, compose the first type of measurement, referred to as the *self-report approach.*

In the second method, or *observational approach,* the person is observed and his behavioral characteristics recorded. Rating scales, anecdotal records, and more recently sociograms are illustrative of instruments employed in this method.

Our goal in this chapter is to help each reader to better understand the use of rating scales, sociometry, and the anecdotal record. The primary purpose is to increase the awareness of the outstanding contribution that physical education can make to a child's social development, particularly when the lesson is planned with that objective in mind.

Measuring Attitudes

We usually consider an attitude as a mood or a feeling toward a person, group, object, situation, or value. The attitude may manifest itself in a type of behavior corresponding to the feeling or conviction evoked by the stimulus. Certainly emotion is involved. Valid appraisal of the attitude can be made when there is a *persistent* disposition to act either positively or negatively toward the stimulus. You, for example, have established attitudes toward such activities as football, bowling, dancing, basketball, playing dominoes, and horseback riding. You may have a reaction pattern to racial problems, to such individuals as your mother, father, coach, and professor, and yes, to this measurement book and its author—let us hope a positive one of the last especially.

Best[2] has outlined several methods which may be employed to obtain opinions from individuals:

1. Asking directly how the individual feels about a subject; for this method one may use a questionnaire or interview.

2. Asking the individual to check from a list the statements with which he agrees.

3. Asking the person to indicate his degree of agreement or disagreement with a series of statements about a controversial subject.

4. Inferring the subject's attitude from his reaction to projective devices through which he may unconsciously reveal his attitudes. The object is to conceal the true purpose of the data-gathering instrument so that a person cannot guess the "correct" answer. The Rorschach inkblot is a popular projective test which requires the talents of the clinical psychologist or psychiatrist for its administration.

One of two methods is usually employed in constructing the attitude scale: the Thurstone and Chave method or the Likert method. Each results in a similar final product and requires responses to statements about a person, group, object, situation, or value.

THURSTONE-CHAVE (METHOD OF EQUAL-APPEARING INTERVALS)

One collects a number of statements (100–150) concerning the particular attitude toward a subject to be evaluated, such as faculty control of athletics, athletic scholarships, and required physical education classes. These statements should vary in the expected responses from strongly agreeing through neutral to strongly disagreeing. The next step is to submit the statements to a panel of fifty or more judges who, working independently, will sort them into eleven piles. Each judge will arrange the statements from one extreme to the other, the statements in pile 1 representing a favorable attitude while those in pile 11 represent an unfavorable one. Hence, the term *equal-appearing* interval, for it is the object to have the statements so spaced by the judges that a continuum exists from pile 1 (most favorable attitude) through 6, the median value (neutral), to pile 11 (most unfavorable).

Upon completion of the judges' efforts, the number of times a particular statement has appeared in a certain pile is tabulated. For example, one statement may have appeared in pile 1 twenty times, in pile 2 thirty times, and in pile 3 twelve times. To calculate the median rank for each statement proceed in the manner as illustrated on p. 37. For example:

Step Intervals	Frequency (f)	Cumulative frequency (cf)
2.5 — 3.4	12	62
1.5 — 2.4	30	50
.5 — 1.4	20	20

$$\frac{\begin{array}{c} 62 \\ .50 \end{array}}{31.0}$$

$$1.5 + \left(\frac{11}{30} \times 1 \right) = 1.87$$

This statement would be given a score value of 1.87 based upon its median position.

In situations in which there has been poor agreement among judges, that is, when a statement has occurred in nearly all piles, that statement is discarded as being ambiguous.

Of the final chosen statements, which will be somewhat fewer than the original number, perhaps twenty to forty hopefully represent the varying intensities of an attitude toward the subject. The list of statements is now presented to the subjects, who are to check *only* those statements with which they *agree*. The score is the median value of the statements checked. When the test is administered, the subject quite naturally remains uninformed as to the median score of each statement. A low score would be associated with agreement and a high score with lack of agreement.

LIKERT METHOD

Shortly after Thurstone published his method for constructing an attitude scale, Likert came forth with a similar method which does not require judges. Correlations between the two methods range from .77 to .92.

The first step is to collect a number of statements that describe either a favorable or an unfavorable attitude toward a particular subject. For each statement there is a given number of possible responses. The individual taking the test must react to *every* statement (unlike the Thurstone instrument, in which the person checks only the statements with which he strongly aggrees).

To measure attitudes toward the physical education program, you might expect a sample of statements as follows:

SA   Strongly agree
A   Agree
U   Undecided (neutral)
D   Disagree
SD   Strongly disagree

SA A U D SD   Physical education should be a required course in high school.

SA A U D SD   A person playing on a varsity or intramural team should not be required to take physical education during that time.

SA A U D SD   Band should be allowed as a substitute for physical education.

Scoring for the Likert method involves assigning a 5 for the attitude that is most desirable and a 1 for that which is least desirable. The test score is the total; the higher the final score, the more favorable the attitude.

Validity and reliability. The primary fault of the attitude scale is the problem of validity. For example, what a person checks on the test as his attitude may not be his *true* feeling. Does a politician kiss babies because he likes them? Actually, he may hate babies, but kissing them gets votes. The real relationship between what a person writes as his attitude and his action elicited by the attitude constitutes genuine validity.

Validity of the attitude scale is obtained either by correlating the test results with those from another test or by using the behavior of the individual as the criterion.

Reliability is determined by constructing alternate forms of the test, or by correlating the odd- and even-numbered items and applying the Spearman-Brown prophecy formula (p. 367).

Validity for attitude scales usually ranges between correlation of .50 and .60; reliability ranges from .77 to .90.

Adams Scale for measuring attitude toward physical education.[1] With second-year university psychology and education students as judges, forty most appropriate statements from an initial lot of 150 were chosen. The forty statements were divided into two test forms, Set I and Set II. Validity was determined by correlating the results of the attitude scale with a cumulative self-rating scale (Set I: $r = .61$; Set II: $r = .69$). A split-half reliability coefficient of .71 was obtained for Set I and Set II. When the two sets are combined (forty items), reliability increases to .84.

Either the first twenty items or the last twenty items may be used, or, if greater reliability is desired, both forms may be given at once. Whatever the case, the following preamble should precede the statements:

> This is a questionnaire to measure your attitude toward physical education as a college subject. There are a number of statements about physical education below, each one followed by a pair of brackets to show two headings, "Agree" and "Disagree." You are asked to check one of these brackets to show whether you agree or disagree with the statement. Please consider each statement carefully and in your answer indicate your present feelings about physical education as you know it.

A sample statement then would appear in this form:

	Agree	Disagree
16. Physical education is my favorite subject	( )	( )

The Statements	*Thurstone Weightings (Not for inclusion in a questionnaire)*
Set I	
1. Physical education gets very monotonous.	3.50
2. I only feel like taking physical education classes now and then.	5.95
3. Physical education should be disposed of.	1.58
4. Physical education is particularly limited in its value.	4.50

The Statements — *Thurstone Weightings*

5. I suppose physical education is all right but I don't much care for it. — 5.03
6. Physical education is the most hateful subject of all. — 1.02
7. I do not want to give up physical education. — 8.64
8. On the whole I think physical education is a good thing. — 8.00
9. People who like physical education are nearly always good to know. — 7.71
10. Anyone who likes physical education is silly. — 2.65
11. Physical education has some usefulness. — 6.45
12. Physical education is *the* ideal subject. — 10.66
13. Physical education develops good character. — 8.92
14. (School) College would be better without physical education. — 2.30
15. Physical education has little to offer. — 9.39
16. Physical education is my favorite subject. — 3.93
17. Physical education gives lasting satisfaction. — 9.60
18. Physical education's good and bad points balance out each other. — 5.99
19. Physical education is a pleasant break. — 7.11
20. Physical education seems useless to me. — 3.08

Set II

21. Physical education only serves the interests of a few people. — 3.19
22. Physical education encourages moral improvement. — 8.64
23. There is no subject as good as physical education. — 10.42
24. Sometimes I think physical education is good and sometimes I think it is useless. — 5.92
25. In physical education we learn many things of no use. — 3.50
26. There is little to be said for or against physical education. — 6.0
27. Physical education is quite good. — 7.34
28. It is a pity we have to do physical education. — 4.64
29. Physical education should be a main part of a child's education. — 9.25
30. Physical education is fundamentally unsound. — 2.09
31. I think physical education is very good. — 9.45
32. Physical education is one of the best subjects I have ever taken. — 10.03
33. Physical education has not yet proved itself indispensable in education. — 5.06
34. Physical education is a deplorable waste of time. — 1.62
35. Physical education has something to commend it. — 6.50
36. I don't like physical education. — 2.79
37. I hate physical education more than anything else. — 1.10
38. I think physical education is good. — 8.26
39. I enjoy physical education if I can succeed in performing. — 7.14
40. Physical education is decreasing in value to society. — 4.05

Scoring. Marks are given for only the "Agree" items checked (the "Disagree" items are ignored). The marks to be given vary from statement to statement. They were derived from the initial sorting by the judges and represent, in refined form, the average position of each statement along the favorable-unfavorable continuum, which is interpreted numerically as ranging from 1 to 11. The marks can be found in the right-hand column alongside the complete list of statements. Thus, if

"Agree" is checked in item number 20, the mark awarded is 3.08. The final score is the sum of all the scores divided by the number of "Agree" items checked (i.e., the average of the item scores). Statement marks should never be printed on the questionnaire itself. A cardboard straight-edge with the appropriate numbers printed and spaced to correspond with the brackets in the questionnaire helps with scoring.

It is optional whether these items are used as a Thurstone and Chave type of scale or as a Likert type of scale. The decision would seem to depend on procedural factors. It is probably a little easier to mark the Thurstone and Chave scale, but it is harder to tally the marks.

Likert Method for Adams Scale. As a Likert type of test, all the items except numbers 3, 10, 11, 18, 24, 26, 33, and 39 should be used. The following preamble is necessary:

> This is a questionnaire to measure your attitude toward physical education as a college subject. There are a number of statements about physical education below, each one followed by a set of "boxes" numbered as follows:

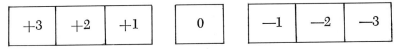

> You are asked to put a mark in *one* of the boxes to show how strongly you agree or disagree with the statement. The numbers in the boxes are there to guide you. This is what they stand for:

> +3 = Very strongly agree   −1 = Disagree
> +2 = Strongly agree   −2 = Strongly disagree
> +1 = Agree   −3 = Very strongly disagree
> 0 = Neither agree nor disagree

> Please consider each statement carefully and in your answer indicate your present feelings about physical education as you know it.

A sample statement then would appear in this form:

16. Physical education is my favorite subject

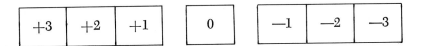

Scoring for this test is rather different. The marks, which range from 6 to 0 for each statement, are weighted so that a response indicating a favorable attitude toward physical education scores higher than one indicating an unfavorable attitude—the more favorable the attitude, the higher the mark. Thus, when the statement is a positive one (numbers 7, 8, 9, 12, 13, 16, 17, 19, 22, 23, 27, 29, 31, 32, 35, and 38), scoring is as follows:

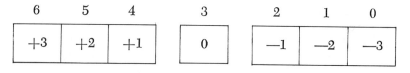

6	5	4	3	2	1	0
+3	+2	+1	0	−1	−2	−3

When the statement is a negative one (numbers 1, 2, 4, 5, 6, 14, 15, 20, 21, 25, 28, 30, 34, 36, 37, and 40), the whole scoring procedure is reversed:

0	1	2	3	4	5	6
+3	+2	+1	0	−1	−2	−3

Again, a scoring key can greatly facilitate marking. A piece of thin cardboard with cut out "windows" bearing the appropriate scores above them is most useful.

Rating Scales

Rating scales that are used in the evaluation of character and personality contain certain descriptive criteria of behavior traits. The rater scores the pupil by assigning a rank usually from 0 to 5, depending upon the frequency with which the pupil exhibits the characteristic of the particular criterion being evaluated. For example, if one were to rate a child on dependability, a score of 5 might be recorded if the youngster were exceptionally dependable; a score of 3 if he were of average dependability; and a 0 for never being dependable.

McCloy Scale. McCloy was responsible for first suggesting a method by which social efficiency of the child might be evaluated in physical education.[12] He listed nine behavior traits: leadership, active qualities, attitudes, self-control, cooperation, sportsmanship, ethics, efficiency, and sociability. Each of these nine behavior traits is further subdivided into more specific behavior actions, which the instructor rates on a scale from 1 to 5, the score of 5 representing exceptionally good behavior. McCloy does not report reliability for this particular scale.

Blanchard Rating Scale. Blanchard, modifying McCloy's work developed a scale to rate twenty-four trait actions.[3] This scale, which appears in Figure 105, was developed for the purpose of measuring character and personality. Reliability of the scale was determined by correlating the teacher and student scores, resulting in an average r of .71. Average validity was reported as the intercorrelation of one trait action with the remaining items in the category of trait actions. The resulting r was .93.

Personal Information:	No Opportunity to Observe	Frequency of Observation					Score
		Never	Seldom	Fairly Often	Frequently	Extremely Often	
Leadership							
1. He is popular with classmates	..	1	2	3	4	5	..
2. He seeks responsibility in the classroom	..	1	2	3	4	5	..
3. He shows intellectual leadership in the classroom	..	1	2	3	4	5	..
Positive Active Qualities							
4. He quits on tasks requiring perseverance	..	5	4	3	2	1	..
5. He exhibits aggressiveness in his relationship with others	..	1	2	3	4	5	..
6. He shows initiative in assuming responsibility in unfamiliar situations	..	1	2	3	4	5	..
7. He is alert to new opportunities	..	1	2	3	4	5	..
Positive Mental Qualities							
8. He shows keenness of mind	..	1	2	3	4	5	..
9. He volunteers ideas	..	1	2	3	4	5	..
Self-Control							
10. He grumbles over decisions of classmates	..	5	4	3	2	1	..
11. He takes a justified criticism by teacher or classmate without showing anger or pouting	..	1	2	3	4	5	..
Cooperation							
12. He is loyal to his group	..	1	2	3	4	5	..
13. He discharges his group responsibilities well	..	1	2	3	4	5	..
14. He is cooperative in his attitude toward the teacher	..	1	2	3	4	5	..
Social Action Standards							
15. He makes loud-mouthed criticisms and comments	..	5	4	3	2	1	..
16. He respects the rights of others	..	1	2	3	4	5	..
Ethical Social Qualities							
17. He cheats	..	5	4	3	2	1	..
18. He is truthful	..	1	2	3	4	5	..
Qualities of Efficiency							
19. He seems satisfied to "get by" with tasks assigned	..	5	4	3	2	1	..
20. He is dependable and trustworthy	..	1	2	3	4	5	..
21. He has good study habits	..	1	2	3	4	5	..
Sociability							
22. He is liked by others	..	1	2	3	4	5	..
23. He makes a friendly approach to others in the group	..	1	2	3	4	5	..
24. He is friendly	..	1	2	3	4	5	..

Figure 105. Blanchard behavior rating scale. (Blanchard, B. E.: A Behavior Frequency Rating Scale for the Measurement of Character and Personality in Physical Education Classroom Situations. Research Quart., 7:56, 1936.)

In using a rating scale, one of the most common difficulties is the presence of the "halo" effect when evaluating character. The so-called "teacher's pet" is apt to be given a higher rating on some traits than he actually deserves. Another common error is referred to as the "generosity error." The rater in this instance is inclined to range each person average or above. This error is multiplied when the agency requesting the rating is only remotely familiar to the rater, such as might occur in the case of the personnel office of some industry. It is suggested that the pupil rate himself on the scale and then a comparison between the instructor's and pupil's ratings be made during a conference with the child. In this way the rating scale becomes a means for bringing attention to desirable habits of social conduct. Then, too, in visiting with the child the instructor may point out instances of application of these desirable behavior traits to situations in everyday living.

Rating scales suffer from lack of validity and reliability. It is impossible to obtain an accurate test of validity because of the nature of the rating scale. Reliability between raters is in the .50 to .60 range, which is quite low. Regardless of the many pitfalls of rating scales they will continue to be used when judgments of one's fellow men are necessary.

To increase the reliability and validity of the rating scale, when possible, employ multiple ratings by several people and rate the person on a comparative basis with the total group. In forming a basis for judgment, try to use as a criterion the overt behavior that appears to be persistent over a period of time, rather than an action that occurs on one occasion.

Sociometric Evaluation

Sociometry is relatively new. Moreno[13] and Jennings[8] pioneered in the field, and their techniques have been adapted for use in industry, business, education, and recreation. This new method of evaluation, which shows great promise for the physical education instructor, can facilitate better understanding and planning for social outcomes in the program.

Moreno defines the sociometric test as an instrument to measure the amount of organization shown by social groups.[13] Kozman defines sociometry as a scientific method of studying groups and examining the interrelationships between the individuals making up these groups.[10] Todd defines sociometry as a quantitative method of studying the organization of groups, affording means of presenting simply and graphically the entire structure of relations existing at a given time among members of a given group.[18] She further claims that the retests permit the teacher to note changes in individual and group status, thus presenting objective evidence of behavior changes, which may be concomitants of guidance and class management. This, then, offers the instructor a comparatively simple technique that may reveal valuable clues basic to effective guidance, efficient group organization, and evaluation.

Kozman indicates that the sociometric test requires an individual to choose his associates from any group of which he is or might become a member.[10] The choices should be based upon specific criteria, such as people with whom he would like to live, study, work, or play. It is emphasized that the question should be selected that relates to an activity that is actually to be undertaken, so that the pupils may gain a respect for the particular process.

For example, the teacher may ask the class to make three preferences for other pupils with whom they would like to be squad-mates. The teacher would also ask the pupils to indicate if there is anyone with whom they would prefer not to participate as a squad-mate. Choices should be kept confidential, and the pupils should be instructed to write the first and last name of each person they select.

Todd suggests two types of sociometric tests that have been found especially useful in physical education classes—the acquaintance volume test and the functional choice test.[18]

Acquaintance volume test. This type of test measures how well pupils become acquainted over a given period of class participation. At the first class meeting each member is asked to write the first and last names of those he knows in the group. Upon completion of the class unit or semester, the test is repeated, and, by simple arithmetical differences, one computes the number of new names that each pupil has added to his list.

Functional choice test. This test is a method of determining who desires to be with whom. Each member of the class is presented with the opportunity of saying whom he or she would like to join in performing group activities. Also, a pupil is permitted to make known whom he would reject.

Reliability and validity of sociometric data. When one is confronted with establishing reliability of sociometric data, some difficulties arise. In measuring such qualities as personal and group relationships, the situation is constantly changing. The relative positions of pupils within a social group fluctuate. This, of course, is to be expected, particularly when some socializing activities are introduced to the group.

In testing reliability of individual preferences, studies have shown the first-level choices are at least twice as stable as secondary and tertiary choices. Also, when determining the reliability of relative group status, based upon total choices received, a greater constancy is noted. As an example, Bonney and Fessenden, in surveying twenty studies relative to reliability, found that the median rank order coefficient was .90 when the time interval of the retests was one week or less apart.[4] Furthermore, it was observed that, when the retest was taken from two to nine weeks later, the median coefficient was .76. In studies where the retest was given three months to a year later, the median rank order coefficient was .65. The decrease in correlations (.90—.76—.65) indicates that an individual's choice status changes as the time interval between test and retest is increased. As Bonney and Fessenden point out, this is to be expected as a result of the dynamic characteriestics of a group.[4]

The validity of sociometric data has been established by two methods. Some investigators feel that if the pupils give honest and sincere responses to the question, then these answers have "face validity"; that is to say, the child is the true and only judge of his feelings toward another classmate. Thus, when one asks, "With whom would you like to go on a picnic?", the child's choice is the pure criterion.

The second method of testing validity is to determine the relationships that exist between sociometric scores and scores on other psychological tests that purport to measure social adjustment.

Bonney and Fessenden report that the research findings derived from self-reporting inventories, teacher ratings of pupils' personal and social behavior, pupils' ratings of each other, projective devices, observa-

Sociometric Test—Tally Sheet					
No. Boys 9 No. Girls 9 Class/Grade Social Dance B9					
School X Junior High					
City Central City					
Date 5/20/50					
Test question: With whom would you most like to work on a committee?					
No. choices requested 3 ; total no. possible 54 ; no. made 48					
No. rejections requested 3 ; total no. possible 54 ; no. made 11					
Name	*Attendance*	*No. Choices Received*		*No. Rejections Received*	
1. Betty Adams		11	2		0
2. Bob Bigelow		11	2	11	2
3. Sally Brown		↺↺↺↺	5	1	1
4. Jean Call		1	1		0
5. George Day		↺↺↺↺	5		0
6. Charles Dean			0		0
7. Jane Doe			0	11	2
8. Frances Dunn	Absent	111	3		0
9. Alice Fine		↺↺↺↺ 11	7		0
10. Mary Graham		111	3		0
11. Jim Kettle		111	3		0
12. Joan Little		111	3		0
13. Nancy Martin			0	11	2
14. Ronald Nester	Absent	11	2		0
15. Bill Page		11	2	1	1
16. Bill Schoop		1111	4	11	2
17. Marvin White		↺↺↺↺ 1	6		0
18. Carl Willets			0	1	1
Total			48		11

Figure 106. Sociometric test tally sheet. (Kozman, Hilda C. (ed.): Group Processes in Physical Education. New York. Harper & Brothers, 1951, p. 200.)

tional records, and the sociometric tests are similar in two respects: (1) when total groups are studied, the relationship between these various methods of personality assessment and sociometric scores are not marked; but (2) when those who are high in the upper quartile relative choice status are compared with those who are low, the findings are quite consistent in showing most frequently chosen individuals to be superior to the infrequently chosen youngster in some psychologically or socially approved types of behavior adjustments or in both.[4]

In applying sociometry to the senior high school physical education program, Todd[17] found sociometrically selected squads more enjoyable and efficient than those grouped by any other method. In this study, sociometry was being used primarily to study the democratic method of class management in physical education. The author found that the increased acquaintance during the semester resulted in a decrease in the number of unpopular and unwanted girls.

Thus one might conclude that the reliability and validity of sociometric tests are quite satisfactory in terms of what they attempt to measure. That is, children who are most frequently selected for the most part exhibit many more socially desirable assets than do those seldom chosen.

Sociometric Tabulation Form

Chosen → / Chooser ↓	1. Betty Adams	2. Bob Bigelow	3. Sally Brown	4. Jean Call	5. George Day	6. Charles Dean	7. Jane Doe	8. Frances Dunn	9. Alice Fine	10. Mary Graham	11. Jim Kettle	12. Joan Little	13. Nancy Martin	14. Ronald Nester	15. Bill Page	16. Bill Schoop	17. Marvin White	18. Carl Willets
1. Betty Adams			1		3				2									
2. Bob Bigelow	3		2													1		
3. Sally Brown	1							3				2						
4. Jean Call					1										3		2	
5. George Day			3	1													2	
6. Charles Dean					2				1	3								
7. Jane Doe		2											3	1				
8. Frances Dunn																		
9. Alice Fine			3								1						2	
10. Mary Graham			2		1											3		
11. Jim Kettle									2			3					1	
12. Joan Little									2								3	1
13. Nancy Martin											2	3				1		
14. Ronald Nester																		
15. Bill Page					2			3								1		
16. Bill Schoop		1						3	2									
17. Marvin White								3	1		2							
18. Carl Willets											3			1		2		
No. of 1st Choices	1	1	1	1	2				2		2	1			2	2	1	
No. of 2nd Choices		1	2		2				4	1	1	1					4	
No. of 3rd Choices	1		2		1			3	1	2		1		2		2	1	
Total	2	2	5	1	5	0	0	3	7	3	3	3	0	2	2	4	6	0

Figure 107. Sociometric tabulation form. (Jennings, Helen: Sociometry in Group Relations. American Council on Education, 1948, p. 18.)

Recording sociometric data   *Sociometric tally sheet.*   Figure 106 illustrates a tally sheet used to reveal at a glance the status of each child in the group. It also indicates the youngsters most frequently chosen as well as the "fringers" or rejected children. In the sample tally sheet, a limited number of pupils were included, to facilitate understanding.

Tabulation form.   Figure 107 illustrates a form designed to show who made the choices and rejections in addition to the same information which is included on the tally sheet.

Kozman[10] suggests other types of tabulating forms that might be constructed to reveal:

1. Number of choices requested and number made.

2. Number of rejections requested and number made.

3. Number of people chosen, mutually chosen, rejected, and mutually rejected.

4. Number of times boys were chosen; number of times girls were chosen; number of choices between boys and girls; number of choices within and between racial groups; and so forth.

5. Rejections for the same items as those given in item 4.

6. Choices reciprocated and not reciprocated, and variations.

The sociogram.   Figure 108 contains a diagram of a sociogram, which is used to reveal the basic social structure of a group. Todd suggests that this sociometric instrument may be used to identify cliques, pairs, threesomes, and gangs as well as to call attention to the unwanted and wanted child.[18]

In plotting the sociogram the usual procedure is to place the popular pupils in the center of the diagram and the lonely or rejected children near the fringes; lines are then drawn of attraction, and of reciprocated and unreciprocated choices between them. Kozman regards the sociogram as the most inclusive of the test tabulation methods and, as such, an important sociometric instrument.[10]

Interpretation of the sociogram may be simplified by selecting one name and analyzing all the lines leading to and from it. Thus the relationships within the group may be studied.

Once the sociometric test results have been analyzed, the instructor can then group or regroup the pupils in accordance with the test data. In so doing, Jennings[8] suggests the following considerations:

1. Give each unchosen or seldom chosen individual his first choice. These individuals have the greatest need for security. Highly chosen individuals are usually secure and can aid others.

2. If there is a pair relationship, give each individual his highest reciprocal choice.

3. If the individual only receives choices from persons he has not chosen, give him his first choice.

4. Be sure that no individual is put with persons who have rejected him.

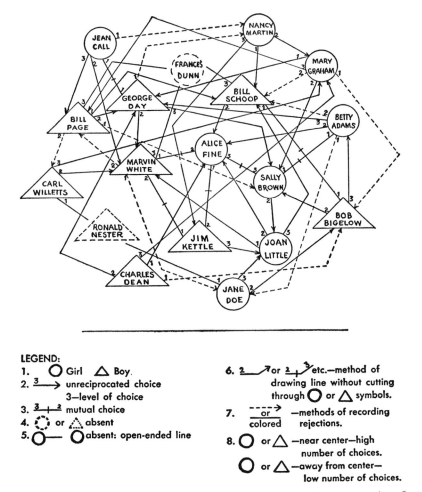

LEGEND:

1. ◯ Girl △ Boy.
2. 3——→ unreciprocated choice
    3—level of choice
3. 3—+—2 mutual choice
4. ◌ or ⬸ absent
5. ◯— ◯ absent: open-ended line

6. 2——↗ or 2—↗ etc.—method of
    drawing line without cutting
    through ◯ or △ symbols.
7. ---→ or —methods of recording
    colored   rejections.
8. ◯ or △ —near center—high
    number of choices.
    ◯ or △ —away from center—
    low number of choices.

Figure 108. Sociogram. (Jennings, Helen: Sociometry in Group Relations. American Council on Education, 1948.)

5. Be sure to give each individual one of his choices.

Sociometric testing appears to be a valuable aid for the physical educator in better understanding group structure and the behavior of pupil members comprising the group.

The following is a study that illustrates the application of techniques of sociometry in grouping pupils in the fifth and sixth grades for physical education activities. In grouping, the first consideration was given to pupils with extremely low scores, and those rated extremely high. The least popular children were placed in groups in which there were at least two or three popular children who accepted them and none who completely rejected them.

These play groups, for the most part, remained intact for the rest of the year. As a result, it was observed that a great improvement occurred in team spirit and organization over results noted in previous years. Bickering was reduced to a minimum. Nearly everyone participated in the activities much more enthusiastically and seemed happier than before. Much of the success of the grouping seemed attributable to the excellent group leaders discovered through the use of the sociometric test. The leaders were selected on the basis of both their quantitative and qualitative test scores.

On retesting the classes at the end of the school year, it was found that the degree of group socialization rose significantly in three out of four classes. These same three groups also improved considerably in terms of mutual attachment. There was a corresponding decrease in negative feelings. Correlations were computed on the test-retest data, and found to range from .228 to .736. Most of the change in relative status occurred among those in the middle range of scores. The very high and low scores remained about the same.

The authors feel that sociometric grouping is definitely an effective method of group organization and control in physical education classes.[5] It makes teachers more conscious of the seriously maladjusted.

The Anecdotal Record

The anecdotal record is a means for objectively recording actual behavior incidents that occur in the gym, on the play fields, or in the classroom. The information contained in such a written report may contribute much toward gaining insight as to peculiarities of conduct exhibited by certain pupils.

Obviously the value of the anecdotal record increases with the number of observations that have been recorded. In this way, certain modes of conduct may reveal patterns of behavior that will give the counselor greater understanding of the child.

Traxler, in discussing the problems associated with use of the anecdotal record, suggests that most teachers are not trained in observation of behavior.[19] To substantiate this point, Shaffer reports a study in which Wikman (1928) had a group of 511 elementary school teachers rank a list of fifty school behavior problems in order of their seriousness.[15] Thirty clinical psychologists also rated these conduct disorders as to seriousness from the point of view of mental hygiene. The teachers considered sex problems and aggressive actions directed against persons and property as most undesirable, while they rated a number of signs of seclusiveness and withdrawal as relatively inconsequential. The psychologists, in startling contrast, deemed the symptoms of unsocial behavior (withdrawing modes of defense) as more insidious than aggressive types because they are likely to escape detection, are more difficult to overcome in treatment, and because they more frequently lead to serious phases of mental disorder.

Also included as a difficulty in use of the anecdotal record is the fact that teachers do not have time to make the observations and record them. Then, too, such measures of evaluation must be expertly summarized and the information applied through careful follow-up procedures in order to derive benefits from the anecdotal record.

Because the physical education program provides a variety of social situations, the anecdotal record can be, however, a very useful evaluative instrument when properly used. Following are several characteristics of a good anecdotal record:

1. The anecdote should be recorded as soon as possible after the incident. Delay in so doing may lead to inaccuracies as well as the forgetting of pertinent facts. The child should be unsuspecting of the record.

2. An accurate, concise statement about the child's behavior with a parenthetical note of the teacher's interpretation should be made.

3. In order to obtain a valid "behavior log," anecdotes should be recorded continually and over a period of time. Certainly, more frequent recordings result in a better understanding of the child. It has been suggested that one record per child each week is ideal.

4. The event should be recorded on a card that can be filed; then at least twice a year a summary of the anecdotes should be made. The behavioral record should follow the child from grade to grade.

Following is an example of the anecdoted record:

Grade 9

3/6/66 Today we began our unit in gymnastics. Bill Smith, very much overweight, was chided by the class because of his failure to chin himself once. Shortly after this episode, Bill asked to be excused as he was sick to his stomach. (Bill not only has a problem with obesity, but he also appears to be very insecure when attempting to perform before a group.)

3/15/66 For the second time in a row Bill has brought a note requesting to be excused from physical education. During conversation Bill admitted he became embarrassed because of his frequent failures to perform successfully before the class. Bill has volunteered to join our adaptive class. (In addition to our working on basic strength and motor skills, Bill's eating habits will require much attention.)

Summary and Conclusions

Rating scales, sociometry, and anecdotal records have been discussed in this chapter as instruments for appraising social development.

The Thurstone and Likert methods of constructing attitude scales are the most commonly employed. The primary problem in using attitude scales is validity. The Adams scale for measuring attitude toward physical education is contained in this chapter and may be used with either high school or college students.

Perhaps one of the most recent and encouraging advances in techniques of evaluation in the area of social efficiency is the use of sociometry. This type of evaluation appears to be extremely well adapted for use in physical education because of the numerous group activities of which the program is composed. In identifying the overly aggressive, the rejected, and the leaders in a group, the instructor is made more aware of group structure and interaction, and hence is better equipped to organize groups effectively and to plan individual programs for those children in need of recognition or a feeling of belonging to the group.

This chapter could hardly be complete without the fine summary paragraph from Gladys Scott's article, "The Contributions of Physical Activity to Psychological Development."[14]

> There is perhaps no area of our professional background that offers more challenge to us than psychological development. The challenge is multiple. We need a better background in general psychology, personality development, social psychology, and cultural anthropology. We need to develop research competencies in these areas and to pursue our understandings of prophylactic and therapeutic contributions of experiences in motor skills. As teachers and administrators, we must be ready to modify our practice in line with new evidence.

BIBLIOGRAPHY

1. Adams, R. S.: Two Scales for Measuring Attitude Toward Physical Education. Research Quart., March, 1963, p. 91.
2. Best, John W.: Research and Education. Englewood Cliffs, New Jersey, Prentice-Hall, Inc., 1959, p. 156.
3. Blanchard, B. E.: A Behavior Frequency Rating Scale for the Measurement of Character and Personality in Physical Education Classroom Situations. Research Quart., Vol. 7, No. 2, May, 1936.
4. Bonney, Merl E., and Fessenden, Seth A.: Manual Bonney-Fessenden Sociograph. California Test Bureau, Los Angeles, California, 1955.
5. Bonney, Warren C., and Burleson, Reba M.: Socializing Techniques. J. A. A. Health, Phys. Educ. & Recreation, March, 1954.
6. Cowell, Charles C.: The Contributions of Physical Activity to Psychological Development. Research Quart., 31:2, 286, Pt. II, March, 1960.
7. Jaeger, Eloise M., and Slocum, Helen M.: Physical Education Teachers Contributions to Guidance in Minnesota Secondary Schools. Research Quart., Vol. 27, No. 1, March, 1956.
8. Jennings, Helen: Sociometry in Group Relations. American Council on Education, 1948.
9. Jones, Harold E.: Motor Performance and Growth. Berkeley, Calif., University of California Press, 1949.

10. Kozman, Hilda C. (ed.): Group Processes in Physical Education. New York, Harper & Brothers, 1951.
11. Kuhlen, Raymond G., and Lee, Beatrice J.:Personality Characteristics and Social Acceptability in Adolescence. J. Educ. Psychol., Vol. 34, No. 6, September, 1943.
12. McCloy, C. H.: Character Building through Physical Education. Research Quart., Vol. 1, No. 3, October, 1930.
13. Moreno, J. L.: Who Shall Survive? A New Approach to the Problem of Human Relationships. Washington, Nervous and Mental Disease Publishing Company, 1934.
14. Scott, Gladys: The Contributions of Physical Activity to Psychological Development. Research Quart., 31:2, 317, Pt. II, May, 1960.
15. Shaffer, L. F.: The Psychology of Adjustment. Boston, Houghton Mifflin Co., 1936.
16. Skubic, Elvera: Studies of Little League and Middle League Baseball. Research Quart., Vol. 27, No. 1, March, 1956.
17. Todd, Frances E.: Democratic Methodology in Physical Education. Doctoral dissertation, Stanford University, 1951.
18. Todd, Frances: Sociometry in Physical Education. J. A. A. Health, Phys. Educ. & Recreation, Vol. 24, May, 1953.
19. Traxler, Arthur E.: The Use of Tests and Rating Devices in the Appraisal of Personality. New York, Educational Records Bureau, 1938.
20. Tryon, Caroline C.: Evaluations of Personality by Adolescents. Society for Research in Child Development, Vol. 4, 1939.

chapter 12

sports
knowledge tests

Evaluation in physical education cannot be complete without the use of knowledge tests. For, as we have stressed throughout, evaluation and measurement serve as a means of determining how successful we as teachers have been in meeting our obectives. Insight as to the pupil's comprehension of the subject matter in sports and health knowledge can be secured only through the use of written tests. The results offer the teacher an opportunity to appraise status and progress of the group or the individual, to mark, and to indicate possible instructional weaknesses in terms of the mental accomplishments.

Knowledge tests may be classified in two types, standardized and teacher-made. Standardized tests are those that have been scientifically constructed and possess an accompanying set of norms. These tests meet the criteria of scientific authenticity, administrative feasibility, and educational application as discussed in Chapter 3. The teacher-made test is the type that you might make out to administer to one of your classes.

Probably the very first sports knowledge test to be published appeared in 1929, and to this day not one commercial educational agency has published a standardized test in physical education. It is not an easy matter to construct a good written test, and perhaps this is one reason why so few appear in the literature. For this very argument, it might be well for us as prospective teachers to gain an understanding of the fundamental principles and procedures involved in constructing written tests. As long as we are in the teaching field, writing and administering knowledge tests will be, or should be, as certain as death and taxes, for they are vitally necessary and extremely complementary to good instruction.

It is definitely beyond the scope of this text to go into a detailed discussion of the manner in which knowledge tests are developed. At the same time one must understand, in a general way, the basic approach that the researcher follows when constructing standardized tests. By so doing a greater comprehension of the test in terms of its applicability, as well as an appreciation for the efforts of the scientist, will be gained. On this basis then, we will first outline principles for making out an examination; next will follow a brief discussion of some statistical approaches used in determining validity and reliability of standardized tests. This will be concluded by presenting an example of how a tennis knowledge examination was actually constructed. The remaining pages of the chapter will be devoted to a brief description of a number of standardized sports and health knowledge tests.

Principles of Writing Knowledge Tests

Writing test items is probably an art as much as it is a science. From your experience in taking examinations you no doubt will agree with this statement. Further evidence of this fact is quite apparent when, on the day following a written test, the instructor goes over his examination with you and begins to answer your questions pertaining to the various test items. Such questions may come from the examinees as, "What did you mean by this word?"; or the examinee may make such statements as, "I thought that the answer was false because of such and such." Perhaps all bedlam breaks loose and the instructor is forced to make concessions because more than one answer applies to the question, or because poorly worded items have created misunderstanding among a number of the pupils. The validity of the examination must be seriously questioned when numerous problems pertaining to the test items arise.

To overcome these obstacles as much as possible in constructing a good examination, the following are a few of the more important principles of writing test questions. They should be adhered to rather closely for good results.

1. The important aspects of the subject matter should be covered in the same relative proportion that they were emphasized in the instructional unit. If 50 per cent of the learning situation dealt with techniques and mechanics, then 50 per cent of the examination should test this area of knowledge.

2. Directions should be explicit and succinct.

3. Ambiguity should be avoided.

4. A large number of items should be included (100 for reliability).

5. The instructor should beware of stereotyped determiners such as "all," "never," "nothing," "always," and "no." These words, when included in the true-false type of examination, are most frequently asso-

ciated with false statements, therefore permitting the examinee to guess the correct answer.

6. Statements should be brief; if possible, not more than twenty-five words should be used.

7. The distribution of scores for the examination should approximate the normal curve.

8. Trivial items should not be included.

There are several kinds of objective test items that are used most frequently in constructing teacher-made examinations. Among them are the recall type and the recognition type of questions. The recall type includes both the simple recall and the completion questions. The recognition type includes matching, multiple-choice, and alternative-response items.

Recall questions. These test items limit the answer to one word or phrase; the questions are economical of space, rather easy to construct, and allow a wide sampling of subject matter. Among the disadvantages are the fact that a number of pupils may give different answers than the one expected, which sometimes makes the item difficult to score, and that it is often hard to construct statements that are demanding of thought and application of knowledge on the student's part. When the completion question is employed, caution must be exercised in wording it, with two particular points in mind. Pupils should be discouraged from memorizing statements in the textbook. (Do not lift a statement from a rule book and merely delete a word or phrase and think it is a good recall question.) The question should also be written without giving clues as to its answer.

Scoring the completion items may prove cumbersome, particularly when a paragraph containing several blanks is employed as a question. To facilitate this procedure, the blank lines, which should be of uniform length, may be numbered and correspondingly numbered blanks placed vertically on the right-hand margin of the paper opposite to the question. Each blank space should require only one word. Sample questions follow:

a. In what country was golf first played?　　　　　　　a. _____
b. Who is the national president of the American Association for Health, Physical Education and Recreation?　　　　　　　　　　　　　　　b. _____
c. A volleyball team is composed of_____members.　c. _____

Recognition questions *Matching.* The matching question usually consists of two columns, one of which is to be paired with a word or phrase in the second; there may be at times more than one column from which the correct answer is to be selected. Or the matching question may be of the incomplete-sentence type. In this latter instance a series of uncompleted sentences appears in column I, while column II contains a group of words or phrases, usually arranged alphabetically, from which the correct answer is to be selected for completing the statement. Lindquist states that this type of question is well adapted to testing in "who," "when," and "where" types of situations or for naming and identifying abilities.[9] Generally speaking, it is wise to have not fewer than six to ten items appearing in column II, and not more than eight to twelve items listed in column I. Column I should be homogeneous, so that guessing can be eliminated to a large extent. Then too, there should always be more answers in column II than there are test items in column I, so that the more difficult questions cannot be answered by a process of elimination rather than by knowledge. Material such as dates and events, rules and examples, and principles and illustrations may be readily adapted for use in the matching question.

Ross and Stanely claim that the principal limitations of this form of question are that the questions are not well adapted to measurement of understanding as distinguished from mere memory, that the questions may include irrelevant clues to the correct response, and that unless skillfully made they are time-consuming for the student.[12] Additional limitations are that the exercises are difficult to construct, particularly in that clues may easily crop up, and that more than one answer may fit a particular item. A sample matching question follows:

DIRECTIONS: Match column I with column II in the spaces provided.
1. Outstanding athletes.

Column I	Column II	
A. Badminton	Patty Berg	D
B. Bowling	Toni Sailer	F
C. Diving	Andrew Bathgate	E
D. Golf	Bob Clotworthy	C
E. Hockey	Helen Wills Moody	H
F. Skiing	Jim Spalding	B
G. Swimming		
H. Tennis		

Multiple-choice. In these questions the pupils select the best item for completing a statement correctly. Two or more responses are included, only one of which is correct, or is significantly better than the others. The item is usually written in the form of a direct question or incomplete statement. Care should be taken in constructing the question to make sure that at least four logical choices are available; less than four permits chance to play a greater part in the final score. To be sure, if a non-logical answer is included in the choices there are not really four possible answers. If it is difficult to get four plausible answers the material would perhaps better fit into another question type. Items of this kind are usually regarded as the most worth-while and most generally applicable type of question in terms of demanding discrimination and judgment on the part of the pupil. In constructing the question the examiner must avoid irrelevant or superficial clues. Direct questions are preferable, avoiding the use of such words as "a" or "an" immediately preceding the group of choices. Such words limit the possible answers to the question. The choices for the correct answers should be arranged in random order throughout the exercise. It cannot be overemphasized that the most important single factor in writing these test items is the ability of the examiner to select the responses so that each one appears as a plausible answer. The primary limitations of the multiple-choice question are that it is difficult to construct and that it requires a considerable amount of space in comparison to other types of questions. An example follows:

> DIRECTIONS: In the space provided, place the correct letter for the word or words that best complete the statement.
> _____ An eagle in golf is the same as: (A) hole in one; (B) one stroke under par; (C) two strokes under par; (D) par for the hole.

Alternative-response. This type of question requires only two possible responses such as true-false, yes-no, or right-wrong. The true-false examination is by far the one most commonly seen. It is applicable to a wide range of subject matter, is objective in scoring, and a broad sampling of knowledge can be tested in a short period of time. The test does, however, have definite limitations, such as the negative suggestion of false statements which may be contrary to the best educational interests of the younger pupil, the encouragement to guessing, and the extreme skill required in its construction. To be reliable and to overcome its limitations to some extent, the true-false test must be lengthy and exceptionally well prepared. Certain authors suggest that fifty questions be the absolute minimum, while no fewer than seventy-five items is preferable.

Ross and Stanely recommend the use of the true-false test for those situations in which other question forms are not applicable, and then that particular care be given to the wording of the items.[12] Approximately one-half of the test should be composed of true statements and one-half of false statements. Here one must be careful not merely to lift sentences from the text or rule book, for this encourages rote memory. Also, tricky and ambiguous statements as well as unfamiliar language should be avoided when writing the items. If extreme care is not employed in constructing these items, you may well find yourself in an embarrassing position of trying to defend a badly written examination. The following are sample questions:

> DIRECTIONS: Circle T if the statement is true, or F if the statement is wholly or partly false.
>
> 1. The instep kick in soccer is the most accurate method of shooting.   T   F
> 2. Substitution in soccer is limited to ten men.   T   F

Scoring the test. It is always a good idea to design the examination to facilitate the correcting procedures. A little forethought in this department pays excellent dividends. First of all the entire examination should be so constructed that it is neat in appearance, easily read, and has sufficient space allowed for recording answers. The directions must be brief and explicit, leaving no doubt whatsoever in the mind of the examinee as to where and how the answer is to be recorded. It is usually easier to correct answers if they appear vertically on the right-hand margin of the paper, rather than on the left. Placing questions into groups of four or five, with triple spacing between the groups, usually facilitates the grading procedure. This system works particularly well with the true-false, yes-no, or right-wrong type of question. The use of letters and numbers for recording the answers in the spaces or parentheses provided for them is a good practice. This eliminates reading or attempting to read the student's handwriting, which in some cases is none too good, to say the least. The completion item does require a written answer, so one should make sure that adequate space is provided; and remember that, since all blanks should be of identical size regardless of the answer, the spaces should be of such length that the largest answer will fit into them. For variety at least, it is prudent to include several types of questions on one examination. When this is done you may wish to equate the test items in the various exercises. Russell has prepared Table 45 for just such a purpose.

In summary it may be stated that the construction of the written objective examination is a complex task. Lindquist, to indicate the difficulty in writing test items, quotes Adkins to the effect that experienced professional item writers regard an output of five to fifteen good achievement test items per day as a satisfactory performance.[9] Further, it is not uncommon for item writers to receive $2.00 or more for the production of a single good test item. The cost of an approved item may range from $3.00 to $10.00, depending upon the content involved and care exercised. Actually, each one of us does not expect to become a test-construction professional. However, it behooves all of us to recognize the need for extreme care and forethought in the process of writing knowledge tests

TABLE 45. *Method of Equating Test Items*

Type of Test	Number of Elements	Score Range	Total Score
True-false	20	0–1	20
Multiple-choice	10	0–2	20
Completion	7	0–3	21
Matching	10	0–2	20

Russell, Charles: Classroom Tests. Boston, Ginn and Co., 1926, p. 185.

for our pupils. As was mentioned earlier, it is impossible to cover in detail the various aspects of test construction in this chapter; for more complete understanding of this subject, the reader is referred to such excellent sources as Lindquist[9] and Ross and Stanely.[12]

Determination of Validity and Reliability of Standardized Tests

From the chapter on test selection we learned that a scientifically constructed test will be both valid and reliable. As the statistical approach to this problem for written tests is somewhat different from the methods employed in constructing physical tests, it is the purpose of this section to describe briefly one method of validating knowledge tests.

Validity of the knowledge test is dependent upon how well the test covers the curriculum, including the proper weighting of the various areas of emphasis, and the wording of the questions. To aid in determining what is referred to as *curricular validity,* at least one or more of the following initial methods may be employed: analysis of textbooks, of courses of study, and of other tests, and the judgment of competent persons. Once the first, or experimental, form of the test is devised, it is administered to a group with instructions for the pupils to question any of the items for wording or clarification. After the papers are scored, statistical techniques are employed to demonstrate validity and reliability of the test in an objective manner. Upon the basis of the statistical evaluation, the test is re-worked and written in its final form. The same statistical procedures for determining validity and reliability of the experimental form are again applied to the final form of the examination.

In the statistical analysis, each item or test question is analyzed first for validity. This is called *item analysis* or *item validity* and is used to determine the worth of the individual questions. The good items are retained, while the poor ones are discarded or rewritten. To evaluate the good and poor items, several statistical methods may be used. One of the simpler ways is to divide the number of correct responses by the number taking the test. This figure is expressed as a percentage and the lower the difficulty rating, the more difficult the question. An ideal situation exists when the items possess a difficulty rating ranging from 10 to 90 per cent, with the majority at about 50 per cent.

The value of an item not only depends upon its degree of difficulty, but also upon its ability to discriminate between the good and poor students. The *index of discrimination,* as it is properly called, tells us whether or not a lower percentage of those pupils who scored high on the test answered a particular question correctly, rather than indicating those who did poorly on the test. A test item discriminates when the good pupils answer it correctly and the poor pupils fail the item. As would be expected, a test item has a negative discrimination index when more of the good pupils than poor pupils fail it. Usually the good papers consist of the top 27 to 30 per cent of the total number taking the test, while the poor papers make up the bottom 27 to 30 per cent. Thus, by analyzing each question, an index of discrimination may be obtained, giving the researcher insight as to the worth of a question in terms of its degree of difficulty and ability to discriminate.

The statistical method of item analysis commonly employed is the *phi coefficient*. Phi is a type of correlation used to determine the relationship between the scores of the good and poor students, and the degree to which the students answered a particular question correctly, the object being to ascertain the discriminatory ability of the individual test items. In summary it can be stated that both curricular analysis and item analysis are the means used to arrive at the total validity of a knowledge test. It might be wise to point out here that regardless of high reliability and validity reported for a test, to be truly valid for your particular use it *must* agree with *your* course content.

To determine the reliability of a written test one of two methods may be used: correlation of the odd-numbered questions against the even-numbered ones, or construction of alternate forms of the same test. Provided the latter method is used, the two forms of the test are administered to two like samples and the results correlated. The first method is most commonly employed in our field, and frequently it is referred to as the *split-halves method*. When this system is employed, you no doubt will read that the r was corrected for actual length of the test. This is reasonably explained by an example. If one has a test of 100 questions and correlates the odd questions against the even, obviously the N would equal fifty. The resulting coefficient is the reliability for half of the test. By adding to the number of questions (N) the reliability of the test is increased. Therefore, the researcher will find it necessary to determine statistically the expected reliability for the actual length of the test (in this case for 100 questions). Usually the Spearman-Brown formula is used as follows in making the computation:

$$r_{wt} = \frac{2r_{ht}}{1 + r_{ht}}$$

r_{wt} = reliability coefficient for the whole test

r_{ht} = reliability of one-half the test computed from the test data.

As an illustration:

$$r_{wt} = \frac{2 \times .70}{1 + .70} = .82$$

Correlation for the entire test as predicted by the Spearman-Brown formula equals .82.

Sample Knowledge Test (Tennis Test for Women)

The Women's Physical Education Department at the University of Washington has appointed grading committees to standardize and improve marking procedures in various sports activities.[1] The tennis test that is reported here was developed for use with college women. The experimental design in constructing this test is a typical procedure employed for developing standardized knowledge tests.

The first step was the administration of an experimental test to eighty-seven students. This original examination contained 100 questions separated, in accordance with content, into the following question types with corresponding curricular emphases:

Part   I. True-False: Position, Timing, Footwork, Fundamental
                Strokes, and Advanced Strokes.
Part   II. Multiple-Choice: Strategy and Court Position.
Part III. Completion: History, Events, and Equipment.
Part IV. Matching: Advanced Strokes.
Part   V. Yes-No: Rules and Scoring.
Part VI. Identification: Court Markings and Strategy.

The experimental test was then administered to the students, who were asked to make notations on items that were questionable. The reliability of the test was computed to be .84, as determined by correlating half of the test against the other half (split-halves method). In order to satisfy the curricular validity, three techniques were used: test items to be included on the original test were determined by an analysis of the knowledge tests already available in the area, by textbooks, and by the minimum essentials set up as standards for teaching by the Women's Department; everything covered on the test was included somewhere in the curriculum; and the percentage of the test items dealing with each phase of the activity agreed as much as possible with the emphasis placed on that particular phase in the course of study.

Item validity was found by dividing the test papers into upper, middle, and lower thirds, according to total score. The percentage of the upper and lower groups who failed each item was calculated. Then the phi coefficient for the item was determined in order to show whether or not the question as worded in the test was useful in discriminating between those who did well on the entire examination and those who did poorly. Items that showed an ability to discriminate between the students who did well and those who did poorly on the examination were retained. The test questions that could not discriminate between the good and the poor student, or those that were questioned by the students, were revised.

Reliability of the revised test was computed on 297 beginning students and 46 intermediate students. The reliability for the beginning class was .82 ± .013; for the intermediate class, .92 ± .015; and for the combined classes, .86 ± .009.

Item validity was determined for the beginning class only, as there were too few students for such a study in the intermediate group. For the final test the group was divided approximately into thirds; the lowest eighty-eight papers and the highest eighty-eight papers constituted the top and bottom groups. The percentage (29.6) that was selected as a natural break in the scores occurred at this point. To compute item validity for the revised test the phi coefficient was employed in the same manner as that used with the experimental form of the test in determining whether or not the questions were discriminatory.

The authors conclude that the knowledge test satisfies most of the criteria for a good test. It is completely objective and can be administered in fifty minutes. By comparing the beginners' scores with the intermediates' scores, it was found that the latter did much better, which contributes to the evidence of the validity of the test. The average number of items missed by the beginners was 48.2 with a standard deviation of 12.5, while the average failed by the intermediates was 29.4 with a standard deviation of 11.5.

Physical Education Knowledge Tests

Badminton.   The faculty women at the University of Washington have developed a test to measure badminton knowledge for beginning college women students.[3] The test contains 106 questions with distribution of emphasis as follows: thirty-one questions on analysis of strokes and techniques, forty-one on rules and scoring, eleven on strategy, and twenty-three dealing with badminton terminology. Curricular validity, item validity, and item difficulty were determined in the usual manner, assuring the test to be statistically valid. Reliability computed by the split-halves method was found to be .90 ± .012, based upon 124 students. The questions are uniformly arranged and a separate score sheet has been devised for ease of handling and correcting papers. The complete examination with the scoring sheet appears in reference 3.

Phillips has constructed a badminton knowledge test for use with college women in classes of varying instructional levels.[11] The test contains forty-five multiple-choice items and fifty-five true-false questions. Based upon 1471 cases, the reliability was found to be .87 for a homogeneous group and .921 for a heterogeneous group when true-false items were corrected for guessing. The difficulty range of the test is from 7 to 93 per cent, with a mean difficulty for the entire test of 50.8 per cent. Norms in terms of T-scores and percentile ranks have been established for both beginners and intermediates and appear in reference 11.

The Research Committee, Central Association for Physical Education of College Women, with M. Gladys Scott as chairman, has devised a test to evaluate both skills and knowledge of badminton for college women. The final form of the written examination contains forty-seven multiple-choice and thirty-three true-false items. The reliability on 100 papers selected at random was computed by the odd-even method and corrected to actual length; a reliability coefficient of .72 was obtained for the true-false items and .79 for the multiple-choice questions. A grading scheme based upon the scores made by 350 players appears in reference 13; also included is a description of the skill test with an accompanying grading scheme as well as a T-scale for both beginning and advanced players.

Golf.   Waglow and Rehling have constructed an objective true-false golf knowledge test to be used for marking students in the required physical education program.[16] The validity of the 100-question test was based upon the fact that the test items were taken from prominent books. The reliability of the test, using odd- against even-numbered questions, was .70 for 100 men. The reliability of the whole test, using the Spearman-Brown formula, was found to be .82. Standards have been developed on the basis of T-scores; also a classification table for assigning letter marks based upon the standard deviation technique appears in reference 16.

Field hockey.   This hockey knowledge test was devised for grades nine to twelve inclusive.[2] Consideration was given to comprehensiveness, administrative efficiency, and flexibility in terms of being easily altered with changing rules. The test, which can be administered in thirty minutes, contains seventy-seven questions made up of short-answer, multiple-choice, and true-false items, and appears in reference 2. Reliability is not reported.

Kelly and Brown have developed a 106-item objective field hockey test designed to be used by women majoring in physical education.[7] Validity of the test was determined by item analysis. In addition, three further approaches to the problem of validity were made as follows: comparison of scores made by experts, majors, and service and lay subjects; correlation of test scores with extent of field hockey experience; and correlation of test scores with instructors, ratings of major students' competence to teach field hockey. Reliability for 209 students, including expert, major, service, and lay, was found to be .89; for the major group alone reliability was reported as .79.

Softball.   Waglow and Stephens developed a softball test for purposes of determining the extent of knowledge and the marking of college students.[17] The test consists of sixty true-false items, twenty-five completion items, five fair or foul ball questions, and ten concerning whether the ball is in play or dead. The odd-even reliability coefficient for 115 cases on the second revision of the complete test was found to be .78. The value of the individual items was determined by a difficulty rating, which was obtained by dividing the number of correct responses by the number who took the test, and by an index of discrimination, which was obtained by computing the percentage of "highs" and "lows" answering the items correctly. Twenty-seven per cent of the sample constituted the "highs" and 27 per cent the "lows." The softball test, norm table for assigning letter marks, and a table of T-scores appear in reference 17.

Swimming. The Research Committee of the Central Association of Physical Education for College Women has devised a valid examination for swimming, which can be used in college swimming classes for the purpose of measuring level of understanding, for classification on the basis of knowledge, and for marking.[14] The complete test appears in reference 14. In the elementary form, there are thirty multiple-choice and twenty-six true-false items; the reliability based upon 100 cases was found to be .888. In the intermediate test there are twenty-two multiple-choice and thirty-six true-false questions; the reliability for 100 cases was reported to be .867.

Tennis. In addition to the tennis knowledge test appearing on page 324, used as an example in test construction, Miller has developed and standardized a tennis knowledge test for appraising achievements of women majoring in physical education.[10] Curricular validity of the test was approached through the analysis of textbooks, courses of study, and judgment of competent persons. Twenty-seven colleges returned 381 completed answer sheets. Twenty-seven per cent of the scores at either end of the distribution were used in determining item validity. Reliability of the test was found to be .90 when the correction-for-chance-success formula was applied in the scoring. Norms in the form of T-scores and percentile ranks based on 612 individuals have been provided in reference 10.

Grouped knowledge tests. French has done a splendid and extensive research assignment in constructing knowledge tests to serve as partial determiners of the technique requirements for women students majoring in physical education at the State University of Iowa.[4] (For those individuals who wish to prepare themselves in the area of knowledge testing the original reference, which was Dr. French's Doctoral Study at the State University of Iowa, is strongly recommended.) The following activities were included: badminton, basketball, body mechanics, canoeing, field hockey, folk dancing, golf, recreational sports (aerial darts, bowling, deck tennis, handball, shuffleboard, table tennis, tetherball), rhythms, soccer, softball, stunts and tumbling, swimming, tennis, track and field, and volleyball. The general methods which are customarily employed in constructing knowledge tests were followed. The procedures in solving the problem consisted of the following steps: (1) clarification of objectives; (2) outlining of courses; (3) planning the distribution of items by content classification; (4) preparation of items; (5) critical evaluation of items; (6) selecting the subjects; and (7) administering the tests. The reliabilities of the tests for the long form are from .70 to .88, while those for the short form range from .61 to .87. The questions in the various tests number from twenty-one to twenty-six. Norms are available for the short forms of the examinations. French suggests that the tests appear adequate for such uses as:

1. A basis for profile charts, indicating areas of strength and weakness for the individual student.

2. A basis for scheduling technique classes according to student needs.

3. An indication of the students' ability to retain information and make applications.

4. Measurement of students' progress by administering the tests before and after the instructional unit.

Hennis has constructed a group of knowledge tests for badminton, basketball, bowling, field hockey, softball, tennis, and volleyball which are suitable for use with the women's instructional program.[6] All tests consist of four-choice multiple-choice type of items. A survey of course content was made preliminary to construction of the seven knowledge tests. Of the 117 colleges and universities surveyed, ninety-seven returned the check lists. The number of students taking the examinations was from 208 in softball to 2291 in tennis. Reliability of the tests ranged from .72 for badminton to .81 for softball. Percentile norms have been devised for each of the seven tests; and any qualified instructor may obtain information concerning the tests from the author at Woman's College of the University of North Carolina in Greensboro.

BIBLIOGRAPHY

1. Broer, Marion, and Miller, Donna Mae: Achievement Tests for Beginning and Intermediate Tennis. Research Quart., 21:303–313, 1950.

2. Dietz, Dorthea, and Frech, Beryl: Hockey Knowledge Test for Girls. J. A. A. Health, Phys. Educ. & Recreation, 11:366, 1940.

3. Fox, Katharine: Beginning Badminton Written Examination. Research Quart., 24:135–146, 1953.

4. French, Esther: The Construction of Knowledge Tests in Selected Professional Courses in Physical Education. Research Quart., 14:406–424, 1943.

5. Hawkes, Herbert E., Lindquist, E. F., and Mann, C. R.: The Construction and Use of Achievement Examinations. Boston, Houghton Mifflin Co., 1936, p. 150.

6. Hennis, Gail M.: Construction of Knowledge Tests in Selected Physical Education Activities for College Women. Research Quart., 27:301–309, 1956.

7. Kelly, Ellen Davis, and Brown, Jane E.: The Construction of a Field Hockey Test for Women Physical Education Majors. Research Quart., 23:233–239, 1952.

8. Langston, Dewey F.: Standardization of a Volleyball Knowledge Test for College Men Physical Education Majors. Research Quart., 26:60–68, 1955.

9. Lindquist, E. F. (Editor):Educational Measurement. Washington, D. C., American Council on Education, 1951, p. 186.

10. Miller, Wilma K.: Achievement Levels in Tennis Knowledge and Skill for Women Physical Education Major Students. Research Quart., 24:81–90, 1953.

11. Phillips, Marjorie: Standardization of a Badminton Knowledge Test for College Women. Research Quart., 17:48–63, 1946.

12. Ross, C. C., and Stanely, Julian C.: Measurement in Today's School. 3rd ed. Englewood Cliffs, New Jersey, Prentice-Hall, Inc., 1954, p. 186.

13. Scott, M. Gladys: Achievement Examinations in Badminton. Research Quart., 12: 242–253, 1941.

14. Scott, M. Gladys: Achievement Examinations for Elementary and Intermediate Swimming Classes. Research Quart., 11:100–111, 1940.

15. Speer, Robert K., and Smith, Samuel: Health Test. Rockville Center, New York, Acorn Publishing Co., 1949.

16. Waglow, I. F., and Rehling, C. H.: A Golf Knowledge Test. Research Quart., 24: 463–470, 1953.

17. Waglow, I. F., and Stephens, Fay: A Softball Knowledge Test. Research Quart., 26:234–243, 1955.

chapter 13
marking in physical education

Youngsters' marks are an extremely important part of the educational program. In addition to the recognized purposes of marks, they probably constitute the single most important instrument of communication between school and parent. Regardless of the value that teachers place on the report card, parents attach a great deal of significance to Johnny's or Mary's marks. Recognizing this fact, school administrators are gradually changing the report card into a much more elaborate instrument. For instance, a card may now contain two or three pages, in which are included marks for aptitude, sociability, attitude, and progress, in addition to the subject or course marks. Also, it is not unusual to find a space for notes written by the homeroom teacher relative to the strengths and weaknesses of the pupil. These may be similar to anecdotal record reports. We can rest assured that for the most part parents carefully study the report card, for it contains meaningful information about their child. Physical educators must come forward with a sound marking system and use to advantage this valuable medium for making clear the aims of their program and profession.

Need for a marking scheme. It is commonly agreed among physical educators that, in most cases, the present practice of marking in physical education leaves much to be desired. For example, in a recent study, conducted among fifty practice teachers who had just returned from their respective schools, it was found that in 80 per cent of the systems the child's mark was based solely on his being present and in uniform daily.[5]

In an earlier study,[9] among twenty-six colleges and universities, the following items were found to be in use as a basis for the mark in physical education:

FACTORS	INCIDENCE (PER CENT)
Attendance	88.46
Effort	84.61
Skill	80.76
Posture	80.76
Improvement in skill	57.67
Physical efficiency	30.76
Improvement shown in physical examination	26.92

As can be observed, the most frequently occurring factor is attendance. One might raise the question, "Should the physical education mark be something more than merely a measure of attendance or absence?"

In addition to promiscuous marking on the basis of uniform and attendance, physical educators frequently resort to the "S" (satisfactory) and "U" (unsatisfactory) method of marking. It might be further mentioned that the "S" appears on the card with such regularity that apparently no one ever fails in physical education.

Careless marking truly belittles the physical educator as well as his profession. It seems almost better to refrain from turning in a mark at all, if it carries little or no meaning.

Problems of marking in physical education. Actually, the instructor is not entirely responsible for the common practices of marking in physical education. This is true because the school administration, in many cases, is unfamiliar with the real concept of physical education, and unknowingly forces upon the physical educator a marking system that is impractical and frequently educationally unsound. In the first place, physical education is not a course like English or spelling, but rather a program made up of many courses. Thus it follows that if the physical educator is expected to mark in a manner similar to that of the English or history teacher, then the pupil should receive a mark for each activity or course. Obviously the common report card does not allow space for such marking. Then, too, if one did comply with this practice, marking would become a tremendous burden, for the physical educator most likely will have 300 to 400 pupils in his classes each week. As a matter of fact, merely placing 300 to 400 marks on report cards four to six times a year is no small job in itself. Hence the teacher is forced to become more interested in getting the physical labor accomplished than in planning and putting into effect a sound marking system. Regulations imposed by the school administrator often result in a very slipshod method of marking, which is far too common in our profession.

As an example, in the author's first school, the principal requested five grades in each subject for every pupil, regardless of the course. The report cards were issued six times each year, and the author taught about 400 pupils. In other words, the author recorded 2000 marks each time the cards came out, or 12,000 grades in a school year! Just the process of recording was a tremendous task, and as a result the marks were based on nothing more than a quick subjective opinion. It would have been better if the author had not placed any marks on the cards, for they meant little or nothing to the pupil, to the parent, or to himself.

Values of a good marking system. To eliminate such problems, it seems advisable to take a rational look at marking and to develop a system that is practical and at the same time informative to pupil, parent, and administrator. By initiating a sound marking system, the prestige of the physical education department could be elevated considerably, for the following reasons:

1. The report card can be the means of informing the parent and the administrator as to the purposes of physical education.

2. The card can illustrate the use of objective and scientific testing methods.

3. The mark can be tangible evidence of the pupil's status in terms of the objectives of physical education. Such marking is sound educationally and can help to direct the parents' interest to the physical education program and its contributions for their child.

Philosophy of marking. Before discussing the principles and steps in formulating a marking scheme, one should first recognize that marking is essentially philosophical in nature. Purposes of marking in a professional school of physical education, for example, are different from the purposes underlying marking in the public school physical education program. In the professional school the grade may be based upon competition within the class; that is to say, the instructor will give so many A's, B's, C's, and D's in accordance with the distribution of the class scores. Such professional marking reflects to a certain extent the academic standards of the college. These standards, whether we like them or not, do protect the profession as well as the value of the degree that the student earns. On the other hand, in the public school the pupil may suffer certain physical or hereditary handicaps that impose restrictions on his performance as well as on his ability to develop such attributes as a high degree of fitness and proficiency in skills. Such factors of individual differences must be recognized and dealt with so that the child will receive a fair and encouraging mark.

In addition to recognizing individual pupil limitations, as in the developmental and remedial phase of the program, the instructor must also determine what he is going to grade upon, the amount of weight that he is going to assign to each component of the mark, in arriving at a total physical education grade. For example, should 50 per cent be assigned to physical fitness and 25 per cent each given to recreational and social fitness? One method of accomplishing the weighting of marks is suggested by Moriarty[8] as follows: Assign each letter grade a number, e.g., A—5; B—4; C—3; D—2; E—1. The total grade, which logically includes knowledge tests, may then be computed in the following manner:

Factors	Weight	Average	Points	
Physical fitness	3	B	3×4	12
Recreational skills	2	A	2×5	10
Social efficiency	1	C	1×3	3
Total				25

The final answer to such questions must be arrived at through sound reasoning by the individual instructor in accordance with the needs peculiar to his particular situation.

To a large extent, insight as to the distribution of emphasis among the selected areas of marking may be gained from testing results. For instance, if the school population is low in recreational skills, then more attention should logically be placed in this area; by the same token, if the majority of the pupils are unusually low in fitness, then more emphasis should probably be placed upon this objective.

Principles of marking. In undertaking the organization and initiation of a marking system, there are certain principles[1] that should be kept in mind:

1. The marking method should conform with that of the school administration. Even though the administrator may allow the physical educator to develop his own methods, the final marks placed on the report card should be of the same kind as those in other subjects. For example, if grades are assigned as A, B, C, D, and F, then all departments within the school should follow this procedure and mark on comparable bases.

2. The mark should be interpreted, so that the methods used in arriving at a given grade are made known to the pupil, the parent, and the school administration. By use of objective methods such as fitness and skill testing, it becomes a simple job to average the marks and to illustrate how the final grade was determined. The greatest value of objective testing and marking is that it leaves little doubt in anyone's mind as to the meaning of the mark.

3. It must be recognized that subjective grading, as well as objective grading, must form a part of the total physical education grade; if not, such measures as attitude, cooperative endeavor, leadership, followership, and sportsmanship would necessarily be eliminated.

McCormick suggests the use of three methods of objective evaluation and two more or less subjective methods designed to measure "attitudes," "effort," and "sportsmanship." The measures suggested are: (1) an initial mid-term physical achievement test; (2) a term's-end re-test of physical achievement; (3) a written examination based upon assignments and posted material regarding sports, objectives of physical education, and what physical fitness is, how achieved, and how maintained; (4) a mid-term instructor's rating of each student's achievement in sportsmanship and performance of the skills offered in the instruction-participation activity program; and (5) a final term's-end instructor's rating similar to the mid-term rating.[7]

Laporte suggests four criteria pertaining to subjective-objective ways of grading: performance of skills; knowledge of rules, general performance, and strategy; social attitudes, including cooperativeness, sportsmanship, leadership, and so forth; posture and bearing.[4]

4. The marking system should be based upon the teacher's objectives. Hence the degree of proficiency that the pupil attains in the stated objectives would constitute the mark. This principle is perhaps one of the most important, for it clearly indicates the areas of physical education that should be measured. If we establish, as our basic objectives, physical fitness, recreational fitness, and social fitness, then we should measure the degree of proficiency that the pupil develops in these areas. The pupil's developed proficiency in the stated objectives should then constitute a major portion of if not the total grade.

5. The mark should reflect the progress that the pupil has made toward achieving the class objectives. The relative portion of the total mark should correlate with the amount of emphasis placed upon each activity.

6. The marking system should not be too time-consuming.

Methods of marking. One may group types of marking into the letter system and the descriptive sentence method.

Letter system. There are five classifications that seem best adapted to the letter system of marking: (1) the per cent system; (2) the numerical standard; (3) the accomplishment quotient; (4) the Sigma scale scores; (5) and the pass or fail. In most instances the first four methods are recorded on the report card in a five-letter division of A, B, C, D, and F. The fifth plan is usually recorded as "S" (satisfactory) and "U" (unsatisfactory).

The per cent system is perhaps the most common, although considered by some authors to be one of the weakest. In this case, the pupil is marked on the basis of 100 per cent. What the 100 implies is difficult to determine (perfect performance? best performance in the class? greatest improvement? or what?).

The numerical standard system is most closely related to the per cent system, for letter grades represent scores such as 95 to 100 (A), 85 to 94 (B), and so on. This method does avoid the difficulty of distinguishing between the performances of, say, 82 and 83. However, the difficulty lies in distinguishing between a C and a B. Certainly the difference between the scores at the extremes of the class division is over-emphasized.

The accomplishment quotient is a method that is no longer recommended in the school system. The basic philosophy underlying this type of marking scheme is that the pupil should be graded according to his or her own potential accomplishment. Even though the pupil in comparison to his classmates attains a high level of proficiency, he should not be marked high unless he is approximating his expected potential.

One of the better systems of marking is based on the Sigma scores. The basis for this grade is derived from a normal curve, which in turn is based upon the distribution of the test scores in a given class. The advantage of the Sigma score method of marking is that the scores are based upon the standard deviation of the data and are comparable from year to year, and from test to test, as well as from pupil to pupil.

Davis and Lawther[3] provide an apt illustration of the use of the Sigma score in marking a skill's test:

> Mean score of a soccer kick for a group of twelve-year-old boys was 75 feet and the standard deviation was 12. If a boy kicks 99 feet, subtract the mean from the score received by the boy and it would be 24. Then divide the score by the standard deviation and the answer is plus 2 sigmas above the mean.

A more complete description for the use of the Sigma score appears in Chapter 3.

The "S" and "U" method of marking places the pupils into two classifications and hence does not adequately indicate the type of work that the pupil is doing. Furthermore, it fails to define pupil status, progress, or retrogression. From the administrator's point of view, such a method prevents the faculty from knowing their own pupils, which in turn limits the efforts of the vocational and educational guidance departments.

Descriptive sentence method. A recent development in marking is a system that seems to be becoming popular in secondary schools. It is the descriptive sentence method, which employs a written analysis by the teacher relative to the status of the pupil. For example:

> A is average in her group in hockey. She has learned the elementary skills very quickly and easily. She seems very interested in physical activities, and she is always willing to take advantage of opportunities for self-improvement. A is a very enthusiastic member of the group, but there are times when she could exert more self-control for the good of the group as a whole.[8]

This type of marking requires time as well as a very skilled observer. Too frequently the report may become quite a burden, particularly in physical education, where the teacher may have to write 300 to 500 such reports every four to six weeks, depending upon the number of pupils and frequency with which the cards are issued.

Developing a marking system. Generally speaking, the objective tests that will be most helpful in formulating a mark will fall in the category of (1) fitness tests, and (2) tests of recreational skills. Measurement in these two areas, which must also include knowledge or paper-and-pencil tests, can practically and effectively constitute the major components of a marking system.

In arriving at a recreational mark, the first step is to determine the courses that will be offered throughout the school year. The activities should be weighted according to their values in contributing to the overall development of the pupil, as well as the amount of time spent on each. A method of evaluation should then be selected, such as skill tests, passing skills (e.g., swimming strokes, and events in tumbling and apparatus), and paper-and-pencil tests.

Another method of marking skills is for the instructor to evaluate subjectively the major skills of a given sport. Say, for example, you wished to give a mark in basketball. The most important skills to master in this game would include dribbling, shooting, passing, and pivoting. A score sheet such as appears in Figure 109 could be carried to class each day during the basketball unit and perhaps three to six pupils could be graded during drills and regular play. The skills might be evaluated on the basis of 0 to 5, and each pupil could be marked a couple of times on the selected skills, which would enable the instructor to average the marks for the final basketball grade.

In selecting the recreational skills for which to assign marks, it is certainly obvious that all activities taught cannot possibly figure into the final mark. Therefore, only those that most significantly contribute to the pupils' recreational development should be included. For example, tennis, golf, swimming, archery, badminton, and the like should receive major emphasis, whereas activities of low organization, such as box hockey, darts, and ping-pong, may not be included at all. In addition to marking on specific sports, some authors suggest marking on general motor ability. However, it seems that if a mark is given for recreational sports and fitness, then the combined score should adequately reflect motor ability. If desired, Cozens' or McCloy's general motor ability tests are examples of instruments that may be used for purposes of marking in this area.

Next, a test of general fitness should be selected and administered at least once each year, but preferably twice—in the fall and in the spring. The test results will then enable the physical educator to mark on status as well as improvement, which is a great motivating device. The selection of the fitness test could be one of motor fitness or a strength test such as Larson's dynamic strength test; or, if equipment is available, the PFI is recommended.

The third category of evaluation is in the social efficiency area.

Baseball Name	Date	Fielding 3	Throwing 2	Batting 4	Running Bases 3	Average 3
Bill Barck						

Code: Excellent 5   Fair 2
Good 4   Poor 1
Average 3

Basketball Name	Date	Dribbling 5	Shooting 4	Passing 4	Play 3	Average 4
Glen Hardesty						

Code: Excellent 5   Fair 2
Good 4   Poor 1
Average 3

Figure 109. Score sheets for subjective marking in sports skills.

Under this objective are included such traits as attitude, appreciations, social graces, modes of conduct, and sportsmanship. Some physical educators feel that uniform and attendance, as previously mentioned, should also be a part of the social fitness mark. However, one should recognize that uniform and attendance fall more logically under the heading of departmental policies rather than items on which to grade. The physical education department should *require* neat and clean uniforms. If the policy is violated, then disciplinary measures should be taken to enforce the regulation. As for attendance, the principal in most cases has a policy that requires a valid excuse for absences. Thus it seems rather difficult, in view of such reasoning, to defend the inclusion of dress and attendance in the grading scheme, even though this is a quite common practice.

Although social fitness is impossible to measure objectively and hence difficult to grade, it is advisable to use an instrument to detect tendencies toward maladjustment. If a social adjustment test cannot be administered, the teacher should be more on the alert for symptoms designating tendencies toward maladjustment. As was mentioned before, the very social character of the activities program permits an excellent opportunity for the observant teacher to notice such problems. The anecdotal record, the rating scales, and the sociometry, as discussed in Chapter 11, are valuable methods for noting atypical behavior among pupils.

McCloy suggests that ratings of character should not be included in the mark, but rather ought to be used for making clear to the teacher the

Achievement Measured	Marks and Equivalent Points					Frequency of Test per Semester
	A	B	C	D	E	
Attendance	12	9	6	3	0	1
*Decathlon or Rhythms	8	6	4	2	0	1
Hygiene Inspections	4	3	2	1	0	3
New Type Tests (Rules, Strategy)	4	3	2	1	0	3
Physical Fitness Test	8	6	4	2	0	1
Posture Tests	4	3	2	1	0	3
Skill-Citizenship Estimate	8	6	4	2	0	3
Stunts Test	8	6	4	2	0	1
Towel and Lock fees	4	3	2	1	0	1

* Decathlon for boys; Rhythms for girls.

Attendance Mark		Equivalent Letter Marks	
0–1 day absent	A	100–87	A
1–2 days absent	B	86–67	B
2–5 days absent	C	66–37	C
5–9 days absent	D	36–14	D
9–more days absent	E	13–0	E

Figure 110. Weighting system for marking in physical education. (Courtesy of Karl Bookwalter, Indiana University.)

pupil's status relative to conduct, habits, and attitudes; also, such ratings can be employed as a guide for the teacher in helping to formulate laboratory experiences in an adequate number and variety.[6] The final decision as to just what will be included in the mark, as well as the distribution of emphasis, must necessarily be left to the individual instructor.

The following marking scheme, which has considerable merit, was developed by Bookwalter.[2] It makes use of a weighing chart as seen in Figure 110. This system works for both boys and girls; however, when marking girls, the rhythms test is substituted for the decathlon. Also contained in the figure are the numerical ranges for assigning letter grades and marks for days of absence. Attendance receives considerable emphasis in the mark. This is because the author of the marking system feels that attendance is of vital importance in physical education, even more so than in the academic classes. As physical education is primarily an activity subject, a social situation missed on one day can never be recalled on another. Furthermore, the organic development lost cannot be made up by a double dose on a later date. Even though this marking system is empirically constructed in terms of weighting, it has worked effectively in a number of situations; for this reason it is presented for your consideration.

Following is an illustration of how a mark would be computed:

WEIGHTED MARK	POINTS
A pupil receives a semester mark of B in attendance (missed class no more than twice)	9
He receives an A in the decathlon	8
Three hygiene inspection marks A, B, B (4 3 3)	10
New type tests A, C, B (4 2 3)	9
Physical fitness test A	8
Posture tests B, B, A (3 3 4)	10
Citizenship A, B, A (8 6 8)	22
Stunt tests A (8)	8
Administrative requirements A (4)	4
Total points	88

Referring to Figure 110, one determines the interval in which the 88 lies. As can be seen, the 88 points correspond to a letter mark of A.

A physical education report card. In view of the difficulties involved in trying to conform to the general marking scheme of a school system, it appears that some good may come from developing a report card specifically for physical education. The advantages of such a card, which would be issued twice each year, far outweigh the small cost and effort involved. A portion of a sample card, designed for use in the girls' program, appears in Figure 111. The original card was made from a durable $8\frac{1}{2} \times 11$ inch sheet of folded cardboard. On the first page appeared the school emblem, name, and the principal's and director's names. Also

TOTAL MARKS

	Se-mester	Total Fitness	Sports	Citi-zenship	Physical Edu. Mark
Freshman	1	A	B	A—	A—
	2				
Sophomore	3				
	4				
Junior	5				
	6				
Senior	7				
	8				

EMPHASIS

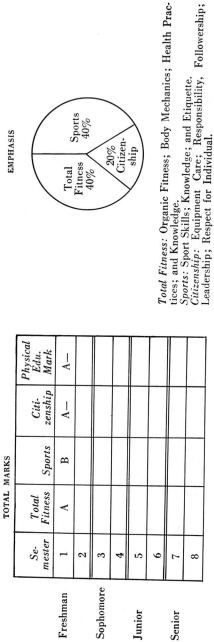

Total Fitness: Organic Fitness; Body Mechanics; Health Practices; and Knowledge.
Sports: Sport Skills; Knowledge; and Etiquette.
Citizenship: Equipment Care; Responsibility, Followership; Leadership; Respect for Individual.

Figure 111. A physical education report card.

ORGANIC FITNESS TEST

Points	PULL-UPS Semester								SIT-UPS Semester								50-YD. RUN Semester								SARGENT JUMP Semester								20-YD. HOP Semester							
	1	2	3	4	5	6	7	8	1	2	3	4	5	6	7	8	1	2	3	4	5	6	7	8	1	2	3	4	5	6	7	8	1	2	3	4	5	6	7	8
100																	√																√							
90	√								√																√															
80																																								
70																																								
60																																								
50																																								
40																																								
30																																								
20																																								
10																																								
0																																								

Check (√) indicates percentile points earned. Marks assigned for average of five tests as follows: 90-100 A; 80-89 B; 70-79 C; 60-69 D.

Figure 111. (Continued.)

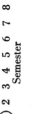

① 2 3 4 5 6 7 8
Semester

Comments:

SPORTS EVALUATION
(Knowledge and Skills)

Teacher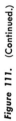

Marie Frailey
Name

First Semester	*Year in School*			
	9	10	11	12
BASKETBALL	A			
SPEEDAWAY	C			
HOCKEY	C			
RECREATIONAL GAMES	A			
FOLK DANCING	—			
BADMINTON	—			
BOWLING	—			
MODERN DANCE	—			
COMBINED GRADE	B			

Figure 111. (Continued.)

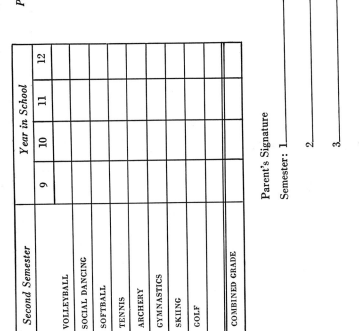

Second Semester	Year in School			
	9	10	11	12
VOLLEYBALL				
SOCIAL DANCING				
SOFTBALL				
TENNIS				
ARCHERY				
GYMNASTICS				
SKIING				
GOLF				
COMBINED GRADE				

Parent

Parent's Signature

Semester: 1 _____   5 _____

2 _____   6 _____

3 _____   7 _____

4 _____   8 _____

Figure 111. (Concluded.)

SAMPLE PHYSICAL FITNESS TESTING SCORE SHEET
(For BOYS 10 Years of Age)

Pupil_____   School_____   Teacher_____

1st test – Circle scores in RED.   2nd test – Circle scores in GREEN.   3rd test – Circle scores in BLUE.
Connect circled scores after each test to show physical fitness profile.

	Sit Ups	Pull Ups	Broad Jump	50 Yard Dash	Shuttle Run	Softball Throw	600 Yards
EXCELLENT	60	6	5'6"	7.6	10.3	122'	2:15
	58	5	5'5"	7.7	10.4	121'	2:17
	56		5'4"		10.5	119'	2:18
				7.8	10.6	117'	2:20
	54		5'3"		10.7	115'	
GOOD	52	4	5'2"	7.9	10.8	113'	2:22
					10.9	111'	2:24
	50		5'1"	8.0	11.0	109'	2:26
					11.1	107'	2:28
	48	3	5'0"	8.1	11.2	105'	2:30
						103'	
	46		4'11"	8.2	11.3	102'	2:32
	44				11.4		2:34
	42			8.3		100'	
	40		4'10"		11.5		2:36
	38	2		8.4	11.6	98'	2:38
SATISFACTORY	36		4'9"		11.7	96'	2:40
	34			8.5		94'	2:42
	32				11.8		2:44
	30		4'8"	8.6	11.9	92'	2:45
	29		4'7"	8.7	12.0	90'	2:47
	28					88'	2:49
	27		4'6"	8.8	12.1		2:51
	26					86'	2:53
POOR	25	1					
	24		4'5"	8.9	12.2	84'	2:55
	23						2:57
	22		4'4"	9.0	12.3	82'	2:58

Note: This score sheet will serve one boy for all three tests during the school year.

Figure 112. The score sheet will serve one boy for three tests. (Youth Fitness Manual; President's Council on Youth Fitness, July, 1961, p. 55.)

on the cover was included a brief note to the parents explaining the purpose and objectives of the program as well as the essentials of the marking system. The back of the card contained a norm table on the motor fitness items used to evaluate the child's physical fitness, similar to the one appearing in Figure 112.

As can be seen from Figure 111, the physical fitness test contains a percentile scale for converting the raw scores to a 0–100 basis. For each of the test items a check is placed at the percentile in which the child

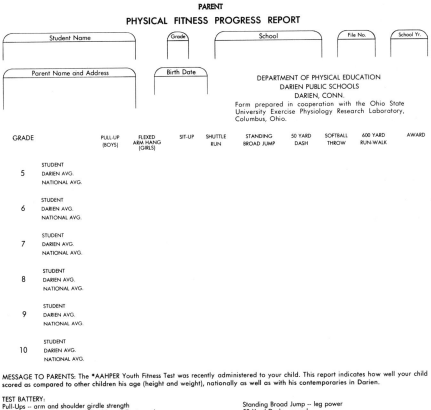

PARENT
PHYSICAL FITNESS PROGRESS REPORT

Student Name | Grade | School | File No. | School Yr.

Parent Name and Address | Birth Date

DEPARTMENT OF PHYSICAL EDUCATION
DARIEN PUBLIC SCHOOLS
DARIEN, CONN.
Form prepared in cooperation with the Ohio State University Exercise Physiology Research Laboratory, Columbus, Ohio.

GRADE		PULL-UP (BOYS)	FLEXED ARM HANG (GIRLS)	SIT-UP	SHUTTLE RUN	STANDING BROAD JUMP	50 YARD DASH	SOFTBALL THROW	600 YARD RUN-WALK	AWARD
5	STUDENT									
	DARIEN AVG.									
	NATIONAL AVG.									
6	STUDENT									
	DARIEN AVG.									
	NATIONAL AVG.									
7	STUDENT									
	DARIEN AVG.									
	NATIONAL AVG.									
8	STUDENT									
	DARIEN AVG.									
	NATIONAL AVG.									
9	STUDENT									
	DARIEN AVG.									
	NATIONAL AVG.									
10	STUDENT									
	DARIEN AVG.									
	NATIONAL AVG.									

MESSAGE TO PARENTS: The *AAHPER Youth Fitness Test was recently administered to your child. This report indicates how well your child scored as compared to other children his age (height and weight), nationally as well as with his contemporaries in Darien.

TEST BATTERY:
Pull-Ups -- arm and shoulder girdle strength
Flexed Arm Hang -- arm and shoulder girdle strength
Sit-ups -- strength of abdominal and hip flexor muscles
Shuttle Run -- speed and change of direction

Standing Broad Jump -- leg power
50 Yard Dash -- speed
Softball Throw -- skill and coordination
600 Yard Run-Walk -- cardiovascular efficiency (heart-lung test)

SCORING: The scoring table above shows three lines under each test item. The student score is the actual score your child received on each test. Also shown is the average score of our Darien youngsters and average score for the nation. The national average and the Darien average allow you to make comparisons with your youngster's score.

AWARDS: The column on the extreme right is used for indicating if your youngster scored sufficiently well to win a fitness award.
Awards are made on the following basis:
1. Presidential - Must score on or above the 85th Percentile on all tests.
2. Gold - Must score on or above the 80th Percentile on all tests.
3. Silver - Must score on or above the 50th Percentile on all tests.
The purpose of giving the test is to determine the physical fitness level of your child and as one measure of the effectiveness of the program in the school. It has no bearing on any grades given on report cards. The Physical Education department is continually modifying its program to give increased emphasis to the more vigorous type activities, especially for children whose performance on the tests fell below average. It is recommended that parents encourage their children to participate regularly in physical activity.

Questions relative to interpretation and what can be done to improve the level of fitness should be directed to the teacher of physical education in your child's school.

*AMERICAN ASSOCIATION FOR HEALTH, PHYSICAL EDUCATION AND RECREATION

Figure 113. Fitness Progress Report employed by Darien Public School System, Darien, Conn.

scored. To obtain the fitness test mark, the five percentile scores are averaged. Notice also that space has been provided for recording a mark in the sports skills area as well as for citizenship. From the circle, which shows the emphasis placed on each category, observe the many factors that go into making up the mark for each of the three areas. Note too that the card is issued twice a year and may be used over a four-year period.

To be sure, this card does not represent a model marking scheme, nor will it necessarily fit every situation. It is merely a guide from which the physical educator may derive ideas for initiating a marking system, or perhaps for improving the one already in effect.

Figure 113 contains a fitness progress report currently in use at Darien, Connecticut. The parent, current physical education teacher and next year's physical education teacher each receive a copy, while one is maintained for the pupil's cumulative record.

These approaches to recording marks in physical education offer excellent opportunities to establish good relations with the parent. In addition, they are also a means of elevating your profession in the eyes of the school administrator as well as in the estimation of the parent and child. They are significantly removed from the "S" and "U" or "P" and "F" basis of marking too frequently practiced in our profession.

As was mentioned earlier, the youngster with a handicap cannot be marked in accordance with the general marking scheme. It is better to evaluate the handicap and decide upon realistic goals for the child to reach. By so doing, standards for marking on an individual basis can be established.

BIBLIOGRAPHY

1. Bahmeier, E. C.: Principles Pertaining to Marking and Reporting Pupil Progress. The School Review, January, 1951.
2. Bookwalter, Karl: Personal correspondence. University of Indiana, 1957. (See also: Marking in Physical Education. J. A. A. Health, Phys. Educ. & Recreation, Vol. 7, No. 1, January, 1936.)
3. Davis, Elwood C., and Lawther, John D.: Successful Teaching in Physical Education. 2nd ed. New York, Prentice-Hall, Inc., 1948, p. 578.
4. Laporte, William Ralph: The Physical Education Curriculum. Los Angeles, Parker and Co., 1951.
5. Mathews, Donald K.: Unpublished data. Washington State College, Pullman, Washington, 1956.
6. McCloy, Charles H., and Young, Norma Dorothy: Tests and Measurements in Health and Physical Education. 3rd ed. New York, Appleton-Century-Crofts, Inc., 1954, p. 285.
7. McCormick, H. J.: A Grading Procedure for the Physical Education Activity Program. J. A. A. Health Phys. Educ. & Recreation, December, 1947.
8. Moriarty, Mary J.: How Shall We Grade Them? J. A. A. Health, Phys. Educ. & Recreation, January, 1951.
9. Wood, Marian: Standards for Determining Semester Grades in Physical Education. Paper read before Society of Directors of Physical Education for College Women at its annual meeting in 1922.

chapter 14

organization and administration of the measurement program

One of the greatest services that the physical educator can render to a community is to care for the physical fitness of its children. In addition to maintaining the fitness of his pupils, the physical educator should seek to identify the sub-fit child, to determine the causes of low fitness, and ameliorate them by devising a program of individual development for the child. In order to fulfill these objectives, measurement is vital.

Components of measurement schedule. The basic components of a measurement schedule include:

1. Selection of test.
2. Skill and techniques in administering the test.
3. Application of results.

For purposes of presentation it seems best to treat each one of these three categories separately. One should keep in mind that the application of the principles involved in the conduct of the measurement program pertains to a small school or a large city system.

Selection of test. Certainly the primary consideration in selecting a test or tests will be the purpose or objective you wish to accomplish. What specifically do you wish to measure: sports skills, motor fitness, strength, nutritional status, mechanical symmetry, cardiovascular fitness, or social status? Is the purpose of the test to classify pupils, to determine student status to measure progress, or to provide an objective means for marking? Once this purpose has been decided upon, the criteria of scientific authenticity (reliability, objectivity and validity) administrative feasibility, and educational application must be applied in making the final decision as to which test you will use.

Skills and techniques in administering the test. The first step that the instructor must take is to orient himself and the pupils as to the proper testing procedures for a given test. This may be done by the instructor's writing out the proper directions as a first step in administering the test. Next, the pupils should be oriented and permitted to practice the tests prior to the time of the actual test day. Not only should the youngsters be taught proper techniques, but they should also be informed as to the reasons for the tests, with the instructor pointing out what the results may mean to them. Obviously, the more complex the test, the more time should be devoted to the training period.

As an illustration, Mathews, in the administration of the PFI, set up an experiment to observe the amount of improvement that might occur using experienced subjects and experienced examiners, as compared with inexperienced subjects and examiners.[2] A group of forty college physical education majors who had not experienced taking the test previously were given it for the first time by examiners selected from a class in tests and measurements. Although the student examiners had never administered the test, they were instructed by experienced testers, as to the proper techniques involved. One week later the same forty subjects, now considered as being oriented, for they had taken the test once, were again administered the PFI test, this time by trained examiners. It was found from this study that the experienced subjects, with trained testers administering the test, increased their scores significantly on every item. There was an average gain of seventeen points for the PFI score.

This experiment has a fault in that it does not indicate which factor contributed most to the difference in scores—the ability of the trained testers or the learning involved in taking the tests. However, the study does illustrate that care must be taken to make certain that the pupils and the examiners know what they are doing.

After the pupils have practiced the tests, the examiners should draw a flow chart on paper. An example appears in Figure 114. This is a diagram of the testing area with each of the testing stations labeled. In constructing such a diagram one should keep in mind the following points:

1. Stations should be arranged in order from the least strenuous test to most strenuous, unless the order is otherwise specified in the test directions.

2. Stations should be clearly marked with numbers or letters.

3. There should be sufficient space around each station to assure that the subject does not feel restricted in taking the test.

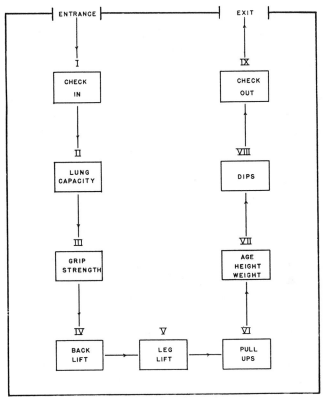

Figure 114. Flow chart for testing area.

4. If one test requires quite a bit of time, it is desirable to have two identical stations in order to have a continuously moving group. For example, in administering the PFI battery it is best to have two leg-lift stations, for this is a slow test to administer.

5. One should not schedule more tests than can be conveniently administered during the testing period. It is better to spend more time and make sure that the pupils have been well tested than to rush through an entire test in one or two days.

It is most helpful to have a practice run once the flow chart or system by which the pupils pass from one station to the next is established on paper. This is like a dress rehearsal before the big event. The instructor should select ten or fifteen pupils and have them go through the test as it is planned to be conducted on the testing day. This is a valuable practice, for it will make obvious the problems that might cause serious delays in the flow of pupils from one testing station to the next. If student leaders are to assist in collecting data, they should be on hand for the practice run so that the instructor can make certain that the tests are being administered properly.

Tests that contain items of endurance, such as runs, continuous sit-ups, or squat jumps, should not be administered without good knowledge of the pupils' condition. It is best to work gradually on each exercise over a period of at least two weeks, giving an opportunity for each youngster to be tested without such complications as stomach upsets or complaints about sore muscles. In this manner you will obtain a more valid test score, because apprehension and inexperience are largely eliminated. You yourself will develop a better understanding of what is to be expected on the testing day, and hence can make more efficient plans.

It should be decided what method is to be used in recording the test scores. There are two ways in which this can be done. One system is to have a "carry card." Each pupil as he enters the testing area receives a card on which appears space for such items as his name, class, age, height, and weight. In addition, each test is listed, enabling the tester to record his test score on the card as the pupil moves from station to station. The second method is to have at each station one sheet on which all the names have been recorded. The only advantage to this latter method is that the pupils do not have access to their test scores.

If one were to administer the AAHPER test to his pupils, it would be primarily as a screening measure. This is true with all tests of the motor fitness variety. That is, the test is sufficiently definitive to select at least three groups of children: the highly fit, the average, and the sub-fit. This of course is the purpose of the test, and once the sub-fit are located a greater variety of tests may be used, including the more definitive tests. For example, Figure 115 contains a record card the author uses in his testing situation for a more thorough evaluation of the child's fitness status. As you can see, it includes many aspects of evaluation in physical education and takes about one and one-half hours to complete. Once all the information is compiled, the physical educator can then decide what type of program should be initiated.

Application of test results. Once the test has been administered it is expected that the techniques, as established in Chapter 3, will be followed for the analysis of the test scores. Usually one will find that approximately 20 per cent of the pupils will be considerably deficient in terms of the general fitness test. These youngsters must then be sorted out for further study and follow-up procedures. There are four steps to be taken in handling this important part of the program:

1. All pertinent information that might have bearing upon the possible cause or causes of the child's low fitness should be collected. Clarke's case study form (Fig. 116) might well be used to gather this information and keep it as a part of the pupil's permanent record on file in the physical education office.

2. A personal interview should be held with the pupil; the purpose is twofold: to establish rapport with the child, and to determine the cause

SUBJECT:_____   Age: _____   _____
                                                 Weight: _____   _____
                                                 Height: _____   _____

I. GENERAL FITNESS:

    A. Physical Fitness Index:

        1. Lung Capacity   _____   _____

        2. Back Strength   _____   _____

        3. Leg Strength   _____   _____

        4. Right Grip Strength   _____   _____

        5. Left Grip Strength   _____   _____

        6. Push-ups   _____   _____

        7. Pull-ups   _____   _____

        8. Arm Strength   _____   _____

        Obtained Strength   _____   _____

        Normal Strength Index   _____   _____

        Physical Fitness Index   _____   _____

    B. Cardiovascular Fitness:
       (Harvard Step Test — short form)
       Index =   _____   _____

    C. Nutritional Status:
       Wetzel Grid   _____   _____

    D. Biceps Girth:
       Right   _____   _____
       Left   _____   _____

    E. Blood Pressure:
       Systolic   _____   _____
       Diastolic   _____   _____

    F. Chest:
       Relaxed   _____   _____
       Inspiration _____   _____

    G. Mechanical Symmetry:

    H. General Coordination:

    I. Motor Fitness:
        1. Explosive Power   _____   _____
        2. Two-minute Sit-ups   _____   _____
        3. Burpee (30 sec.)   _____   _____
        4. Pull-ups   _____   _____
        5. Dips   _____   _____

Figure 115. Record form for refined evaluation of general fitness.

II. MOTOR ABILITY:

III. BODY TYPE:

RECOMMENDATIONS:

Figure 115. (Continued.)

or causes of his low level of fitness. The Clarke health-habit questionnaire has been especially prepared to survey the child's health habits (Fig. 117). This questionnaire may be filled out by the physical educator as he interviews the child, or the older pupils may fill out the forms by themselves. In establishing rapport, use may be made of the commonly known fact that girls want to be beautiful and boys desire to be strong, with a well-proportioned physique. These, then, can be wise avenues of approach used by the instructor in establishing a willingness on the part of the boy or girl to improve his fitness level.

Case-Study Data Sheet

I. *Physical Objective Test Data*

Date of Test									
Strength Index									
Normal Strength Index									
Physical Fitness Index									
PFI Deviation from proportional									

II. *Somatotype:* ....

III. *Academic Status*

Intelligence quotient: ....

Scholastic Record:

1. Date: .... Record:...

2. Date: .... Record: ....

3. Date: .... Record: ....

IV. *Individual PFI - Somatotype - I.Q. Synthesis:*

V. *Weight Record*

Date									
Height									
Weight									
Per Cent Above or Below Normal									
Gain or loss in weight									

VI. *Mechanical and Functional Impairment*

VII. *Medical Examination*

	Date	Summary of Findings	Physician
Examination prior to Physical Fitness Test			
Re-Examination			
Re-Examination			

VIII. *Recent Illnesses, Accidents, and Operations*

Date	Condition	Physician's Recommendation

Figure 116. Clarke case-study form. (Courtesy of H. H. Clarke, University of Oregon.)

IX. *Faulty Health Habits*

Date	Faulty Habits	Recommendations	Interviewer

X. *Social Adjustment*

XI. *Posture Appraisal*

XII. *Nurse's Report*
(Indicate economic status of family)

XIII. *Physical Fitness Council*
(Give date and summary of suggestions)

XIV. *Clinical or Other Services*
(Give date and explanation of services)

XV *Treatment, and Results*

XVI. *Summary of Case*

Figure 116. (Continued.)

3. Once the physical educator ascertains the cause or causes of low fitness, an individual program on the basis of the findings should be initiated. This at first may appear difficult to get launched because of the frequently overcrowded schedule of the physical educator. However, there are ways to get a developmental and remedial program started if there is a strong desire on the part of the instructor to do so.

In the first place, we should recognize the fact that those children who are seriously deficient in skills ability should in some instances be kept out of the regular physical education program. The most obvious reason for this is that it avoids a very undesirable social situation for the pupil in question as well as for the entire class. No youngster wants to be ridiculed by his own age group; and this may happen in a physical education class. As an illustration, let us suppose that a class in apparatus is being conducted and the pupils are performing "skin-the-cat" on the horizontal bar. One of the pupils is an obese youngster who does not have the arm strength to hold his body up, let alone perform a skill on the bar. When his turn comes his failure provides an excellent opportunity for his group to chide him. This can easily result in an emotional jolt for the child. It is not a good situation for either the child or the group. Then, too, in relays sometimes the children are permitted to choose sides. Have you ever heard, "Oh, we don't want him; he can't run"? We must recognize that it is not good to allow such harmful social situations to develop. They can be overcome by creating a special class for the sub-fit pupils.

Health-Habit Questionnaire
(Second Revision)

Name: ....   Grade: .... Date: ....
        (Print last name first)

Instructions: Please answer as carefully and accurately as you can each of the following questions concerning your health habits. You are asked for this information in order that your physical education teacher may help you to improve your physical condition. Your answers will be kept confidential.

1. How many hours do you sleep each night?...................... Is your sleep restful?.....................................

   Do you sleep with your windows open at night?.......... Are you warm at night (especially in the winter)?.......

2. Are you usually rested and refreshed in the morning?................................. Drowsy?...........................

   Are you sleepy during the day?............................... In class?.............. When studying?............... ....

   Do you take a nap during the day?........................... How often? .... For how long?.....................

   Do you work and play without being more than comfortably tired mentally or physically at bed time?.....Fatigued?....

   Do you get to sleep easily at night?..................................... If not, why?...

3. Are your living conditions congenial?.....Depressing?....Do you have a room for yourself?.....Bed for yourself?.....

4. Are you often "on edge", nervous, or jittery?........................ Is it difficult for you to relax?...................

   Are you subject to worries?.......... Moods?.......... Usually cheerful?.......... Are you really happy?............

5. How far do you live from school?............................ How do you get to school?...............................

   What time do you leave in the morning?........................ When, home at night?...................................

   How much time do you usually study at home each school day?...

   How much time do you usually work at outside employment (or chores) each school day?...........................

   What do you do?...

6. Do you have a hobby?.......... What is it?...

   How many hours per day of physical activity do you usually get outside of school hours?.......What do you do?......

   What organizations do you belong to?...

   What social activities do you participate in with mixed groups (boys and girls)?.............. How often?..........

   What extra-curricular school activities do you take part in?..
   ....

   What do you do with your spare time?...
   ....

7. Please check (X) the frequency with which you have the following?

	Never	Seldom	Occasionally	Often
a. Headaches				
b. Colds				
c. Sore throat				
d. Ear ache				
e. Indigestion				
f. Bad breath				
g. Coated tongue (bad taste)				
h. Pimples or skin eruptions				
i. Boils				
j. Twitching face and eyelids				
k. Eye strain				
l. Sinus infections				
m. Foot trouble				
n. Joint pains				

Do you wear glasses?.......... If so, when were they last tested?.............. Do you hear well?...................

Figure 117. Clarke health-habit questionnaire. (Courtesy of H. H. Clarke, University of Oregon.)

To get such a program in operation, one high school used the varsity team members as leaders in working with the developmental and remedial classes, a device similar to the buddy system. The coach and director of physical education noted through the measurement program that some of their athletes had limited strength, which could be improved by a progressive resistance exercise program. Thus, by teaming the athletes with the sub-fit children, a developmental and remedial program was put into effect simultaneously.

Not until the system had been in operation for a couple of weeks were the coach and director in for a pleasant surprise. They observed a

8. Do you eat three meals a day regularly?......Is your appetite good?......Do you eat at the school cafeteria at noon?...

Carry your lunch?.......... Go home for lunch?.......... What do you usually eat at noon?...........................

....

Do you eat between meals? (Check) Never .... Seldom .... Often .... Usually ....

What do you eat between meals?...

9. How often do you usually eat each of the following kinds of food (check):

	Very Seldom	Once Each Week	Three Times Each Week	Once Each Day	Twice Each Day	Three Times Each Day
a. Meat (including fish and eggs)						
b. Green vegetables (spinach, cabbage, lettuce, etc.)						
c. Other vegetables (carrots, peas, beans, beets, etc.)						
d. Potatoes						
e. Rice, Macaroni						
f. Pie, cake, pastry						
g. Candy, sweets						
h. Fresh fruit						
i. Salads						
j. Oranges, tomatoes						
k. Dried fruits (prunes, apricots, figs, etc.)						
l. Cereals						
m. Pork						
n. Fried foods						
o. Whole wheat foods						

10. How many glasses of water do you usually drink daily?........How many glasses of milk?......Tea?......Coffee?..

11. Are you troubled with constipation?........................ What do you do to correct it?................................

12. Do you smoke?............... If so, how much daily?..

Do you drink alcoholic beverages? .... If so, what?..................... How often?........... How much?........

13. How often do you visit the dentist?.................... How often do you usually clean your teeth?.....................

14. Have you been vaccinated?............ Immunized for diphtheria?..................... Typhoid?..........................

What other immunizations?...

15. Are you parents healthy and physically fit?............... If not, what is the reason?................................

What is the physical stature of your father?   Tall................. Medium................. Short ....
                                                Fat................. Average................. Thin ....

What is the physical stature of your mother?   Tall................. Medium................. Short ....
                                                Fat................. Average................. Thin ....

16. Do you desire to be strong and physically fit (boys)?......... Do you wish to be attractive (girls)?...............

Are you satisfied with your present physical condition?..

If your *Physical Fitness Index* is low, can you account for it?............. How?..

....

Summary of Interview: ....

Produced by
Fred Medart Products, Inc.
St. Louis, Mo.

Figure 117. (Continued.)

definite improvement in outlook and behavior in a number of athletes. Apparently they were taking their newly acquired responsibilities seriously and as a result were developing desirable, mature qualities of leadership and appreciation.

Some children may take part in the regular program and at the same time be receiving additional help. Obviously, the final judgment as to whether or not the child should be kept out of the regular program entirely is dependent upon the individual case, and what particular part of the program is being taught. For example, in activities where weight is an asset, as in a tug-of-war, our obese pupil would be desired by all as the anchor man.

4. There are times when a physical educator will come across a child with a poor fitness score and, because of the complexity of the symptoms, will not be able to determine clearly the cause of the low fitness. When such cases present themselves, it is the physical educator's duty to call upon the various specialists in the school and the community to aid in determining the seat of the trouble and to take steps for its amelioration. Frequently, much can be gained through the organization of a *fitness council*.

Physical fitness, as described in Chapter 1, because of its broad implications, is not only the concern of the physical educator but also of all specialists working in the school educational program. On this basis, then, all personnel in the school whose background and training would contribute to understanding the general fitness of the child should be organized as a group or a committee. Greater insight and understanding of the children's needs would be gleaned by the coordinated efforts of these specialists. Hence a more effective approach to the solution of a given problem could be made.

This group of experts should meet only when there is a need. That is, when the physical educator discovers, through his measurement program, a pupil whose fitness problem does not have any immediately apparent cause. In this case the available records of the child would be brought before this panel of specialists for consultation and recommendation of a course of action.

In addition to the physical educator, the council should consist of at least the following experts: the guidance director, the school nurse, the dietician or home economics teacher, the classroom teacher, a physician, a parent, and the principal.

The *guidance director,* or *counselor,* is a key person in the measurement program. He will have in his files pertinent data on the pupils, collected by such school personnel as the principal, the nurse, and the classroom teacher, and data from his own testing program. This material would include such information as the results of the medical examination, academic index, anecdotal records, and personality test scores. Actually, the guidance office might be compared to a central intelligence agency since it functions as a center where all the available information concerning a pupil may be found.

In most instances the guidance director gathers useful information about the child, but does not necessarily counsel or guide each youngster. Guidance is left up to the individual teachers; and, because of his unique position, the physical educator and the guidance director can effectively join forces in "seeing through Johnny, and seeing Johnny through."

The *school health nurse* is also a very important person in this measurement scheme, for she is the liaison between the school, the physician, and the parent. In addition to rendering follow-up services, she is vital in serving as a medical consultant to the physical educator.

The *dietician* or *home economics teacher* can contribute information relative to diet and other nutritional problems that may be basic to the cause of low fitness among some children. Too frequently the valuable services of this specialist are overlooked in the measurement program.

Because the *classroom teacher* has charge of the pupil as much as six hours a day, she has the opportunity to become most familiar with a child's behavior characteristics and home background. As a result she is a valuable source in gaining more insight relative to a particular child's problems.

The *physician* is of value in determining the pupils who should be referred for a medical examination to ascertain causes of low fitness. He will aid in deciding whether a child should be placed in a restricted program and in selecting the activities that should be included in the developmental and remedial portions of the physical education program.

A *parent* should be on the council to represent the interests of all the mothers and fathers. He or she can contribute in terms of parental reaction to the program and help in disseminating information relative to the purposes and actions of the council to such agencies as the Parent-Teacher Association.

The *school administrator* or *principal* has as his chief concern the cooperative efforts of his entire staff in accomplishing the aims of education. Therefore he is in position to aid in coordinating the entire program of the council.

Thus, the function of the fitness or health council, whatever the name may be, is to study the data that have been gathered on a particular child and recommend proper action in ameliorating the unsatisfactory condition. For example, the council might recommend that a child be referred to a medical specialist for examination. If the family was hard pressed, then the council would aid in locating financial help. Thus the duty of this group of specialists is twofold: to recommend procedures for locating cause or causes of low fitness, and to follow up the recommendation to see that action is forthcoming.

The medical examination. Many school systems require that a medical examination be administered at the beginning of each school year. At this time children who should not participate in a strenuous

SPECIAL ADAPTATIONS OF PHYSICAL EDUCATION TO
MEET INDIVIDUAL NEEDS

_____School

To Dr._____Family Physician   Date_____

Regarding the physical education activities of your patient_____

_____, we shall appreciate your cooperation in filling out

this blank and returning it at your earliest convenience to_____

_____, principal of_____School.

All pupils registered in the schools are required by the Education Law to attend courses of instruction in physical education. These courses are required to be adapted to meet individual pupil needs. This means that a pupil who is unable to participate in the entire program should have his activities modified to meet and/or improve his condition.

Specific activities are provided for children who are below par physically and require special attention for the following conditions:

(Check the condition which applies to this pupil)

_____Postoperative   _____Defective posture (functional)

_____Convalescent   _____Flabby musculature

_____Faulty nutrition   _____Foot defects

_____Early fatigue   _____Others (specify)

_____Cardiac

The following is a general list of activities included in the physical education program:

V = Vigorous; M = Mild; N = None

V	M	N		V	M	N	
			Apparatus				Swimming
			Athletics				Recreational sports
			Dual combat				Marching tactics
			Self-testing stunts				Quiet games
			Calisthenics and free exercises				Corrective exercises
			Mimetics				Rest
			Rhythms and dances				
			Running games				

This is to certify that I have examined_____

and recommend that he should participate only in the activities that are checked

above for a period of _____ weeks.

Remarks:_____

_____

_____Family Physician   Date_____

Note. This report will be attached to the child's school health record and a duplicate made for the physical education office.

Figure 118. Questionnaire for children with medical excuses.

physical education program are screened out. However, just because the physician has found cause to exclude a child from physical education is not sufficient reason for the youngster to be placed on the shelf and forgotten. Rather, the physical educator should work with the medical specialist to determine if a less strenuous program might be established for the child, depending, of course, upon the condition or illness. Figure 118 contains a questionnaire that may prove useful with children who have received medical excuses. Quite frequently there are situations in which the child would gain much if the physical educator and the medical people would more closely coordinate their efforts.

Selection of tests in the program.   Tests in physical education may be classified into eight areas, as follows: physiological; body mechanics; nutrition; strength; motor fitness; general motor ability; skills, and social evaluation. Certainly the physical educator must limit his choice of tests relevant to the needs in the program. However, he should include as a minimum some type of evaluation in the areas of general physical fitness and body mechanics.

Once tests of general fitness and body mechanics screening evaluation have been administered, the youngsters who are found to be deficient constitute for the most part the developmental and remedial group. It is with this group that more definitive measurements relative to the deficiency may be applied. Such evaluation might include nutritional tests, physiological tests, and the more specific measures found in the area of body mechanics.

Skill and knowledge tests, as was stated earlier, are to be used for marking, classification, equating teams, and determining progress. As there are tests for almost every skill, it is recommended that only the major activities in the program be evaluated in order to expedite the measurement scheme.

The use of rating scales and similar tests for evaluating social efficiency should be used with prudence. However, the characteristics included in the rating scales may effectively be used as a criterion in the subjective evaluation of children's behavior patterns. Those youngsters who have an apparent unsatisfactory level of adjustment should be more carefully observed. It is with these youngsters that the anecdotal record may prove helpful in determining the cause or causes of maladjustment, and provide useful information in constructing a program for the child. It seems doubtful, in respect to the advantages that would be forthcoming, that a rating sheet should be kept on every child. Perhaps the most practical method of evaluating group structure and individual status, for the physical educator, is use of sociometric tests.

BIBLIOGRAPHY

1. Barrow, Harold M.: The ABC's of Testing. Journal AAHPER, May-June 1962, pp. 35–37.
2. Mathews, Donald K.: Comparison of Testers and Subjects in Administering Physical Fitness Index Tests. Research Quart., 24:442–445, 1953.

appendix A

table of square roots of numbers from 1 to 1000

Using the Table

To find the square root of 220, look down the number column and read the square root directly opposite the number. For example, on page 408, you will find that the square root of 220 is 14.832. To find the square root of 3.75, look up 375 under the number column. Record the number under the square root column opposite, moving the decimal point one place to the left. The square root of 375 (p. 409) is 19.363. The square root of 3.75 is 1.9363. To find the square root between two whole numbers you must interpolate. For example, to find the square root of 37.5:

$$
\begin{array}{ll}
\text{Square root of 38} & = 6.164 \\
\text{Square root of 37} & = -6.083 \\
\hline
& .081
\end{array}
$$

$$.5 \times .081 = .0405$$

$$
\begin{array}{ll}
\text{Square root of 37.5} = & 6.083 \\
+ & .0405 \\
\hline
& 6.1235
\end{array}
$$

Number	Square root	Number	Square root
1	1.000	51	7.141
2	1.414	52	7.211
3	1.732	53	7.280
4	2.000	54	7.348
5	2.236	55	7.416
6	2.449	56	7.483
7	2.646	57	7.550
8	2.828	58	7.616
9	3.000	59	7.681
10	3.162	60	7.746
11	3.317	61	7.810
12	3.464	62	7.874
13	3.606	63	7.937
14	3.742	64	8.000
15	3.873	65	8.062
16	4.000	66	8.124
17	4.123	67	8.185
18	4.243	68	8.246
19	4.359	69	8.307
20	4.472	70	8.367
21	4.583	71	8.426
22	4.690	72	8.485
23	4.796	73	8.544
24	4.899	74	8.602
25	5.000	75	8.660
26	5.099	76	8.718
27	5.196	77	8.775
28	5.292	78	8.832
29	5.385	79	8.888
30	5.477	80	8.944
31	5.568	81	9.000
32	5.657	82	9.055
33	5.745	83	9.110
34	5.831	84	9.165
35	5.916	85	9.220
36	6.000	86	9.274
37	6.083	87	9.327
38	6.164	88	9.381
39	6.245	89	9.434
40	6.325	90	9.487
41	6.403	91	9.539
42	6.481	92	9.592
43	6.557	93	9.644
44	6.633	94	9.695
45	6.708	95	9.747
46	6.782	96	9.798
47	6.856	97	9.849
48	6.928	98	9.899
49	7.000	99	9.950
50	7.071	100	10.000

Number	Square root	Number	Square root
101	10.050	151	12.288
102	10.100	152	12.329
103	10.149	153	12.369
104	10.198	154	12.410
105	10.247	155	12.450
106	10.296	156	12.490
107	10.344	157	12.530
108	10.392	158	12.570
109	10.440	159	12.610
110	10.488	160	12.649
111	10.536	161	12.689
112	10.583	162	12.728
113	10.630	163	12.767
114	10.677	164	12.806
115	10.724	165	12.845
116	10.770	166	12.884
117	10.817	167	12.923
118	10.863	168	12.961
119	10.909	169	13.000
120	10.954	170	13.038
121	11.000	171	13.077
122	11.045	172	13.115
123	11.091	173	13.153
124	11.136	174	13.191
125	11.180	175	13.229
126	11.225	176	13.266
127	11.269	177	13.304
128	11.314	178	13.342
129	11.358	179	13.379
130	11.402	180	13.416
131	11.446	181	13.454
132	11.489	182	13.491
133	11.533	183	13.528
134	11.576	184	13.565
135	11.619	185	13.601
136	11.662	186	13.638
137	11.705	187	13.675
138	11.747	188	13.711
139	11.790	189	13.748
140	11.832	190	13.784
141	11.874	191	13.820
142	11.916	192	13.856
143	11.958	193	13.892
144	12.000	194	13.928
145	12.042	195	13.964
146	12.083	196	14.000
147	12.124	197	14.036
148	12.166	198	14.071
149	12.207	199	14.107
150	12.247	200	14.142

Number	Square root	Number	Square root
201	14.177	251	15.843
202	14.213	252	15.875
203	14.248	253	15.906
204	14.283	254	15.937
205	14.318	255	15.969
206	14.353	256	16.000
207	14.387	257	16.031
208	14.422	258	16.062
209	14.457	259	16.093
210	14.491	260	16.125
211	14.526	261	16.155
212	14.560	262	16.186
213	14.595	263	16.217
214	14.629	264	16.248
215	14.663	265	16.279
216	14.697	266	16.310
217	14.731	267	16.340
218	14.765	268	16.371
219	14.799	269	16.401
220	14.832	270	16.432
221	14.866	271	16.462
222	14.900	272	16.492
223	14.933	273	16.523
224	14.967	274	16.553
225	15.000	275	16.583
226	15.033	276	16.613
227	15.067	277	16.643
228	15.100	278	16.673
229	15.133	279	16.703
230	15.166	280	16.733
231	15.199	281	16.763
232	15.232	282	16.793
233	15.264	283	16.823
234	15.297	284	16.852
235	15.330	285	16.882
236	15.362	286	16.912
237	15.395	287	16.941
238	15.427	288	16.971
239	15.460	289	17.000
240	15.492	290	17.029
241	15.524	291	17.059
242	15.556	292	17.088
243	15.588	293	17.117
244	15.620	294	17.146
245	15.652	295	17.176
246	15.684	296	17.205
247	15.716	297	17.234
248	15.748	298	17.263
249	15.780	299	17.292
250	15.811	300	17.321

Number	Square root	Number	Square root
301	17.349	351	18.735
302	17.378	352	18.762
303	17.407	353	18.788
304	17.436	354	18.815
305	17.464	355	18.841
306	17.493	356	18.868
307	17.521	357	18.894
308	17.550	358	18.921
309	17.578	359	18.947
310	17.607	360	18.974
311	17.635	361	19.000
312	17.664	362	19.026
313	17.692	363	19.053
314	17.720	364	19.079
315	17.748	365	19.105
316	17.776	366	19.131
317	17.804	367	19.157
318	17.833	368	19.183
319	17.861	369	19.209
320	17.889	370	19.235
321	17.916	371	19.261
322	17.944	372	19.287
323	17.972	373	19.313
324	18.000	374	19.339
325	18.028	375	19.363
326	18.055	376	19.391
327	18.083	377	19.416
328	18.111	378	19.442
329	18.138	379	19.468
330	18.166	380	19.494
331	18.193	381	19.519
332	18.221	382	19.545
333	18.248	383	19.570
334	18.276	384	19.596
335	18.303	385	19.621
336	18.330	386	19.647
337	18.358	387	19.672
338	18.385	388	19.698
339	18.412	389	19.723
340	18.439	390	19.748
341	18.466	391	19.774
342	18.493	392	19.799
343	18.520	393	19.824
344	18.547	394	19.849
345	18.574	395	19.875
346	18.601	396	19.900
347	18.628	397	19.925
348	18.655	398	19.950
349	18.682	399	19.975
350	18.708	400	20.000

Number	Square root	Number	Square root
401	20.025	451	21.237
402	20.050	452	21.260
403	20.075	453	21.284
404	20.100	454	21.307
405	20.125	455	21.331
406	20.149	456	21.354
407	20.174	457	21.378
408	20.199	458	21.401
409	20.224	459	21.424
410	20.248	460	21.448
411	20.273	461	21.471
412	20.298	462	21.494
413	20.322	463	21.517
414	20.347	464	21.541
415	20.372	465	21.564
416	20.396	466	21.587
417	20.421	467	21.610
418	20.445	468	21.633
419	20.469	469	21.656
420	20.494	470	21.679
421	20.518	471	21.703
422	20.543	472	21.726
423	20.567	473	21.749
424	20.591	474	21.772
425	20.616	475	21.794
426	20.640	476	21.817
427	20.664	477	21.840
428	20.688	478	21.863
429	20.712	479	21.886
430	20.736	480	21.909
431	20.761	481	21.932
432	20.785	482	21.954
433	20.809	483	21.977
434	20.833	484	22.000
435	20.857	485	22.023
436	20.881	486	22.045
437	20.905	487	22.068
438	20.928	488	22.091
439	20.952	489	22.113
440	20.976	490	22.136
441	21.000	491	22.159
442	21.024	492	22.181
443	21.048	493	22.204
444	21.071	494	22.226
445	21.095	495	22.249
446	21.119	496	22.271
447	21.142	497	22.293
448	21.166	498	22.316
449	21.190	499	22.338
450	21.213	500	22.361

Number	Square root	Number	Square root
501	22.383	551	23.478
502	22.405	552	23.495
503	22.428	553	23.516
504	22.450	554	23.537
505	22.472	555	23.558
506	22.494	556	23.580
507	22.517	557	23.601
508	22.539	558	23.622
509	22.561	559	23.643
510	22.583	560	23.664
511	22.605	561	23.685
512	22.627	562	23.707
513	22.650	563	23.728
514	22.672	564	23.749
515	22.694	565	23.770
516	22.716	566	23.791
517	22.738	567	23.812
518	22.760	568	23.833
519	22.782	569	23.854
520	22.804	570	23.875
521	22.825	571	23.896
522	22.847	572	23.917
523	22.869	573	23.937
524	22.891	574	23.958
525	22.913	575	23.979
526	22.935	576	24.000
527	22.956	577	24.021
528	22.978	578	24.042
529	23.000	579	24.062
530	23.022	580	24.083
531	23.043	581	24.104
532	23.065	582	24.125
533	23.087	583	24.145
534	23.108	584	24.166
535	23.130	585	24.187
536	23.152	586	24.207
537	23.173	587	24.228
538	23.195	588	24.249
539	23.216	589	24.269
540	23.238	590	24.290
541	23.259	591	24.310
542	23.281	592	24.331
543	23.302	593	24.352
544	23.324	594	24.372
545	23.345	595	24.393
546	23.367	596	24.413
547	23.388	597	24.434
548	23.409	598	24.454
549	23.431	599	24.474
550	23.452	600	24.495

Number	Square root	Number	Square root
601	24.515	651	25.515
602	24.536	652	25.534
603	24.556	653	25.554
604	24.576	654	25.573
605	24.597	655	25.593
606	24.617	656	25.612
607	24.637	657	25.632
608	24.658	658	25.652
609	24.678	659	25.671
610	24.698	660	25.690
611	24.718	661	25.710
612	24.739	662	25.729
613	24.759	663	25.749
614	24.779	664	25.768
615	24.799	665	25.788
616	24.819	666	25.807
617	24.839	667	25.826
618	24.860	668	25.846
619	24.880	669	25.865
620	24.900	670	25.884
621	24.920	671	25.904
622	24.940	672	25.923
623	24.960	673	25.942
624	24.980	674	25.962
625	25.000	675	25.981
626	25.020	676	26.000
627	25.040	677	26.019
628	25.060	678	26.038
629	25.080	679	26.058
630	25.100	680	26.077
631	25.120	681	26.096
632	25.140	682	26.115
633	25.159	683	26.134
634	25.179	684	26.153
635	25.199	685	26.173
636	25.219	686	26.192
637	25.239	687	26.211
638	25.259	688	26.230
639	25.278	689	26.249
640	25.298	690	26.268
641	25.318	691	26.287
642	25.338	692	26.306
643	25.357	693	26.325
644	25.377	694	26.344
645	25.397	695	26.363
646	25.417	696	26.382
647	25.436	697	26.401
648	25.456	698	26.420
649	25.475	699	26.439
650	25.495	700	26.458

Number	Square root	Number	Square root
701	26.476	751	27.404
702	26.495	752	27.423
703	26.514	753	27.441
704	26.533	754	27.459
705	26.552	755	27.477
706	26.571	756	27.495
707	26.589	757	27.514
708	26.608	758	27.532
709	26.627	759	27.550
710	26.646	760	27.568
711	26.665	761	27.586
712	26.683	762	27.604
713	26.702	763	27.622
714	26.721	764	27.641
715	26.739	765	27.659
716	26.758	766	27.677
717	26.777	767	27.695
718	26.796	768	27.713
719	26.814	769	27.731
720	26.833	770	27.749
721	26.851	771	27.767
722	26.870	772	27.785
723	26.889	773	27.803
724	26.907	774	27.821
725	26.926	775	27.839
726	26.944	776	27.857
727	26.963	777	27.875
728	26.981	778	27.893
729	27.000	779	27.911
730	27.019	780	27.928
731	27.037	781	27.946
732	27.055	782	27.964
733	27.074	783	27.982
734	27.092	784	28.000
735	27.111	785	28.018
736	27.129	786	28.036
737	27.148	787	28.054
738	27.166	788	28.071
739	27.185	789	28.089
740	27.203	790	28.107
741	27.221	791	28.125
742	27.240	792	28.142
743	27.258	793	28.160
744	27.276	794	28.178
745	27.295	795	28.196
746	27.313	796	28.213
747	27.331	797	28.231
748	27.350	798	28.249
749	27.368	799	28.267
750	27.386	800	28.284

Number	Square root	Number	Square root
801	28.302	851	29.172
802	28.320	852	29.189
803	28.337	853	29.206
804	28.355	854	29.223
805	28.373	855	29.240
806	28.390	856	29.257
807	28.408	857	29.275
808	28.425	858	29.292
809	28.443	859	29.309
810	28.460	860	29.326
811	28.478	861	29.343
812	28.496	862	29.360
813	28.513	863	29.377
814	28.531	864	29.394
815	28.548	865	29.411
816	28.566	866	29.428
817	28.583	867	29.445
818	28.601	868	29.462
819	28.618	869	29.479
820	28.636	870	29.496
821	28.653	871	29.513
822	28.671	872	29.530
823	28.688	873	29.547
824	28.705	874	29.563
825	28.723	875	29.580
826	28.740	876	29.597
827	28.758	877	29.614
828	28.775	878	29.631
829	28.792	879	29.648
830	28.810	880	29.665
831	28.827	881	29.682
832	28.844	882	29.698
833	28.862	883	29.715
834	28.879	884	29.732
835	28.896	885	29.749
836	28.914	886	29.766
837	28.931	887	29.783
838	28.948	888	29.799
839	28.965	889	29.816
840	28.983	890	29.833
841	29.000	891	29.850
842	29.017	892	29.866
843	29.034	893	29.883
844	29.052	894	29.900
845	29.069	895	29.916
846	29.086	896	29.933
847	29.103	897	29.950
848	29.120	898	29.967
849	29.138	899	29.983
850	29.155	900	30.000

Number	Square root	Number	Square root
901	30.017	951	30.838
902	30.033	952	30.854
903	30.050	953	30.871
904	30.067	954	30.887
905	30.083	955	30.903
906	30.100	956	30.919
907	30.116	957	30.935
908	30.133	958	30.952
909	30.150	959	30.968
910	30.166	960	30.984
911	30.183	961	31.000
912	30.199	962	31.016
913	30.216	963	31.032
914	30.232	964	31.048
915	30.249	965	31.064
916	30.265	966	31.081
917	30.282	967	31.097
918	30.299	968	31.113
919	30.315	969	31.129
920	30.332	970	31.145
921	30.348	971	31.161
922	30.364	972	31.177
923	30.381	973	31.193
924	30.397	974	31.209
925	30.414	975	31.225
926	30.430	976	31.241
927	30.447	977	31.257
928	30.463	978	31.273
929	30.480	979	31.289
930	30.496	980	31.305
931	30.512	981	31.321
932	30.529	982	31.337
933	30.545	983	31.353
934	30.561	984	31.369
935	30.578	985	31.385
936	30.594	986	31.401
937	30.610	987	31.417
938	30.627	988	31.432
939	30.643	989	31.448
940	30.659	990	31.464
941	30.676	991	31.480
942	30.692	992	31.496
943	30.708	993	31.512
944	30.725	994	31.528
945	30.741	995	31.544
946	30.757	996	31.559
947	30.773	997	31.575
948	30.790	998	31.591
949	30.806	999	31.607
950	30.822	1000	31.623

appendix B

suggested laboratory exercises

The highlight of the measurement course manifests itself in the laboratory, where each student is offered an opportunity to practice test administration under the trained eye of the professor. The objectives of this experience include:

1. Opportunity to select a test or tests with a specific purpose to be accomplished.

2. Preparing oneself to administer the test properly and efficiently.

3. Responsibility for preparing the test area, which includes organizing equipment, securing score cards, and drawing up directions.

4. Orienting the students to be tested.

5. Analyzing the test data for meaningful results.

6. Reporting to class on the test results, and suggesting how they might be applied in the construction of a physical education program.

The pedagogical approach to the laboratory program varies, depending upon the instructor. For example, this is the way in which the author conducts his tests and measurement laboratories:

After the lecture in which classification of testing instruments is presented, time is spent discussing in some detail the types of tests included in each of the classifications. The discussion always emphasizes the use of test results in the physical education program. Testing for the sake of testing is a waste of time.

Once the students have gained a fair understanding of the classification, two or three students are assigned an area of testing, e.g., strength, cardiovascular, motor fitness, motor ability, nutrition, skill, or body mechanics. These students then become responsible for selecting a test or tests to be administered, and for the complete organization and administration of the laboratory. After the data are gathered, the students responsible for the laboratory analyze their data by elementary statistical procedures and present the results to the class during the concluding days of the course. They are required to indicate how a physical education program might be modified in light of the test results. Not only does this give them experience in completely following through with a testing problem, but it also affords a neat summary of the entire course, permitting the class to see in a more objective way the manner in which the various tests fit into the physical education curriculum.

From data recorded as a result of tests administered in the laboratory, the students can be given practical and first-hand experience in use of their statistical procedures, and at the same time gain fundamental insight into the interrelationships of a number of test variables. Figure 119 illustrates a chart for recording such data. Sample problems for use of these data are as follows:

1. What is the relationship between leg strength and explosive power? Correlate leg lift with Sargent jump. If there is a high correlation, what significance does this have in track and field, football, and basketball?

2. Rank the students in class on the McCloy arm strength scores and then do likewise with the Rogers arm strength scores. Compute a rank difference correlation. If the relationship is low, account for it. Note the emphasis on weight in the McCloy formula, whereas the Rogers formula mathematically declares "if you are going to be large you must be strong."

3. Is the number of dips you can do related to the number of pull-ups, push-ups?

4. How well does the AAHPER test correlate with the DGWS, PFI, JCR, or Army Air Force Tests?

5. Does the Strength Index correlate well with the other so-called tests of motor ability—Newton, Humiston, Scott, Cozens?

6. Cureton found that men who habitually stand with their center of gravity more forward have straighter upper backs than do those who hold their weight less forward. Is this true of your classmates?

7. Cureton also found that men who score high on fitness stand with their weight relatively farther forward. Do your data indicate this?

8. Are leg strength and speed in running related? Explosive power and running speed?

9. If you administer a skill test, such as a badminton test, have the class play a round-robin tournament, and modify the scoring system to save time. Compute a correlation, using ρ, between the standings and the test scores. Is this a study of objectivity, reliability, or validity?

10. Do those who score high on the Brady volleyball test have better explosive power?

TEST ITEMS									
Neilson & Cozens Classification Index									
300-Yard Shuttle									
DGWS									
Squat Thrusts									
Standing Broad Jump									
Vertical Jump									
Push-ups									
PFI									
Strength Index									
Lung Capacity									
Left Grip									
Right Grip									
Back Lift									
Leg Lift									
Arm Strength (McCloy)									
Arm Strength (Rogers)									
Dips									
Pull-ups									
Center of Gravity									
Harvard Step Test									
Brady Volleyball									
AAHPER Test									
Cozens Athletic Ability									
Humiston Motor Ability									
Barrow Motor Ability									
Scott Motor Ability									
McCloy Classification Index									
NAME									

Figure 119. Chart for recording results of Tests and Measurements Laboratory.

11. Someone has suggested the substitution of the jump and reach test for the standing broad jump as a measure of explosive power, because it is more difficult to perform the latter. Do your classmates make relatively the same scores on each?

12. What is lung capacity? Is it related to any of the variables you have measured in class? Some people think it should not be included in a fitness battery, such as the PFI. What do you think? List arguments for and against.

13. Are the results of the Harvard step test (a test of cardiovascular endurance) related to the results of any other tests you have administered? Would you expect them to be related to the results of a 300-yard shuttle test?

14. Squat thrusts done in thirty seconds are supposedly a measure of agility; Barrow's zigzag run and Cozens' dodging run also are measures of agility. Are they related?

15. If one were to rank players in volleyball according to their ability and then correlate the rankings with the scores, would it be a study of validity, reliability, or objectivity? What method of correlation would you use?

16. If one person were to administer the Dyer tennis test to the same group on two successive days, and then correlate the results, would this be a study of reliability, objectivity, or validity? How would you calculate the objectivity of the test results?

17. Calculate the reliability and objectivity of a cardiovascular test.

appendix C

the New Britain system

CHARLES T. AVEDISIAN
Director of Physical Education
Darien, Connecticut

JOSEPH A. BEDARD
Director of Guidance Services
New Britain Public Schools,
New Britain, Connecticut

In the New Britain secondary schools there are a number of boys (830) who deviate from the normal in relation to the physical fitness index tests which have been administered in recent years. These boys have been aptly described in various ways. Some common terms utilized to describe them are: handicapped, crippled, atypical, retarded, deviant, and exceptional. On a more practicable level, our concern is with 471 students who deviate from the normal physical fitness score of 90 to 99, which is the New Britain norm developed on the basis of 3493 cases. In other words, these boys have special educational needs and life problems, which causes them to be classified as EXCEPTIONAL.

The research indicates that, of over four million exceptional children in the country who are attending schools, only eleven per cent receive services in terms of special classes. Here at this point the responsibility and challenge to teachers and administrators in physical education, to the school superintendents of schools, and to the boards of education remains of paramount importance in the endeavor to meet the needs of all youth in a democratic society.

The regular class program of physical education—required of all students by state law—is open to all students who have no special restrictions placed upon them or their activities. Our exceptional students either cannot successfully participate in physical education activities, or are not safe.

The modus operandi in our schools as it involves the physical education program for boys is predicated on the simple fact that students, regardless of whether they are classed as SUB-STRENGTH, NORMAL, SUPERIOR, or GIFTED should not be excused from the class program. Over-protection for the sub-strength is an old mistake still practiced by some parents and teachers. The denial of a program of physical education which will enable them to achieve the optimum development of which they are capable is not consistent with a free society which endeavors to provide a place for all children in any democratic education, especially public education. More emphasis on a student's ability than on his disability will tie him in with his peers instead of creating a vacuum of indifference and hostility.

Meaningful experiences in physical education will provide a sensible program and create new and imposing demands for teachers and the administrative staffs. This means that an effective program of coordination that involves medical staff, the parent, community groups (semi-public and private agencies) needs to be developed. Profitable time can be spent by teachers of physical education with a teacher of special education who by virtue of his special training can guide the academic and vocational education of exceptional students—or as we term them, the SUB-STRENGTH.

Professional physical educators and the research in the field substantiate the use of the term ADAPTED PHYSICAL EDUCATION for those who need "individualized physical education." Simply stated, this descriptive term is used because a student's success or failure depends to a certain extent upon the program which taps his limitations or capabilities, the careful planning of varied experiences within this realm, and, of course, the influence and extent of the enrichment of the student's present and future life as a direct result of these experiences. Thus, an adapted physical education can lay claim to including any or all of the following: improved physical fitness; psychological adjustment; social adjustment; recreational fitness, in the light of acquisition of sports skills with carry-over for later life; increased self-confidence and personal security. (Fig. 120).

DEFINITION OF EXCEPTIONAL STUDENTS

In the New Britain secondary schools, students are classed as exceptional on the basis of sub-strength classification, deaf, hard of hearing, speech problems, the orthopedically handicapped, the epileptic, socially retarded, mentally retarded, and the gifted. Also in physical education we have included cerebral palsied, cardiopathic, malnourished among the delicate; and the various delinquent and behavior problem boys are

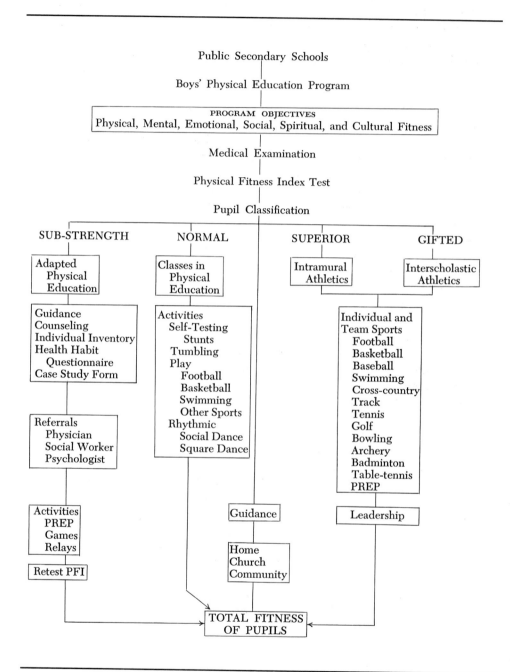

Figure 120. Adapted physical education program for boys, New Britain, Connecticut, public school system. Prepared by Charles T. Avedisian and Joseph A. Bedard.

placed in the category of the emotionally or socially maladjusted. Thus boys in physical education are categorized as exceptional when they manifest differences in mental, emotional, or behavior traits, which means that in the interest of equal educational opportunity, special provisions should be provided for their proper education.

THE NUMBER OF EXCEPTIONAL STUDENTS

The number of cases, according to the latest available records, in the United States, is an estimated 23 million persons who are handicapped to some extent by disease, accidents, maladjustments, or war. However, since we are concerned with a local situation, the figures are: 471 students who deviate from the normal physical fitness index test scores, out of a possible 3493 cases. These boys are not necessarily to be classed as suffering from heart disease, nor as epileptics, mentally retarded, and the like. However, they are sub-par physically and need to have a program that will meet their needs. The United States Office of Education reports that 441,820 who are exceptional students attended residential schools, day schools, and classes during 1947-1948. Yet 89 per cent of the estimated 4,000,000 exceptional children are attending regular schools. Many exceptional students are still without the special instruction they should have. In New Britain, our initial venture in providing for their needs in physical education is via two periods per week in junior and senior high schools, and integrated classes at the senior high level. Thus instruction needs to be improved and expanded because the load per class is not what it should be.

PHYSICAL EDUCATION AND THE EXCEPTIONAL CHILD

The handicapped child must be granted help in overcoming his disability as well as acquiring a general education in the public schools. Certain adjustments and adaptations in the program must be made. The regular class program of physical education is designed for the students who have no restrictions on their activity. On this basis there are two courses of action. First, *excuse the student* and the second has been to *place him in a "corrective program."* These are not the answers to a student's total needs or the potentialities of the entire school for the need of the students.

To excuse a student from physical education is the safe way out, but it does not meet his needs since it becomes costly to him in the long run. The inference here is not to say that physical educators advocate placing a child in a program of physical education which will aggravate an injury, cause frustration, or to make him do things which are beyond his ability.

Simply stated, we feel that excusing him is not meeting his needs. As a student in a free society where endeavors are made to live and grow with his peers in the same age group, the handicapped student must still live others. A student seeks assistance from the school and feels let down when an oversimplified solution to his problem, such as excusing him from activity, is initiated by people from whom he seeks valuable help. Study halls and the like are not the answer to engaging in selected physical activities with his peers in his own social group. Summary dismissal from participating in any kind of physical education activity for the handicapped student is not universally accepted in our schools today nor is it compatible with modern educational philosophy and its procedures. New Britain secondary schools have already sought an answer to this approach with the ADAPTED PHYSICAL EDUCATION program. The initial program of physical education—the class type which is required by state law—with one set of activities is not the answer. The adapted program provides for the special needs of the handicapped and those who are classed as sub-strength, since they need this educational experience more than those who are normal. Varied needs emphasize a call for a program that can meet individual needs of students in which all may participate. A balanced educational program—physical education in particular—must provide opportunities to all students, which, in itself, means more planning, personnel, time and inspirational teaching. Exceptional children must have the same opportunities as others if they are to have the provisions for equal education under our concept of democratic education to "seek and gain from every part of the curriculum that which is available to them."

CORRECTIVE CONCEPT AND ITS INADEQUACIES

In many schools the CORRECTIVE type of physical education had a poor connotation in that it gave people the mistaken notion of correcting remedial conditions on the basis of special exercises. Research indicates that students cannot all be classed in the category of this concept. Many students cannot have a disability remedied through corrective exercises. In some cases, chronic illness, spastic cases, poliomyelitis, partial vision, poor hearing, various kinds of heart disorders, bone and joint injuries, and mental and emotional disturbances should not be required to take corrective exercises unless prescribed by a physician in writing. The list is long. These children should have rest, relaxation, and the like, and even restricted adapted physical education activities only after the teacher of physical education has consulted with the school physician or the student's physician. As pointed out by Stone:

> Some progress has been made in providing for handicapped children. Yet the present program leaves much to be desired. Handicapped students have all the desires and ambitions of the physically

normal. These are intensified by the handicapping condition. An outlet must be found. They need the same opportunities as non-handicapped with the following controls: adapted to the individual, medical guidance, based on educational principles. It is important that the handicapped have an experience in physical education.[1]

In far too many schools the medical phase is neglected because the medical examination is not complete in itself. Also, a corrective exercises program, as pointed out earlier, is too narrow in its approach; there is a complete lack of follow-up study; and corrective exercise as an entity in itself is not a solution. The needs of the child must be thought of and practiced in a program of Adapted Physical Education in terms of the total child. Physical education has much to offer to all children, especially with students whose needs are greater than others—the handicapped students.

THE BROADER PROGRAM—THE REAL CHALLENGE

If the age of total fitness—physical, mental, emotional, social, cultural, and spiritual—is to have any meaning for our students, then more adequate opportunities and experiences must be provided for the handicapped. A student who enrolls in a public school should have the same opportunity for maximum growth and development. Thus physical education must extend its horizon from the corrective concept of physical education to one that is individualized to all students.

No matter what the limitations, all students have certain capacities, needs, and interests, which, in essence, means that the handicapped student's needs are greater. They are not different!! What do these students who are handicapped want? They want acceptance by their peers and suitable recognition on the basis of what they earn. From this may evolve security, which is a direct result of acceptance in the process of growing up and living with friends in school. In spite of the difficulties in arriving at these goals, the handicapped student is one who is willing to work harder for the "normality" which seems to come so easily to others.

Thus in our concept of physical education we have discarded the use of the terms corrective, restricted, remedial, developmental, and rehabilitative. These terms are suggestive of many outmoded approaches: the stigma of definite differences in students, the need for permanent excuses from physical education and the natural tendency for withdrawal. Is it not better to have a student tell his parent that he is engaging in an Adapted Physical Education program of games, conditioning exercises and relays? Is it not wiser to have a program of swimming, rest, relaxation, and many other activities suited to his needs at the time of his participation? An oversolicitous approach, pampering, and excuses, are harmful to the handicapped. Thus there is needed an appropriate kind of terminology which emphasizes the student's abilities, limitations, and the degree to which there is sensible planning of student experience within this range. What does this involve? It involves closer relationship between teacher, student, and parent. An insight on the part of the teacher is needed for a thorough understanding of the total personality of the student and all his immediate needs. In the field of counseling and guidance this is known as the "personal point of view."

All of the professional research indicates the use and need of the term ADAPTED PHYSICAL EDUCATION as the most widely used and acceptable.

THE VALUE OF ADAPTED PHYSICAL EDUCATION

There are many potentialities in Adapted Physical Education which can help any handicapped student realize his goal of worthwhile citizenship both in his school life and in a rewarding adult life. Guidance techniques can help him become "intelligent and realistic" regarding the nature of his condition. They can be aided in establishing goals capable of being reached. They may learn how to protect the condition from being aggravated. In cases of permanent disability their adjustment is furthered by acquiring sports and game skills and knowledges which permit them to participate with others in selected play situations with reasonable success. Psychological and social values can result from the restoration of confidence gained through improvement or adjustment, from the development of a feeling of security stemming from improved physical function and increased capacity for recreational activities.[2]

The gains for the student in later years are of tremendous value. New friendships and socially stimulating situations while in school will pave the way for a happy student. The experience of American physical education has shown that favorable attitude towards wholesome participation in recreational sports by any student means a richer and more satisfying living both in the present and future life of the student.

---

1. Eleanor B. Stone: Physical Handicapped Children in Our Schools. J. A. A. Health, Phys. Educ. & Recreation, February, 1947, p. 67.
2. Arthur S. Daniels: Adapted Physical Education. New York, Harper & Brothers, 1954.

TABLE 46.   *Total PFI Test Scores, New Britain, Connecticut, Public Schools, 1955, 1956, 1957 (Junior and Senior High School Boys)*

Distribution of Scores				Percentile Ratings	
Score	f			PFI Score	Percentile
160–169	2			140+	100
				139	99
150–159	7		A	134	98
				129	97
140–149	35			127	96
				125	95
130–139	107		B	117	90
				112	85
120–129	227			108	80
				104	75
110–119	511		C+	101	70
				98	65
100–109	789			95	60
				93	55
90–99	1026	MEDIAN	C	90	50
				88	45
80–89	1074			85	40
				83	35
70–79	808		C−	80	30
				77	25
60–69	505			74	20
				70	15
50–59	202		D	65	10
				59	5
40–49	71			56	4
				54	3
30–39	17		E	51	2
				44−	1
20–29	3				
	N = 5,384				

A	Gifted	127 and above
B	Superior	107 to 126
C+	High Average	96 to 106
C	Average	85 to 95
C−	Low Average	72 to 84
D	Sub-strength	55 to 71
E	Referrals	54 and below

appendix D

norms for AAHPER youth fitness test

Determine the classification index from either Table 25 or 26 and enter on appropriate chart to find percentile score. For example, a child is 128 months old, 53 inches tall and weighs 68 pounds. From Table 25 the sum of the exponents would equal six. As a result the child would fall into Class A. If this youngster were a boy and performed 60 sit-ups, his percentile score would equal 70. This may be interpreted to mean that 30 per cent of the sample from which the norms were constructed scored more than 60 sit-ups whereas 70 per cent scored fewer.

Flexed Arm Hang: Girls
Percentile Scores Based on Classification Index/Test Scores in Seconds

Percentile	A	B	C	D	E	F	G	H	HSG*	Percentile
100th	72	70	80	64	61	61	64	40	76	100th
95th	39	35	35	28	31	30	17	17	34	95th
90th	29	27	27	22	23	21	13	14	25	90th
85th	24	22	23	18	20	18	11	11	20	85th
80th	21	19	20	15	17	14	11	9	17	80th
75th	18	17	18	13	14	13	9	7	14	75th
70th	16	15	16	11	12	11	8	6	13	70th
65th	14	13	14	10	11	10	7	5	11	65th
60th	12	11	12	9	9	9	6	4	10	60th
55th	11	10	10	8	8	8	5	2	8	55th
50th	10	8	9	7	7	7	4	2	8	50th
45th	9	7	8	6	6	6	3	2	6	45th
40th	8	6	7	6	5	5	2	1	6	40th
35th	7	6	6	5	4	4	2	1	4	35th
30th	6	5	5	4	3	3	1	1	4	30th
25th	5	4	4	3	3	2	0	0	2	25th
20th	4	4	3	2	2	1	0	0	2	20th
15th	3	2	2	1	1	0	0	0	1	15th
10th	2	2	1	0	0	0	0	0	0	10th
5th	1	0	0	0	0	0	0	0	0	5th
0	0	0	0	0	0	0	0	0	0	0

Classification Index

* HSG: High School Girls.

Sit-ups: Girls

Percentile Scores Based on Classification Index/Test Scores in Number of Sit-Ups

Percentile	Classification Index									Percentile
	A	B	C	D	E	F	G	H	HSG	
100th	50	50	50	50	50	50	50	50	50	100th
95th	50	50	50	50	50	50	50	50	50	95th
90th	50	50	50	50	50	50	50	50	50	90th
85th	50	50	50	50	50	50	49	48	50	85th
80th	50	50	50	50	50	50	43	43	41	80th
75th	50	50	50	50	50	49	38	39	38	75th
70th	46	50	50	47	47	44	35	35	35	70th
65th	40	46	50	40	40	40	32	34	32	65th
60th	38	40	45	37	37	36	30	30	30	60th
55th	34	35	40	33	34	34	29	29	29	55th
50th	31	32	35	31	31	31	25	27	26	50th
45th	30	30	31	30	29	30	25	25	25	45th
40th	26	27	30	27	26	27	22	23	24	40th
35th	24	26	25	25	24	25	20	21	21	35th
30th	22	22	23	22	21	23	20	20	20	30th
25th	20	20	20	20	20	21	17	18	18	25th
20th	17	18	18	18	19	20	15	15	16	20th
15th	15	16	16	16	15	16	13	14	14	15th
10th	10	13	11	13	13	13	10	12	12	10th
5th	8	9	8	10	9	10	8	9	8	5th
0	1	2	0	0	0	0	1	3	0	0

Shuttle Run: Girls
Percentile Scores Based on Classification Index/Test Scores in Seconds and Tenths

Percentile	A	B	C	D	E	F	G	H	HSG	Percentile
100th	8.5	8.8	9.0	8.9	9.0	9.0	8.3	9.3	8.0	100th
95th	9.5	10.0	10.0	9.9	10.0	10.0	10.1	10.1	10.0	95th
90th	10.2	10.5	10.2	10.2	10.2	10.2	10.3	10.5	10.2	90th
85th	10.7	10.8	10.5	10.5	10.5	10.5	10.5	10.6	10.4	85th
80th	11.0	11.0	10.8	10.8	10.6	10.5	10.6	10.8	10.6	80th
75th	11.0	11.0	11.0	11.0	10.8	10.7	10.8	10.9	10.8	75th
70th	11.1	11.2	11.0	11.0	11.0	10.9	11.0	11.0	10.9	70th
65th	11.3	11.4	11.2	11.1	11.0	11.0	11.0	11.1	11.0	65th
60th	11.5	11.6	11.4	11.3	11.1	11.0	11.2	11.3	11.0	60th
55th	11.6	11.7	11.5	11.4	11.3	11.2	11.3	11.5	11.1	55th
50th	11.8	11.8	11.5	11.6	11.5	11.4	11.5	11.6	11.3	50th
45th	12.0	11.9	11.7	11.8	11.7	11.5	11.7	11.8	11.4	45th
40th	12.0	12.0	11.9	12.0	12.0	11.7	11.8	12.0	11.5	40th
35th	12.2	12.0	12.0	12.0	12.0	11.9	12.0	12.2	11.7	35th
30th	12.5	12.2	12.0	12.1	12.1	12.0	12.0	12.4	11.8	30th
25th	12.6	12.4	12.2	12.3	12.3	12.2	12.3	12.5	12.0	25th
20th	12.9	12.5	12.5	12.6	12.5	12.5	12.5	13.0	12.1	20th
15th	13.0	12.9	12.7	12.9	12.9	13.0	12.9	13.0	12.5	15th
10th	13.5	13.1	13.0	13.3	13.2	13.5	13.3	13.5	13.0	10th
5th	14.4	14.0	13.8	14.0	14.0	14.0	14.0	14.0	13.6	5th
0	16.2	19.8	17.0	16.0	17.6	18.5	17.0	17.3	20.0	0

Standing Broad Jump: Girls

Percentile Scores Based on Classification Index/Test Scores in Feet and Inches

Percentile	A	B	C	D	E	F	G	H	HSG	Percentile
					Classification Index					
100th	7' 0"	7'10"	7'10"	7' 0"	7'10"	8' 2"	7' 4"	7' 4"	7' 8"	100th
95th	5' 8"	6' 0"	6' 2"	6' 1"	6' 4"	6' 3"	6' 3"	6' 5"	6' 7"	95th
90th	5' 5"	5' 8"	5'11"	5'11"	6' 0"	6' 1"	6' 0"	6' 2"	6' 4"	90th
85th	5' 3"	5' 6"	5' 8"	5' 8"	5'10"	5'11"	5' 9"	5'11"	6' 1"	85th
80th	5' 2"	5' 4"	5' 7"	5' 7"	5' 8"	5' 9"	5' 7"	5' 8"	6' 0"	80th
75th	5' 1"	5' 3"	5' 5"	5' 5"	5' 7"	5' 7"	5' 6"	5' 7"	5'10"	75th
70th	5' 0"	5' 2"	5' 4"	5' 4"	5' 6"	5' 6"	5' 5"	5' 6"	5' 9"	70th
65th	4'11"	5' 1"	5' 2"	5' 3"	5' 4"	5' 4"	5' 4"	5' 4"	5' 8"	65th
60th	4' 9"	5' 0"	5' 1"	5' 2"	5' 2"	5' 3"	5' 3"	5' 3"	5' 7"	60th
55th	4' 8"	4'11"	5' 0"	5' 1"	5' 1"	5' 2"	5' 2"	5' 1"	5' 6"	55th
50th	4' 7"	4'10"	4'11"	5' 0"	5' 0"	5' 1"	5' 0"	5' 0"	5' 4"	50th
45th	4' 6"	4' 8"	4'10"	4'11"	4'11"	5' 0"	5' 0"	4' 9"	5' 3"	45th
40th	4' 5"	4' 7"	4' 9"	4' 9"	4'10"	4'11"	4'10"	4' 9"	5' 2"	40th
35th	4' 4"	4' 6"	4' 8"	4' 8"	4' 8"	4' 9"	4' 9"	4' 8"	5' 0"	35th
30th	4' 4"	4' 5"	4' 6"	4' 7"	4' 7"	4' 7"	4' 7"	4' 6"	4'11"	30th
25th	4' 2"	4' 4"	4' 5"	4' 5"	4' 6"	4' 6"	4' 6"	4' 5"	4'10"	25th
20th	4' 0"	4' 2"	4' 3"	4' 4"	4' 4"	4' 4"	4' 5"	4' 4"	4' 8"	20th
15th	3'10"	4' 0"	4' 2"	4' 2"	4' 2"	4' 2"	4' 2"	4' 2"	4' 6"	15th
10th	3' 9"	3'11"	4' 0"	4' 0"	4' 0"	4' 0"	4' 0"	4' 0"	4' 4"	10th
5th	3' 6"	3' 7"	3' 7"	3'11"	3' 8"	3' 9"	3' 9"	3' 7"	4' 0"	5th
0	3' 1"	2' 8"	3' 0"	2'11"	2'11"	2'11"	3' 1"	2'11"	3' 0"	0

50-Yard Dash: Girls
Percentile Scores Based on Classification Index/Test Scores in Seconds and Tenths

Percentile	Classification Index									Percentile
	A	B	C	D	E	F	G	H	HSG	
100th	6.5	6.0	6.0	6.0	6.0	5.9	6.0	6.0	6.0	100th
95th	7.0	7.0	7.0	7.2	7.0	7.0	7.3	7.2	7.0	95th
90th	7.4	7.5	7.3	7.4	7.2	7.2	7.5	7.4	7.2	90th
85th	7.6	7.6	7.5	7.6	7.5	7.4	7.6	7.5	7.4	85th
80th	7.8	7.8	7.7	7.7	7.6	7.5	7.8	7.6	7.6	80th
75th	8.0	7.9	7.8	7.9	7.7	7.6	7.8	7.8	7.7	75th
70th	8.0	8.0	7.9	7.9	7.8	7.8	7.9	7.9	7.8	70th
65th	8.2	8.0	8.0	8.0	7.9	7.9	8.0	8.0	7.9	65th
60th	8.3	8.2	8.0	8.0	8.0	7.9	8.0	8.1	8.0	60th
55th	8.5	8.3	8.2	8.1	8.1	8.0	8.1	8.2	8.0	55th
50th	8.5	8.4	8.3	8.2	8.2	8.1	8.3	8.2	8.1	50th
45th	8.7	8.5	8.4	8.3	8.3	8.3	8.4	8.4	8.3	45th
40th	8.8	8.6	8.5	8.4	8.4	8.4	8.4	8.5	8.4	40th
35th	9.0	8.8	8.6	8.5	8.5	8.5	8.6	8.6	8.5	35th
30th	9.0	8.9	8.8	8.7	8.6	8.7	8.8	8.8	8.7	30th
25th	9.0	9.0	9.0	8.9	8.8	8.9	9.0	9.0	8.9	25th
20th	9.2	9.1	9.1	9.0	9.0	9.0	9.1	9.2	9.0	20th
15th	9.6	9.2	9.2	9.1	9.2	9.4	9.3	9.4	9.1	15th
10th	10.0	9.5	9.5	9.5	9.5	9.7	9.7	9.6	9.5	10th
5th	10.0	10.0	9.8	10.0	10.0	10.5	10.4	10.0	10.3	5th
0	11.5	11.6	11.3	12.0	14.0	15.7	13.0	11.0	18.0	0

Softball Throw: Girls
Percentile Scores Based on Classification Index/Test Scores in Feet

Percentile	A	B	C	D	E	F	G	H	HSG	Percentile
				Classification Index						
100th	167	136	133	135	141	159	143	168	183	100th
95th	78	85	90	101	106	111	111	120	121	95th
90th	71	77	85	93	99	102	102	112	110	90th
85th	66	73	80	87	92	97	100	104	103	85th
80th	63	69	76	81	87	92	92	102	98	80th
75th	58	65	73	78	84	88	90	99	93	75th
70th	55	62	71	74	80	85	87	92	90	70th
65th	52	60	68	71	76	81	85	85	86	65th
60th	51	57	65	69	74	78	81	82	82	60th
55th	50	55	61	65	70	75	78	80	80	55th
50th	48	51	59	63	67	72	75	77	75	50th
45th	46	50	57	60	64	70	73	75	74	45th
40th	45	47	54	58	61	67	70	72	71	40th
35th	42	45	52	57	60	65	67	70	69	35th
30th	40	43	49	54	56	61	65	66	66	30th
25th	38	41	46	50	53	58	60	63	63	25th
20th	34	39	44	46	50	54	58	60	60	20th
15th	32	36	40	44	47	50	53	57	55	15th
10th	30	30	37	40	43	46	48	51	50	10th
5th	19	26	32	35	39	38	44	44	45	5th
0	8	10	18	18	21	20	20	21	8	0

600-Yard Run-Walk: Girls
Percentile Scores Based on Classification Index/Test Scores in Minutes and Seconds

Percen-tile	A	B	C	D	E	F	G	H	HSG	Percen-tile
100th	1'46"	1'42"	1'46"	1'39"	1'40"	1'50"	1'55"	2' 4"	1'45"	100th
95th	2' 4"	2'10"	2'11"	2'10"	2'11"	2'13"	2'13"	2'19"	2'10"	95th
90th	2'15"	2'16"	2'17"	2'17"	2'19"	2'18"	2'22"	2'25"	2'18"	90th
85th	2'22"	2'22"	2'22"	2'23"	2'24"	2'25"	2'25"	2'30"	2'24"	85th
80th	2'25"	2'26"	2'26"	2'26"	2'27"	2'29"	2'30"	2'33"	2'27"	80th
75th	2'30"	2'30"	2'29"	2'30"	2'32"	2'33"	2'35"	2'38"	2'32"	75th
70th	2'34"	2'33"	2'32"	2'33"	2'36"	2'37"	2'40"	2'41"	2'35"	70th
65th	2'36"	2'36"	2'36"	2'37"	2'40"	2'40"	2'44"	2'46"	2'38"	65th
60th	2'41"	2'39"	2'39"	2'40"	2'43"	2'43"	2'47"	2'50"	2'42"	60th
55th	2'45"	2'43"	2'43"	2'45"	2'46"	2'47"	2'50"	2'55"	2'45"	55th
50th	2'47"	2'47"	2'45"	2'48"	2'50"	2'50"	2'54"	2'59"	2'48"	50th
45th	2'51"	2'49"	2'49"	2'51"	2'55"	2'55"	2'59"	3' 4"	2'52"	45th
40th	2'56"	2'51"	2'53"	2'55"	3' 0"	2'59"	3' 3"	3'10"	2'55"	40th
35th	3' 0"	2'55"	2'59"	3' 0"	3' 2"	3' 2"	3' 6"	3'13"	3' 0"	35th
30th	3' 5"	3' 1"	3' 3"	3' 7"	3' 6"	3' 9"	3'12"	3'16"	3' 3"	30th
25th	3' 9"	3' 7"	3'11"	3'11"	3'12"	3'13"	3'17"	3'21"	3' 9"	25th
20th	3'13"	3'13"	3'18"	3'16"	3'17"	3'18"	3'25"	3'29"	3'15"	20th
15th	3'18"	3'20"	3'25"	3'24"	3'25"	3'26"	3'43"	3'39"	3'24"	15th
10th	3'30"	3'30"	3'40"	3'38"	3'45"	3'40"	3'52"	3'48"	3'35"	10th
5th	3'45"	3'49"	3'59"	3'59"	4' 4"	4' 0"	4' 7"	4'11"	3'56"	5th
0	4'30"	4'47"	5' 0"	4'53"	5'10"	5'10"	5'50"	5'30"	6'40"	0

Pull-Ups: Elementary and Jr. High School Boys
Percentile Scores Based on Classification Index/Test Scores in Number of Pull-Ups

Percen-tile	A	B	C	D	E	F	G	H	Percen-tile
				Classification Index					
100th	16	20	16	15	18	20	17	24	100th
95th	10	8	8	9	9	11	12	12	95th
90th	8	7	7	7	8	9	10	10	90th
85th	7	6	6	6	6	8	10	10	85th
80th	5	6	5	5	5	7	8	9	80th
75th	6	5	4	5	5	6	7	8	75th
70th	5	5	4	4	4	6	6	7	70th
65th	5	4	3	4	3	5	5	7	65th
60th	4	4	3	3	3	4	5	6	60th
55th	4	3	3	3	2	4	4	6	55th
50th	3	3	2	2	2	3	4	5	50th
45th	3	3	2	2	2	3	3	5	45th
40th	3	2	1	1	1	2	2	4	40th
35th	2	2	1	1	1	2	2	3	35th
30th	2	2	1	1	1	1	1	3	30th
25th	1	1	0	0	0	1	1	2	25th
20th	1	1	0	0	0	0	0	1	20th
15th	0	0	0	0	0	0	0	1	15th
10th	0	0	0	0	0	0	0	0	10th
5th	0	0	0	0	0	0	0	0	5th
0									0

Sit-Ups: Elementary and Jr. High School Boys
Percentile Scores Based on Classification Index/Test Scores in Number of Sit-Ups

Percentile	A	B	C	D	E	F	G	H	Percentile
100th	100	100	100	100	100	100	100	100	100th
95th	100	100	100	100	100	100	100	100	95th
90th	100	100	100	100	100	100	100	100	90th
85th	100	100	100	100	100	100	100	100	85th
80th	78	83	90	100	100	100	100	100	80th
75th	70	71	75	99	99	100	100	100	75th
70th	60	60	61	78	81	99	99	100	70th
65th	54	55	55	70	73	85	95	99	65th
60th	50	50	50	60	64	70	76	90	60th
55th	50	50	50	52	57	60	70	78	55th
50th	50	45	47	50	50	55	65	70	50th
45th	40	40	40	50	50	50	56	64	45th
40th	38	36	36	41	49	49	51	60	40th
35th	32	32	32	40	41	42	50	52	35th
30th	30	30	30	35	39	39	47	50	30th
25th	27	27	28	30	35	35	40	43	25th
20th	24	24	25	28	30	30	35	39	20th
15th	21	21	22	23	25	26	30	34	15th
10th	19	18	17	20	22	22	25	30	10th
5th	14	13	12	14	16	17	14	23	5th
0	6	1	0	0	0	0	0	5	0

Classification Index

Shuttle Run: Elementary and Jr. High School Boys
Percentile Scores Based on Classification Index/Test Scores in Seconds and Tenths

Percentile	Classification Index								Percentile
	A	B	C	D	E	F	G	H	
100th	9.0	9.0	8.0	9.0	8.5	8.5	9.0	8.3	100th
95th	10.0	10.0	9.9	9.8	9.8	9.4	9.5	9.1	95th
90th	10.2	10.1	10.0	10.0	10.0	9.6	9.5	9.4	90th
85th	10.3	10.3	10.1	10.0	10.0	9.8	9.8	9.5	85th
80th	10.5	10.5	10.4	10.2	10.1	10.0	9.9	9.6	80th
75th	10.7	10.5	10.5	10.3	10.2	10.0	10.0	9.7	75th
70th	10.9	10.7	10.6	10.5	10.4	10.1	10.1	9.8	70th
65th	11.0	10.8	10.7	10.6	10.5	10.3	10.2	9.9	65th
60th	11.0	10.9	10.9	10.8	10.6	10.4	10.3	10.0	60th
55th	11.0	11.0	11.0	10.9	10.8	10.5	10.4	10.1	55th
50th	11.2	11.0	11.0	11.0	10.9	10.5	10.5	10.2	50th
45th	11.2	11.1	11.2	11.0	11.0	10.7	10.6	10.3	45th
40th	11.4	11.4	11.3	11.1	11.0	10.8	10.8	10.4	40th
35th	11.5	11.5	11.5	11.3	11.2	11.0	10.9	10.5	35th
30th	11.6	11.8	11.6	11.4	11.4	11.1	11.0	10.6	30th
25th	11.8	12.0	11.8	11.5	11.5	11.2	11.3	10.8	25th
20th	12.0	12.0	12.0	11.7	11.7	11.5	11.6	11.0	20th
15th	12.2	12.2	12.0	12.0	12.0	11.8	11.8	11.3	15th
10th	12.6	12.5	12.2	12.3	12.2	12.0	12.0	11.7	10th
5th	13.2	13.0	13.0	12.8	12.6	12.6	12.8	12.1	5th
0	15.0	20.0	15.7	13.0	14.3	14.5	22.0	16.0	0

Standing Broad Jump: Elementary and Jr. High School Boys
Percentile Scores Based on Classification Index/Test Scores in Feet and Inches

Percentile	Classification Index								Percentile
	A	B	C	D	E	F	G	H	
100th	6' 8"	6'10"	7' 2"	10' 0"	7' 9"	8'10"	8' 8"	8' 9"	100th
95th	6' 0"	6' 2"	6' 4"	6' 7"	6' 9"	7' 2"	7' 6"	7'11"	95th
90th	5'10"	5'11"	6' 2"	6' 3"	6' 6"	6'11"	7' 2"	7' 7"	90th
85th	5' 8"	5'10"	6' 0"	6' 2"	6' 4"	6' 9"	7' 0"	7' 6"	85th
80th	5' 7"	5' 9"	5' 9"	6' 0"	6' 2"	6' 8"	6'11"	7' 4"	80th
75th	5' 6"	5' 7"	5' 9"	5'11"	6' 0"	6' 6"	6' 9"	7' 3"	75th
70th	5' 5"	5' 6"	5' 7"	5'10"	6' 0"	6' 4"	6' 8"	7' 1"	70th
65th	5' 4"	5' 6"	5' 6"	5' 9"	5'10"	6' 3"	6' 5"	6'11"	65th
60th	5' 2"	5' 4"	5' 5"	5' 8"	5' 9"	6' 1"	6' 4"	6'10"	60th
55th	5' 2"	5' 3"	5' 4"	5' 6"	5' 8"	6' 0"	6' 2"	6' 8"	55th
50th	5' 1"	5' 2"	5' 3"	5' 6"	5' 6"	5'11"	6' 1"	6' 7"	50th
45th	5' 0"	5' 1"	5' 2"	5' 5"	5' 6"	5'10"	5'11"	6' 6"	45th
40th	4'11"	5' 0"	5' 1"	5' 4"	5' 4"	5' 8"	5'10"	6' 5"	40th
35th	4'10"	4'11"	5' 0"	5' 2"	5' 3"	5' 6"	5' 9"	6' 3"	35th
30th	4' 8"	4'10"	4'11"	5' 1"	5' 1"	5' 5"	5' 7"	6' 1"	30th
25th	4' 7"	4' 8"	4'10"	5' 0"	5' 0"	5' 3"	5' 5"	5'11"	25th
20th	4' 6"	4' 7"	4' 9"	4'10"	4'10"	5' 1"	5' 2"	5' 9"	20th
15th	4' 4"	4' 5"	4' 6"	4' 8"	4' 8"	4'11"	4'11"	5' 5"	15th
10th	4' 3"	4' 3"	4' 4"	4' 5"	4' 6"	4' 7"	4' 6"	5' 2"	10th
5th	4' 0"	4' 0"	4' 1"	4' 2"	4' 3"	4' 3"	4' 2"	4'10"	5th
0	3' 0"	3' 0"	2' 2"	2'10"	2'10"	1' 8"	2' 2"	3' 2"	0

50-Yard Dash: Elementary and Jr. High School Boys
Percentile Scores Based on Classification Index/Test Scores in Seconds and Tenths

Percentile	Classification Index								Percentile
	A	B	C	D	E	F	G	H	
100th	6.8	6.0	6.0	6.0	5.8	5.9	5.8	5.8	100th
95th	7.2	7.0	7.0	6.8	6.7	6.5	6.4	6.1	95th
90th	7.4	7.2	7.1	7.0	6.9	6.7	6.6	6.3	90th
85th	7.6	7.4	7.2	7.0	7.0	6.9	6.7	6.4	85th
80th	7.7	7.5	7.4	7.2	7.1	7.0	6.9	6.5	80th
75th	7.8	7.6	7.5	7.3	7.2	7.0	6.9	6.6	75th
70th	7.9	7.7	7.5	7.4	7.3	7.1	7.0	6.6	70th
65th	8.0	7.8	7.7	7.5	7.4	7.2	7.0	6.7	65th
60th	8.0	7.9	7.8	7.6	7.5	7.3	7.1	6.8	60th
55th	8.1	8.0	7.9	7.7	7.5	7.4	7.2	6.9	55th
50th	8.2	8.0	7.9	7.8	7.7	7.5	7.2	7.0	50th
45th	8.3	8.0	8.0	7.9	7.8	7.5	7.4	7.0	45th
40th	8.4	8.2	8.0	8.0	7.9	7.6	7.5	7.0	40th
35th	8.5	8.3	8.2	8.0	8.0	7.8	7.6	7.1	35th
30th	8.6	8.5	8.4	8.2	8.1	8.0	7.7	7.2	30th
25th	8.7	8.6	8.5	8.3	8.2	8.1	7.9	7.4	25th
20th	9.0	8.8	8.7	8.4	8.4	8.2	8.0	7.5	20th
15th	9.0	9.0	8.9	8.6	8.5	8.3	8.3	7.3	15th
10th	9.2	9.0	9.1	9.0	9.0	8.6	8.6	8.0	10th
5th	10.0	9.6	9.5	9.4	9.2	9.0	9.2	8.5	5th
0	11.0	11.9	10.8	10.9	12.0	11.6	12.0	9.6	0

Softball Throw: Elementary and Jr. High School Boys
Percentile Scores Based on Classification Index/Test Scores in Feet

Percen-tile	Classification Index								Percen-tile
	A	B	C	D	E	F	G	H	
100th	155	175	245	195	239	228	228	242	100th
95th	123	141	151	160	169	188	198	219	95th
90th	115	130	142	150	159	180	190	209	90th
85th	113	123	136	144	152	172	181	200	85th
80th	108	120	131	140	148	167	175	195	80th
75th	105	115	128	135	145	162	170	190	75th
70th	101	112	124	132	141	158	166	188	70th
65th	99	109	121	128	138	153	165	183	65th
60th	96	106	119	125	135	150	161	179	60th
55th	93	105	115	121	131	145	158	176	55th
50th	90	101	112	120	127	141	153	171	50th
45th	89	98	110	116	125	138	150	166	45th
40th	85	96	108	114	121	135	146	162	40th
35th	82	94	104	110	118	132	141	159	35th
30th	80	91	100	107	115	125	139	154	30th
25th	75	87	97	104	113	121	131	149	25th
20th	72	81	93	100	108	118	128	142	20th
15th	69	78	89	93	104	110	124	138	15th
10th	63	73	84	87	95	102	115	127	10th
5th	57	65	75	78	86	89	102	110	5th
0	36	14	30	31	55	25	25	44	0

600-Yard Run-Walk: Elementary and Jr. High School Boys
Percentile Scores Based on Classification Index/Test Scores in Minutes and Seconds

Percen-tile	Classification Index								Percen-tile
	A	B	C	D	E	F	G	H	
100th	1'30"	1'27"	1'32"	1'29"	1'34"	1'35"	1'30"	1'25"	100th
95th	1'53"	1'56"	1'56"	1'52"	1'51"	1'48"	1'44"	1'38"	95th
90th	2'6"	2'3"	2'2"	1'59"	1'57"	1'51"	1'46"	1'42"	90th
85th	2'10"	2'8"	2'6"	2'3"	2'0"	1'54"	1'50"	1'44"	85th
80th	2'12"	2'11"	2'9"	2'6"	2'2"	1'57"	1'52"	1'46"	80th
75th	2'15"	2'14"	2'11"	2'10"	2'5"	1'59"	1'54"	1'48"	75th
70th	2'19"	2'16"	2'13"	2'12"	2'8"	2'2"	1'56"	1'51"	70th
65th	2'22"	2'19"	2'16"	2'14"	2'11"	2'4"	1'59"	1'52"	65th
60th	2'24"	2'21"	2'19"	2'16"	2'15"	2'5"	2'0"	1'55"	60th
55th	2'28"	2'24"	2'21"	2'18"	2'16"	2'8"	2'3"	1'56"	55th
50th	2'31"	2'27"	2'24"	2'22"	2'19"	2'10"	2'5"	1'59"	50th
45th	2'34"	2'30"	2'28"	2'24"	2'22"	2'12"	2'9"	2'1"	45th
40th	2'36"	2'34"	2'31"	2'27"	2'26"	2'15"	2'11"	2'4"	40th
35th	2'40"	2'37"	2'34"	2'30"	2'29"	2'19"	2'14"	2'8"	35th
30th	2'42"	2'41"	2'38"	2'35"	2'32"	2'23"	2'18"	2'12"	30th
25th	2'45"	2'44"	2'41"	2'40"	2'36"	2'27"	2'24"	2'16"	25th
20th	2'49"	2'53"	2'45"	2'46"	2'43"	2'32"	2'30"	2'23"	20th
15th	2'54"	3'1"	2'50"	2'55"	2'53"	2'40"	2'38"	2'29"	15th
10th	3'1"	3'9"	3'2"	3'7"	3'3"	2'55"	2'56"	2'41"	10th
5th	3'21"	3'33"	3'14"	3'30"	3'21"	3'21"	3'15"	3'11"	5th
0	4'16"	5'4"	4'34"	5'6"	5'8"	5'0"	4'25"	5'14"	0

Pull-Ups: High School Boys
Percentile Scores Based on Classification Index / Test Scores in Number of Pull-Ups

Percentile	Classification Index			Percentile
	C	B	A	
100th	20	25	32	100th
95th	14	16	15	95th
90th	12	14	12	90th
85th	10	12	12	85th
80th	10	12	10	80th
75th	9	11	10	75th
70th	8	10	9	70th
65th	7	10	9	65th
60th	7	9	8	60th
55th	6	9	7	55th
50th	5	8	7	50th
45th	5	7	6	45th
40th	4	7	6	40th
35th	4	6	5	35th
30th	4	6	5	30th
25th	3	5	4	25th
20th	3	4	3	20th
15th	2	4	2	15th
10th	1	3	1	10th
5th	0	2	0	5th
0	0	0	0	0

Sit-Ups: High School Boys
Percentile Scores Based on Classification Index/Test Scores in Number of Sit-Ups

Percentile	Classification Index			Percentile
	C	B	A	
100th	100	100	100	100th
95th	100	100	100	95th
90th	100	100	100	90th
85th	100	100	100	85th
80th	100	100	100	80th
75th	100	100	100	75th
70th	100	100	100	70th
65th	100	100	99	65th
60th	100	99	91	60th
55th	91	97	80	55th
50th	75	83	74	50th
45th	65	71	67	45th
40th	60	65	60	40th
35th	55	55	55	35th
30th	50	50	50	30th
25th	45	48	49	25th
20th	39	42	41	20th
15th	35	39	37	15th
10th	31	34	32	10th
5th	26	26	26	5th
0	8	8	5	0

Shuttle Run: High School Boys
Percentile Scores Based on Classification Index / Test Scores in Seconds and Tenths

Percentile	Classification Index			Percentile
	C	B	A	
100th	8.3	8.0	8.0	100th
95th	9.2	9.0	9.0	95th
90th	9.4	9.1	9.0	90th
85th	9.6	9.2	9.2	85th
80th	9.7	9.3	9.3	80th
75th	9.8	9.5	9.4	75th
70th	9.9	9.5	9.5	70th
65th	9.9	9.6	9.6	65th
60th	10.0	9.7	9.6	60th
55th	10.0	9.8	9.7	55th
50th	10.1	9.9	9.8	50th
45th	10.2	10.0	10.0	45th
40th	10.2	10.0	10.0	40th
35th	10.4	10.1	10.1	35th
30th	10.5	10.2	10.2	30th
25th	10.6	10.3	10.4	25th
20th	10.9	10.5	10.6	20th
15th	11.0	10.8	10.9	15th
10th	11.2	11.1	11.1	10th
5th	11.7	11.4	11.5	5th
0	15.0	15.0	16.6	0

Standing Broad Jump: High School Boys
Percentile Scores Based on Classification Index/Test Scores in Feet and Inches

Percentile	Classification Index			Percentile
	C	B	A	
100th	8'11"	8'10"	9' 8"	100th
95th	7' 9"	8' 2"	8' 6"	95th
90th	7' 6"	7'11"	8' 3"	90th
85th	7' 5"	7' 9"	8' 0"	85th
80th	7' 3"	7' 7"	7'11"	80th
75th	7' 0"	7' 6"	7' 9"	75th
70th	6'10"	7' 5"	7' 7"	70th
65th	6' 9"	7' 3"	7' 6"	65th
60th	6' 8"	7' 1"	7' 5"	60th
55th	6' 6"	7' 0"	7' 4"	55th
50th	6' 5"	7' 0"	7' 3"	50th
45th	6' 3"	6'10"	7' 1"	45th
40th	6' 2"	6' 9"	7' 0"	40th
35th	6' 0"	6' 7"	6'11"	35th
30th	5'10"	6' 6"	6' 9"	30th
25th	5' 8"	6' 5"	6' 7"	25th
20th	5' 6"	6' 4"	6' 6"	20th
15th	5' 3"	6' 1"	6' 3"	15th
10th	5' 0"	5'10"	6' 0"	10th
5th	4'10"	5' 5"	5' 7"	5th
0	2'10"	4' 6"	3' 7"	0

50-Yard Dash: High School Boys
Percentile Scores Based on Classification Index/Test Scores in Seconds and Tenths

Percentile	Classification Index			Percentile
	C	B	A	
100th	6.0	5.6	5.6	100th
95th	6.3	6.0	6.0	95th
90th	6.4	6.1	6.1	90th
85th	6.5	6.2	6.2	85th
80th	6.6	6.3	6.2	80th
75th	6.7	6.4	6.3	75th
70th	6.9	6.5	6.4	70th
65th	7.0	6.5	6.4	65th
60th	7.0	6.5	6.5	60th
55th	7.1	6.6	6.6	55th
50th	7.1	6.7	6.6	50th
45th	7.2	6.8	6.7	45th
40th	7.3	6.8	6.8	40th
35th	7.4	6.9	6.8	35th
30th	7.5	7.0	6.9	30th
25th	7.6	7.1	7.0	25th
20th	7.8	7.2	7.0	20th
15th	8.0	7.3	7.2	15th
10th	8.1	7.5	7.3	10th
5th	8.6	7.9	7.7	5th
0	10.4	10.0	10.6	0

Softball Throw: High School Boys
Percentile Scores Based on Classification Index/Test Scores in Feet

Percentile	Classification Index			Percentile
	C	B	A	
100th	209	270	291	100th
95th	199	225	246	95th
90th	185	215	231	90th
85th	180	207	222	85th
80th	174	201	216	80th
75th	171	196	210	75th
70th	166	192	206	70th
65th	164	188	201	65th
60th	159	182	196	60th
55th	156	179	192	55th
50th	152	174	187	50th
45th	148	170	183	45th
40th	145	167	180	40th
35th	143	165	175	35th
30th	140	157	170	30th
25th	127	150	165	25th
20th	123	147	159	20th
15th	111	139	153	15th
10th	105	130	145	10th
5th	88	109	129	5th
0	43	31	30	0

600-Yard Run-Walk: High School Boys
Percentile Scores Based on Classification Index/Test Scores in Minutes and Seconds

Percentile	Classification Index			Percentile
	C	B	A	
100th	1'29"	1'25"	1'23"	100th
95th	1'40"	1'32"	1'31"	95th
90th	1'41"	1'35"	1'34"	90th
85th	1'44"	1'37"	1'36"	85th
80th	1'46"	1'39"	1'38"	80th
75th	1'50"	1'41"	1'40"	75th
70th	1'52"	1'43"	1'42"	70th
65th	1'53"	1'45"	1'44"	65th
60th	1'55"	1'47"	1'45"	60th
55th	1'57"	1'49"	1'47"	55th
50th	1'58"	1'51"	1'49"	50th
45th	2' 1"	1'53"	1'51"	45th
40th	2' 3"	1'55"	1'54"	40th
35th	2' 5"	1'58"	1'57"	35th
30th	2' 8"	2' 1"	2' 0"	30th
25th	2'12"	2' 5"	2' 3"	25th
20th	2'16"	2' 9"	2' 8"	20th
15th	2'22"	2'15"	2'14"	15th
10th	2'34"	2'25"	2'22"	10th
5th	2'45"	2'37"	2'39"	5th
0	3'12"	4'34"	4'45"	0

Percentile Scores for College Women

Percentile	Modified Pull-Up	Sit-Up	Shuttle Run	Standing Broad Jump	50-Yard Dash	Softball Throw	600-Yard Run-Walk
100th	40	50	7.5	7'10"	5.4	184	1:49
95th	39	43	10.2	6'6"	7.3	115	2:19
90th	38	35	10.5	6'3"	7.6	103	2:27
85th	33	31	10.7	6'1"	7.7	96	2:32
80th	30	29	10.9	5'11"	7.8	90	2:37
75th	28	27	11.0	5'10"	7.9	86	2:41
70th	26	25	11.1	5'8"	8.0	82	2:44
65th	24	24	11.2	5'7"	8.1	79	2:48
60th	22	22	11.3	5'6"	8.2	76	2:51
55th	21	21	11.5	5'5"	8.3	73	2:54
50th	20	20	11.6	5'4"	8.4	70	2:58
45th	18	19	11.7	5'3"	8.6	67	3:01
40th	17	18	11.9	5'2"	8.7	65	3:05
35th	16	16	12.0	5'0"	8.8	62	3:08
30th	15	15	12.1	4'11"	9.0	59	3:13
25th	13	14	12.2	4'10"	9.1	57	3:18
20th	12	13	12.4	4'8"	9.2	54	3:23
15th	11	11	12.6	4'7"	9.4	51	3:29
10th	9	9	12.9	4'5"	9.7	47	3:38
5th	7	7	13.4	4'1"	10.1	42	3:53
0	0	0	17.3	2'3"	13.7	5	5:29

Percentile Scores for College Men

Percen-tile	Pull-Up	Sit-Up	Shuttle Run	Standing Broad Jump	50-Yard Dash	Softball Throw	600-Yard Run-Walk
100th	20	100	8.3	9'6"	5.5	315	1:12
95th	12	99	9.0	8'5"	6.1	239	1:35
90th	10	97	9.1	8'2"	6.2	226	1:38
85th	10	79	9.1	7'11"	6.3	217	1:40
80th	9	68	9.2	7'10"	6.4	211	1:42
75th	8	61	9.4	7'8"	6.5	206	1:44
70th	8	58	9.5	7'7"	6.5	200	1:45
65th	7	52	9.5	7'6"	6.6	196	1:47
60th	7	51	9.6	7'5"	6.6	192	1:49
55th	6	50	9.6	7'4"	6.7	188	1:50
50th	6	47	9.7	7'3"	6.8	184	1:52
45th	5	44	9.8	7'1"	6.8	180	1:53
40th	5	41	9.9	7'0"	6.9	176	1:55
35th	4	38	10.0	6'11"	7.0	171	1:57
30th	4	36	10.0	6'10"	7.0	166	1:59
25th	3	34	10.1	6'9"	7.1	161	2:01
20th	3	31	10.2	6'7"	7.1	156	2:05
15th	2	29	10.4	6'5"	7.2	150	2:09
10th	1	26	10.6	6'2"	7.5	140	2:15
5th	0	22	11.1	5'10"	7.7	125	2:25
0	0	0	13.9	4'2"	9.1	55	3:43

appendix E

norms for Kirchner Motor Fitness Test

X denotes the raw score, while T is the scaled score. Each score represents the minimum performance to obtain the ratings "poor" through "superior." The four scores at the bottom of the norms for each age group were obtained by totaling the T-scores for each item in the test battery. For example, Billy, aged six years, obtained the following raw scores:

Test item	Raw score (X)	T-score
Standing broad jump	42 inches	55
Bench push-ups	31	65
Curl-ups	14	55
Squat jumps	13	46
30-yard dash	5.4 seconds	65
	Total $=$	286

He therefore would be classified as "good" on the test battery.

Norms for Kirchner Motor Fitness Test*

	Standing Broad Jump (inches)		Bench Push-ups		Curl-ups		Squat Jumps		30-yd. Dash (seconds)	
	X	T	X	T	X	T	X	T	X	T
Boys: 6 years										
Superior	50	66	31	65	28	65	30	65	5.4	65
Good	42	55	19	55	14	55	20	55	5.9	61
Average	36	46	10	45	6	46	13	46	6.9	45
Below av.	35	44	9	43	5	44	12	44	7.0	41
Poor	27	33	4	34	1	34	6	34	7.8	34
	Superior 326		Good 281		Average 228		Below av. 227		Poor 179	
Boys: 7 years										
Superior	54	65	36	65	38	65	39	65	5.2	65
Good	47	55	21	55	19	55	25	55	5.7	57
Average	40	46	12	46	9	45	15	45	6.5	45
Below av.	39	44	11	44	8	44	14	44	6.6	43
Poor	32	34	5	34	2	34	7	33	7.1	34
	Superior 325		Good 277		Average 227		Below av. 226		Poor 177	
Boys: 8 years										
Superior	60	65	40	65	44	65	47	65	4.9	66
Good	51	55	23	55	23	55	28	55	5.3	56
Average	44	46	12	45	11	45	17	45	5.9	46
Below av.	43	44	11	43	10	44	16	44	6.0	43
Poor	35	33	5	34	3	34	8	34	6.8	34
	Superior 326		Good 276		Average 227		Below av. 226		Poor 176	
Boys: 9 years										
Superior	63	66	36	65	43	65	47	66	4.7	68
Good	54	56	22	55	25	55	31	55	5.2	55
Average	47	45	12	45	13	45	19	45	5.6	45
Below av.	46	44	11	43	12	44	18	44	5.7	44
Poor	37	33	4	34	4	34	9	34	6.4	34
	Superior 329		Good 276		Average 225		Below av. 224		Poor 175	
Boys: 10 years										
Superior	66	66	38	65	46	65	47	67	4.5	65
Good	58	55	23	55	30	55	35	55	4.9	55
Average	50	45	13	45	17	45	21	45	5.5	46
Below av.	49	44	12	44	16	44	20	44	5.6	43
Poor	40	34	4	33	6	34	10	34	6.1	34
	Superior 328		Good 275		Average 226		Below av. 225		Poor 174	

* X=raw score; T = T-score and totals at bottom of columns for each age group are sums of T-scores.

	Standing Broad Jump (inches)		Bench Push-ups		Curl-ups		Squat Jumps		30-yd. Dash (seconds)	
	X	T	X	T	X	T	X	T	X	T
				Boys: 11 years						
Superior	70	66	40	65	49	67	47	66	4.3	67
Good	61	55	24	55	35	55	40	56	4.7	56
Average	53	45	13	45	20	46	24	45	5.2	45
Below av.	52	44	12	44	19	44	23	44	5.3	42
Poor	44	34	4	34	7	34	10	34	5.9	33
	Superior 331		Good 277		Average 226		Below av. 225		Poor 176	
				Boys: 12 years						
Superior	73	65	40	65	45	66	49	68	4.2	66
Good	63	55	23	55	35	55	36	55	4.7	56
Average	54	45	12	45	20	45	21	45	5.2	46
Below av.	53	43	11	44	19	44	20	44	5.3	44
Poor	45	34	3	33	6	34	8	34	5.9	33
	Superior 330		Good 276		Average 226		Below av. 225		Poor 174	
				Girls: 6 years						
Superior	47	66	27	65	27	65	32	65	5.6	65
Good	40	55	16	55	14	55	21	55	6.3	55
Average	33	45	9	46	6	45	13	45	7.0	45
Below av.	26	34	8	44	5	43	12	44	7.1	44
Poor	32	43	2	33	1	33	6	34	8.0	33
	Superior 326		Good 275		Average 228		Below av. 227		Poor 179	
				Girls: 7 years						
Superior	52	66	30	65	33	65	39	65	5.2	65
Good	45	55	17	55	18	55	25	55	5.9	56
Average	37	45	9	45	8	45	16	45	6.6	45
Below av.	36	43	8	44	7	43	15	44	6.7	42
Poor	30	34	2	32	2	33	7	33	7.4	34
	Superior 326		Good 276		Average 225		Belowav. 224		Poor 177	
				Girls: 8 years						
Superior	56	65	30	65	36	65	44	65	4.8	65
Good	48	55	18	55	20	55	28	55	5.5	55
Average	41	55	9	45	10	45	17	45	6.2	46
Below av.	40	44	8	44	9	44	16	44	6.3	44
Poor	33	34	2	32	2	32	8	34	7.0	34
	Superior 325		Good 275		Average 225		Below av. 224		Poor 174	

	Standing Broad Jump (inches)		Bench Push-ups		Curl-ups		Squat Jumps		30-yd. Dash (seconds)	
	X	T	X	T	X	T	X	T	X	T
Girls: 9 years										
Superior	58	65	29	65	40	65	45	65	4.7	65
Good	50	55	16	55	22	55	30	55	5.2	55
Average	43	45	8	46	11	45	19	45	5.8	45
Below av.	42	44	7	44	10	44	18	44	5.9	43
Poor	35	34	2	33	2	32	9	34	6.6	34
	Superior 325		Good 275		Average 226		Below av. 225		Poor 177	
Girls: 10 years										
Superior	63	66	30	66	43	65	44	65	4.7	65
Good	54	55	16	55	26	55	32	55	4.9	57
Average	46	45	7	45	14	45	20	45	5.8	45
Below av.	45	44	6	43	13	44	19	44	5.9	41
Poor	38	34	1	32	4	34	10	34	6.3	34
	Superior 327		Good 277		Average 225		Below av. 224		Poor 174	
Girls: 11 years										
Superior	67	65	29	65	44	65	45	65	4.3	65
Good	58	55	15	55	28	55	34	55	4.9	55
Average	49	45	7	46	16	45	21	45	5.4	48
Below av.	48	44	6	44	15	44	20	44	5.5	44
Poor	39	34	2	34	5	34	9	34	6.0	34
Girls: 12 years										
Superior	68	66	30	65	42	65	46	65	4.6	65
Good	58	55	14	55	26	55	30	55	5.0	57
Average	49	45	6	46	15	46	17	45	5.4	48
Below av.	48	44	5	44	14	44	16	44	5.5	44
Poor	40	34	1	32	5	34	6	34	6.4	34

norms for Oregon motor fitness test

Oregon Motor Fitness Norms
Scoring Table
For Girls Grades 4, 5 and 6

Std. Pts. Based on T-Score	Arm-Flexed Hang in Seconds			Standing Broad Jump in Inches			Number of Crossed-Arm Curl-Ups		
	4th	5th	6th	4th	5th	6th	4th	5th	6th
100	69	65	77	91	104	102	130	120	149
98	66	63	75	89	103	101	126	117	145
96	64	61	72	87	101	99	122	114	140
94	61	59	70	86	99	97	118	110	136
92	59	56	67	84	97	95	114	106	131
90	57	54	62	83	95	93	110	103	127
88	54	52	62	81	93	91	106	99	122
86	52	50	60	79	92	89	102	95	118
84	49	48	57	78	90	87	98	92	113
82	47	46	55	76	88	85	94	88	109
80	44	44	52	75	86	84	90	84	104
78	42	42	50	73	84	82	86	81	100
76	40	40	47	71	82	80	82	77	95
74	37	38	44	70	81	78	78	73	91
72	35	35	42	68	79	76	74	70	86
70	32	33	39	67	77	74	70	66	82
68	30	31	37	65	75	72	66	63	77
66	27	29	34	63	73	70	62	59	73
64	25	27	32	62	72	68	58	55	68
62	23	25	29	60	70	67	54	51	64
60	20	23	27	59	68	65	50	48	60
58	18	21	24	57	66	63	46	45	55
56	15	19	22	55	64	61	42	41	51
54	13	16	19	54	62	59	38	38	46
52	10	14	17	52	61	57	34	34	42
50	8	12	14	51	59	65	30	30	37
48	5	10	12	49	57	53	26	27	33
46	3	8	9	47	55	51	22	23	28
44	1	6	7	46	53	50	18	19	24
42		4	4	44	51	48	14	16	20
40		2	1	42	50	46	10	12	16
38				41	48	44	6	8	11
36				39	46	42	3	4	6
34				38	44	40	1	1	1
32				36	42	38			
30				34	41	36			
28				33	39	35			
26				31	37	33			
24				30	35	31			
22				28	33	29			
20				26	31	27			
18				25	30	25			
16				23	28	23			
14				22	26	21			
12				20	24	19			
10				18	22	18			
8				17	20	16			
6				15	19	14			
4				14	17	12			
2				12	15	10			
1				11	14	9			

GENERAL INSTRUCTIONS TO TEACHERS

1. The motor fitness tests are to be taken by only those individuals who are physically able to participate in the regular program of physical education.
2. In no instance should pupils be permitted to perform any test more than is necessary to get one hundred points. Performance should be stopped on any test if, in the opinion of the instructor, the pupil is overtaxing himself.
3. Individuals should be acquainted with the tests in advance of the testing period and sufficient practice should be allowed for thorough understanding of the execution of the tests.
4. Time should be provided for a few minutes warm-up at the beginning of each test period.
5. All equipment and facilities necessary for the administration of the tests should be prepared before the testing period begins.
6. Establish a policy of strictly enforcing all rules and regulations in scoring and administering the test.

Oregon Motor Fitness Norms
Scoring Table
For Boys Grades 4, 5 and 6

Std. Pts. Based on T-Score	Standing Broad Jump in Inches			Number of Push-Ups			Number of Sit-Ups		
	4th	5th	6th	4th	5th	6th	4th	5th	6th
100	97	100	106	55	43	39	131	153	158
98	95	99	104	53	41	37	127	148	153
96	93	97	102	51	40	36	123	143	147
94	91	95	100	50	39	35	118	138	142
92	90	94	98	48	37	34	114	133	137
90	88	92	97	46	36	33	110	128	132
88	86	90	95	44	34	32	106	123	127
86	85	88	93	42	33	30	102	118	122
84	83	87	91	40	32	29	97	113	117
82	81	85	90	38	30	28	93	108	112
80	80	83	88	36	29	27	89	103	107
78	78	82	86	35	27	26	85	98	102
76	76	80	84	33	26	25	81	93	97
74	74	78	83	31	25	23	76	88	92
72	73	77	81	29	23	22	72	83	87
70	71	75	79	27	22	21	68	78	81
68	69	73	77	25	21	20	64	73	76
66	68	72	75	23	19	19	60	68	71
64	66	70	74	22	18	18	56	63	66
62	64	68	72	20	16	16	51	58	61
60	63	66	70	18	15	15	47	53	56
58	61	65	68	16	13	14	43	48	51
56	59	63	67	14	12	13	39	43	46
54	57	61	65	12	11	12	35	38	41
52	56	60	63	10	9	10	30	33	36
50	54	58	61	9	8	9	26	28	31
48	52	56	60	7	6	8	22	23	26
46	51	55	58	5	5	7	18	18	21
44	49	53	56	3	4	6	14	13	16
42	47	51	54	1	2	5	9	8	11
40	46	49	53		1	3	5	4	6
38	44	48	51			2	1	1	2
36	42	46	49			1			
34	41	44	47						
32	39	43	45						
30	37	41	44						
28	35	39	42						
26	34	38	40						
24	32	36	38						
22	30	34	37						
20	29	33	35						
18	27	31	33						
16	25	29	31						
14	24	27	30						
12	22	26	28						
10	20	24	26						
8	18	22	24						
6	17	21	23						
4	15	19	21						
2	13	17	19						
1	12	16	18						

Oregon Motor Fitness Norms
Scoring Table
For Girls Grades 7, 8 and 9

Std. Pts. Based on T-Score	Arm-Flexed Hang in Seconds			Standing Broad Jump in Inches			Number of Crossed-Arm Curl-Ups		
	7th	8th	9th	7th	8th	9th	7th	8th	9th
100	76	76	107	100	101	105	105	105	121
98	74	74	104	99	100	104	103	103	118
96	72	72	100	98	99	102	101	101	114
94	70	70	97	97	98	101	98	98	111
92	68	68	93	96	97	100	95	95	107
90	66	66	90	95	96	99	92	92	104
88	64	64	86	93	95	98	89	89	100
86	62	62	83	92	94	97	86	86	97
84	60	60	79	90	92	95	83	83	93
82	58	58	76	88	90	93	80	80	90
80	56	56	72	86	88	91	77	77	86
78	54	54	69	85	87	90	74	74	83
76	52	52	65	83	86	89	71	71	79
74	50	50	60	82	84	87	68	68	76
72	48	48	58	80	82	85	65	65	72
70	46	46	55	78	80	83	62	62	69
68	44	44	51	76	78	81	59	59	65
66	42	42	48	75	77	80	56	56	62
64	40	40	44	73	75	78	53	53	58
62	38	38	41	72	74	77	50	50	55
60	36	36	37	70	72	75	47	47	51
58	34	34	34	68	70	73	44	44	48
56	32	32	30	66	68	71	41	41	44
54	30	30	27	65	67	70	38	38	41
52	28	28	23	63	65	68	35	35	37
50	26	26	20	61	63	66	32	32	34
48	24	24	17	59	61	64	29	29	31
46	22	22	14	58	60	62	26	26	28
44	20	20	12	56	58	60	23	23	25
42	18	18	10	55	56	58	21	21	23
40	16	16	9	53	54	56	19	19	21
38	14	14	8	51	53	55	17	17	19
36	12	12	7	49	51	53	15	15	17
34	11	11	7	48	50	51	13	13	15
32	9	9	6	46	48	49	11	11	13
30	8	8	6	45	46	47	9	9	11
28	6	6		43	44	45	7	7	10
26	5	5	5	41	42	43	6	6	9
24	3	3		39	39	41	5	5	8
22	1	1	4	38	38	40	4	4	7
20			3	36	36	39	3	3	6
18			2	35	35	38	2	2	5
16			1	33	33	36	1	1	3
14				32	32	35			2
12				30	30	33			1
10				29	29	32			
8				27	27	30			
6				26	26	29			
4				24	24	27			
2				23	23	26			
1				22	22	25			

Oregon Motor Fitness Norms
Scoring Table
For Boys Grades 7, 8, and 9

Std. Pts. Based on T-Score	Jump and Reach in Inches			Number of Pull-Ups			Potato Race in Seconds		
	7th	8th	9th	7th	8th	9th	7th	8th	9th
100	29	30	34	18	20	23	21	22	20
98	28	29	33	17	19	22	22	23	21
96						21	23	24	22
94	27	28	32	16	18	20			
92							24	25	23
90	26	27	31	15	16	19	25		
88						18	26	26	24
86	25	26	30	14	15	17			
84			29			16	27	27	25
82	24	25	28	13	14	15			
80	23						28	28	26
78	22	24	27	12	13	14	29		
76				11			30	29	27
74	21	23	26	10	12	13			28
72						12	31	30	29
70	20	22	25	9	11	11			
68	19	21	24				32	31	30
66	18	20	23	8	10	10			
64					9		33	32	31
62	17	19	22	7	8	9	34	33	
60						8	35	34	32
58	16	18	21	6	7	7			
56		17	20				36	35	33
54	15			5	6	6			
52			19			5	37	36	34
50		16	18	4	5	4	38		
48							39	37	35
46	14	15	17	3	4	3			
44							40	38	36
42	13	14	16	2	3	2			37
40	12	13		1		1	41	39	38
38	11	12	15		2.				
36							42	40	39
34	10	11	14		1		43		
32			13				44	41	40
30	9	10	12					42	
28							45	43	41
26	8	9	11						
24							46	44	42
22	7	8	10				47		
20							48	45	43
18	6	7	9						
16							49	46	44
14	5	6	8						
12		5	7				50	47	45
10	4	4	6						46
8		3					51	48	47
6	3	2	5				52		
4		1	4				53	49	48
2									
1	2		3				54	50	

Oregon Motor Fitness Norms
Scoring Table
For Girls Grades 10, 11, and 12

Std. Pts. Based on T-Score	Arm-Flexed Hang in Seconds			Standing Broad Jump in Inches			Number of Crossed-Arm Curl-Ups		
	10th	11th	12th	10th	11th	12th	10th	11th	12th
100	104	105	106	105	106	106	121	123	123
98	101	102	103	104	105	105	118	120	120
96	97	98	99	102	104	104	114	116	116
94	94	95	96	101	103	103	111	113	113
92	90	91	92	100	102	102	107	109	109
90	87	88	89	99	101	101	104	106	106
88	83	84	85	98	100	100	100	102	102
86	80	81	82	97	99	99	97	99	99
84	76	77	78	95	97	97	93	95	95
82	73	74	75	93	95	95	90	92	92
80	69	70	71	91	93	93	86	88	88
78	66	67	68	90	92	92	83	85	85
76	62	63	64	89	91	91	79	81	81
74	59	60	61	87	89	89	76	78	78
72	55	56	57	85	87	87	72	74	74
70	52	53	54	83	86	86	69	71	71
68	48	49	50	81	85	84	65	67	67
66	45	46	47	80	83	82	62	64	64
64	41	42	43	78	80	80	58	60	60
62	38	39	40	77	78	78	55	57	57
60	34	35	36	75	76	76	51	53	53
58	31	32	33	73	74	74	48	50	50
56	27	28	29	71	71	71	44	46	46
54	24	25	25	70	70	70	41	43	43
52	20	21	20	68	68	68	37	39	39
50	17	18	17	66	67	67	34	36	36
48	13	14	15	64	65	65	31	33	33
46	11	12	13	62	63	64	28	30	30
44	9	10	11	60	61	62	25	27	27
42	7	8	9	58	60	61	23	25	25
40	6	7	8	56	58	59	21	23	23
38	5	6	7	55	57	58	19	21	21
36				53	55	56	17	19	19
34	4	5	6	51	53	54	15	17	17
32				49	51	52	13	15	15
30	3	4	5	48	50	51	11	13	13
28				47	49	50	9	12	12
26	2	3	4	45	47	48	8	11	11
24	1			43	45	46	7	10	10
22		2	3	42	45	45		9	9
20		1		41	43	44	6	8	8
18			2	40	42	43	5	7	7
16			1	38	40	41	3	6	6
14				37	39	40	2	5	5
12				35	37	38	1	4	4
10				34	36	37		3	3
8				32	34	35		1	1
6				31	33	34			
4				29	31	32			
2				28	30	30			
1				27	29				

Oregon Motor Fitness Norms
Scoring Table
For Boys Grades 10, 11, and 12

Std. Pts. Based on T-Score	Jump and Reach in Inches			Number of Pull-Ups			Potato Race in Seconds		
	10th	11th	12th	10th	11th	12th	10th	11th	12th
100	36	38	41	23	27	28	21	21	23
98	35	37	40	22	26	27	22	22	24
96	34		39			26	23	23	
94	33	36	38	21	25	25			
92					24		24	24	25
90	32	35	37	20	23	24			
88		34	36		22	23	25	25	26
86	31	33	35	19	21	22			
84				18			26	26	27
82	30	32	34	17	20	21			
80	29	31	33		19	20	27	27	
78	28	30	32	16	18	19			
76				15		18	28	28	28
74	27	29	31	14	17	17			
72			30		16		29	29	29
70	26	28		13	15	16			
68		27	29	12		15	30	30	30
66	25	26	28	11	14	14			
64					13	12	31	31	
62	24	25	27	10	12	12			
60	23		26		11		32		31
58	22	24	25	9	10	11			
56				8		10	33	32	32
54	21	23	24	7	9	9			
52		22			8		34	33	33
50	20	21	23	6	7	8			
48			20	5		7	35	34	34
46	19	20	21	4	6	6			
44	18				5	5	36	35	
42	17	19	20	3	4	4			
40			19				37	36	35
38	16	18	18	2	3	3			
36				1			38		36
34	15	17	17		2	2			
32		16			1	1	39	37	
30	14	15	16						
28	13		15				40	38	37
26	12	14	14						
24							41	39	38
22	11	13	13						
20			12				42	40	39
18	10	12	11						
16		11					43	41	40
14	9	10	10						
12									
10	8	9	9						
8	7		8				44	42	41
6	6	8	7						
4	5	7	6				45	43	42
2									
1			5						

index